Endothelin

Contemporary Biomedicine

Endothelin: *Molecular Biology, Physiology, and Pathology*
Edited by *Robert F. Highsmith,* 1998
Cellular Cancer Markers
Edited by *Carleton T. Garrett and Stewart Sell,* 1995
Serological Cancer Markers
Edited by *Stewart Sell,* 1992
The Red Cell Membrane
Edited by *B. U. Raess and Godfrey Tunnicliff,* 1990
Handbook of the Hemopoietic Microenvironment
Edited by *Mehdi Tavassoli,* 1989
Leukolysins and Cancer
Edited by *Janet H. Ransom and John R. Ortaldo,* 1988
Methods of Hybridoma Formation
Edited by *Arie H. Bartal and Yashar Hirshaut,* 1987
Monoclonal Antibodies in Cancer
Edited by *Stewart Sell and Ralph A. Reisfeld,* 1985
Calcium and Contractility: *Smooth Muscle*
Edited by *A. K. Grover and E. E. Daniel,* 1984
Carcinogenesis and Mutagenesis Testing
Edited by *J. F. Douglas,* 1984
The Human Teratomas: *Experimental and Clinical Biology*
Edited by *Ivan Damjanov, Barbara B. Knowles,
and Davor Solter,* 1983
Human Cancer Markers
Edited by *Stewart Sell and Britta Wahren,* 1982
Cancer Markers: *Diagnostic and Developmental Significance*
Edited by *Stewart Sell,* 1980

Endothelin

Molecular Biology, Physiology, and Pathology

Edited by

Robert F. Highsmith

University of Cincinnati College of Medicine
Cincinnati, OH

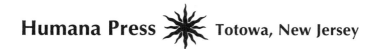

Humana Press Totowa, New Jersey

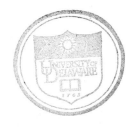

© 1998 Humana Press Inc.
999 Riverview Drive, Suite 208
Totowa, New Jersey 07512

For additional copies, pricing for bulk purchases, and/or information about other Humana titles, contact Humana at the above address or at any of the following numbers: Tel.: 973-256-1699; Fax: 973-256-8341; E-mail: humana@mindspring.com or visit our Website: http://humanapress.com

This publication is printed on acid-free paper.∞
ANSI Z39.48-1984 (American National Standards Institute) Permanence of Paper for Printed Library Materials.

Cover illustration:

Cover design by Patricia F. Cleary.

Photocopy Authorization Policy:

Printed in the United States of America. 10 9 8 7 6 5 4 3 2 1

Library of Congress Cataloging in Publication Data

Endothelin: molecular biology, physiology, and pathology/edited by Robert F. Highsmith.
    p.   cm.—(Contemporary biomedicine)
  Includes index.
  ISBN 0-89603-436-4 (alk. paper)
  1. Endothelins—Physiological effect. 2. Endothelins—Pathophysiology.   3. Endothelins
—Receptors. I. Highsmith, Robert F. II. Series.
  [DNLM: 1. Endothelins—physiology. 2. Receptors, Endothelin—physiology. QU 68
E5654 1998]
QP552.E54E536   1998
612'.015756—dc21
DNLM/DLC
for Library of Congress   97-36783
                                                   CIP

Preface

The vascular endothelium continuously lines the intimal surface of all blood vessels. Just a few years ago, this structure was thought to be a mere passive barrier to diffusion of solutes and other nutrients. We now recognize these cells as a widely dispersed "organ system" that, because of its unique location in the vasculature, is ideally situated to play many key roles in cardiovascular physiology and pathology. For example, we know that the endothelium orchestrates the inflammatory response and participates in thrombosis, angiogenesis, atherosclerosis, and mechanotransduction—sensing forces at the blood–vessel wall interface and making appropriate responses to alter gene expression and release vasoactive molecules.

Knowledge of the role of the endothelium in coagulation and fibrinolysis was followed by the landmark discovery that the endothelial cell expresses molecules that potently influence the contractile state of the underlying vascular smooth muscle. The vasoactive tone of these muscle cells determines blood flow to any given organ. In terms of physiologic regulation of vasomotor tone via the release of endothelium-derived vasoactive factors, perhaps the best-characterized molecule is the inert gas, nitric oxide (NO), and its biosynthetic enzyme, nitric oxide synthase (NOS). Indeed, the ability of the endothelium to alter gene expression of NOS resulting in the rapid release of NO, a short-lived and potent vasodilator, most likely represents an important regulator of blood flow whose perturbation may underlie numerous cardiovascular pathologies.

Another milestone discovery, made in the mid-1980s, was that the endothelial cell also releases a peptidergic factor that is the most potent and long-lasting endogenous vasoconstrictor yet described. The activity of this factor was soon attributed to the 21-amino acid peptide, endothelin, derived from a larger precursor molecule by proteolysis. We also quickly learned of its unique structure, being homologous to only the sarafotoxins present in snake venom, that at least three different genes encode the expression of endothelin in the human genome, and that multiple receptor subtypes mediate different responses to the peptide. Likewise, despite considerable confusion in early reports, great progress has been made in unraveling endothelin's mechanism of action in smooth muscle and other tissues.

v

Since abnormal increases in vasomotor tone clearly underlie a wide variety of vasospastic disorders, as well as hypertension, it was not surprising that the discovery of endothelin set off a wave of intense investigation, mostly basic science in nature, but with some clinical prospects as well, into the molecular biology and cell biology of endothelin. Several national and international symposia were focused on the peptide and the number of scientific publications concerned with endothelin dramatically increased to a peak in 1988 and since have fallen gradually to a more stable rate. Understandably, the rush to publish quickly and the flurry of non-peer-reviewed symposia articles allowed some erroneous conclusions to creep into the literature that have taken some time to purge. I believe that now is a good time to reevaluate the facts regarding endothelin, and to stimulate thought about what functions this molecule may play. Indeed, continued scientific interest in endothelin is sustained by our inability to define a physiologic role for this peptide; nor do we know very much about the extent to which endothelin underlies the disease process.

The purpose of *Endothelin: Molecular Biology, Physiology, and Pathology* is to focus on summarizing progress in selected areas of endothelin research that are now well documented. Because of continuing progress, the book is not comprehensive or all-inclusive, but provides factual information and authenticated interpretation at an appropriate time in the short history of endothelin research, in addition to provoking serious thought about where research should go in the future. The authors have been selected from both academic and industrial settings to provide a well-rounded international perspective. The contributors are authorities in their field as well as active bench scientists. The volume should be a useful source of information to basic scientists and informed clinicians, who very likely may be treating disorders in the future with drugs that are designed to alter the action or expression of the endothelin molecule.

I greatly appreciate the timely contributions of the authors and the excellent secretarial assistance of Linda Saslow. Most importantly, I acknowledge the pioneering observations of my former graduate student, Dr. Kristine Hickey (Agricola), whose doctoral dissertation and early publications planted the seed from which all knowledge about endothelin has grown.

Robert F. Highsmith

Contents

Preface v

List of Contributors ix

Ch. 1. Endothelin Receptor Subtypes and Tissue Distribution
         David M. Pollock 1
Ch. 2. Molecular Biology of the Endothelin Receptors
         Jonathan A. Lee, Eliot H. Ohlstein,
                Catherine E. Peishoff, and John D. Elliott 31
Ch. 3. Molecular Biology of Endothelin-Converting Enzyme
                (ECE)
         Ryoichi Takayanagi, Keizo Ohnaka, Wei Liu,
                Takeshi Ito, and Hajime Nawata 75
Ch. 4. Endothelin Receptor-Signaling Mechanisms in Vascular
                Smooth Muscle
         E. Radford Decker and Tommy A. Brock 93
Ch. 5. Mechanisms of Endothelin-Induced Mitogenesis
                in Vascular Smooth Muscle
         Thomas Force 121
Ch. 6. The Renal and Systemic Hemodynamic Actions
                of Endothelin
         Robert O. Banks, David M. Pollock,
                and Jacqueline Novak 167
Ch. 7. The Development of Specific Endothelin-Receptor
                Antagonists
         Timothy D. Warner 189
Ch. 8. Pathophysiological Role of Endothelin and Potential
                Therapeutic Targets for Receptor Antagonists
         David P. Brooks, Diane K. Jorkasky, Martin I. Freed,
                and Eliot H. Ohlstein 223

Index 269

Contributors

ROBERT BANKS • *Department of Molecular and Cellular Physiology, College of Medicine, University of Cincinnati, OH*
TOMMY A. BROCK • *Texas Biotechnology Corporation, Houston, TX*
DAVID BROOKS • *SmithKline Beecham Pharmaceuticals, King of Prussia, PA*
E. RADFORD DECKER • *Texas Biotechnology Corporation, Houston, TX*
JOHN D. ELLIOTT • *SmithKline Beecham Pharmaceuticals, King of Prussia, PA*
THOMAS FORCE • *Cardiac Unit, Massachusetts General Hospital East, Charlestown, MA*
MARTIN I. FREED • *SmithKline Beecham Pharmaceuticals, King of Prussia, PA*
TAKESHI ITO • *Third Department of Internal Medicine, Faculty of Medicine, Kyushu University, Fukuoka, Japan*
DIANE K. JORKASKY • *SmithKline Beecham Pharmaceuticals, King of Prussia, PA*
JONATHAN A. LEE • *SmithKline Beecham Pharmaceuticals, King of Prussia, PA*
WEI LIU • *Third Department of Internal Medicine, Faculty of Medicine, Kyushu University, Fukuoka, Japan*
HAJAME NAWATA • *Third Department of Internal Medicine, Faculty of Medicine, Kyushu University, Fukuoka, Japan*
JACQUELINE NOVAK • *Department of Physiology and Biophysics, University of Mississippi, Jackson, MS*
ELIOT H. OHLSTEIN • *SmithKline Beecham Pharmaceuticals, King of Prussia, PA*
KEIZO OHNAKA • *Third Department of Internal Medicine, Faculty of Medicine, Kyushu University, Fukuoka, Japan*
CATHERINE E. PEISHOFF • *SmithKline Beecham Pharmaceuticals, King of Prussia, PA*
DAVID M. POLLOCK • *Vascular Biology Center, Medical College of Georgia, Augusta, GA*
RYOICHI TAKAYANAGI • *Third Department of Internal Medicine, Faculty of Medicine, Kyushu University, Fukuoka, Japan*
TIMOTHY D. WARNER • *The William Harvey Research Institute, The Medical College of St. Bartholomew's Hospital, London, UK*

Endothelin

Chapter 1

Endothelin Receptor Subtypes and Tissue Distribution

David M. Pollock

1. Introduction

Subsequent to the realization that endothelial cells are important regulators of vascular, immunological, and probably many other functions, endothelial cell biology has rapidly expanded into a distinct discipline. Numerous endothelial-derived factors have been identified as important contributors in the regulation of vascular tone, including relaxing or contracting substances, such as prostacyclin, nitric oxide, and endothelin.

In 1985, Hickey and colleagues *(1)* reported their discovery that endothelial cells release a peptidergic endothelium-derived constricting factor that produced a sustained contraction in isolated coronary vessels. This factor was purified and cloned in the monumental work of Yanagisawa et al. *(2)* published in 1988. This set off an explosion of research into what these authors described as a family of 21 amino-acid peptides named endothelin (ET). Inoue and colleagues *(3)* published their analysis of human genomic DNA that revealed the existence of three distinct genes encoding three ET isopeptides: ET-1, ET-2, and ET-3. The only isoform thought to be constitutively released from endothelial cells is ET-1, which is believed to play an important role in regulating vascular function. ET-1 is synthesized as the result of a series of proteolytic cleavages of the initial gene product. A unique endothelin-converting enzyme (ECE) is thought to

From: *Endothelin: Molecular Biology, Physiology, and Pathology*
Edited by R. F. Highsmith © Humana Press Inc., Totowa, NJ

remove 18 amino acids from the C-terminus of the immediate precursor referred to as big ET-1. Our knowledge is extremely limited in terms of tissue-specific localization of ECEs. Several receptor subtypes have been identified as mediating the actions of the various ET isopeptides. This chapter will cover what is currently known about the classification of various receptor subtypes and will review the tissue distribution of the receptor subtypes, including some information about the localization of ET isopeptides.

2. ET Receptor Subtypes

2.1. ET_A and ET_B Receptor Subtypes

Multiple receptor subtypes for endothelin have been identified in pharmacological studies both in vitro and in vivo. As evidenced in the study by Yanagisawa et al. *(2)*, at least two receptor subtypes may be responsible for the biphasic nature of the hemodynamic response to iv injection of ET-1: a transient hypotension followed by a sustained increase in arterial pressure. ET-1 and ET-2 are more active than ET-3 as pressor agents and as constrictors of many isolated vascular preparations *(3)*. ET-1 and ET-3 have similar potencies in terms of transient hypotensive effects that are thought to be mediated by the release of nitric oxide and/or prostaglandins *(4,5)*. These results led to the initial subclassification of ET receptors as ET_A (ET-1-selective located on vascular smooth muscle) and ET_B (nonisopeptide-selective located on endothelial cells), which are generally responsible for vasoconstriction and vasodilation, respectively.

ET_A and ET_B receptors were first cloned from bovine and rat tissues, respectively *(6,7)*. Cells transfected with either ET_A or ET_B receptors possess binding characteristics consistent with the ET_A and ET_B classification. There is considerable homology (>90%) between human and bovine or rat ET_A receptors based on their DNA sequence while the ET_B receptor has slightly less, roughly 88%, sequence identity between human and rat receptors. Within a given species, the degree of homology between ET_A and ET_B receptors is roughly 55%. Both ET_A and ET_B receptors are members of the G protein-coupled superfamily of receptors. Multiple effector pathways are activated and are the subject of Chapter 4.

A variety of ligands have been widely used as pharmacological tools for characterizing endothelin receptors (*see* Chapter 7). Much of the receptor identification has been performed by contrasting the binding characteristics of ET-1 vs ET-3 in membrane preparations extracted from various tissues or comparing potencies of these isopeptides in vitro. The sarafotoxins are a family of snake-venom peptides that have a high degree of sequence homology with the endothelins and are often used as endothelin agonists; sarafotoxin 6c is similar to ET-3 in its high affinity for the ET_B receptor and low affinity for the ET_A subtype. Subsequent to the publishing of the DNA sequence of the ET_A and ET_B receptors, mRNA-expression studies have helped in the localizing of receptor subtypes. In the second half of this chapter, a discussion of tissue localization of endothelin peptides and their receptors will be based on this variety of methodology.

The International Union of Pharmacology Committee on Receptor Nomenclature and Drug Classification has recently provided a consensus view of the ET_A / ET_B nomenclature *(8)*. However, the two receptor model appears insufficient to explain the growing amount of biochemical and pharmacological evidence for additional receptor subtypes, primarily the studies using recently developed receptor-selective and nonselective ligands.

2.2. Subtypes of the ET_B Receptor: ET_{B1} and ET_{B2}

Originally it was thought that the ET_A receptor mediated all of the vasoconstrictor properties of ET-1 and that ET-1-induced vasodilation was owing to nitric oxide release stimulated via the ET_B receptors located on the vascular endothelium. Soon after specific ET_A receptor antagonists, such as BQ-123 and FR139317, became available, it was observed that non-ET_A receptors mediate at least some of the vasoconstrictor actions of ET-1. Infusion of BQ-123 intravenously into the rat will completely prevent the rise in mean arterial pressure and hematocrit produced by a simultaneous infusion of relatively high doses of ET-1 *(9)*. However, ET-1-induced decreases in renal blood flow and glomerular filtration rate were totally unaffected even when the doses of BQ-123 were higher than that required to block the systemic actions of ET-1. Binding studies and other in vitro experiments revealed that the renal vasculature and several other arterial and venous circulations contain ET_B receptor-mediated constrictor elements *(10–12)*. Several binding and mRNA expression studies have now confirmed the existence of ET_B receptors in vascular smooth muscle. In fact, infusion of ET_B agonists will elicit a hypertensive response in most species.

Many investigators have proposed the existence of ET receptors that do not conform to the initial ET_A/ET_B classification. For example, it appears as though the ET_B receptor responsible for non-ET_A-mediated vasoconstriction may represent a subtype of the ET_B receptor based on pharmacological evidence. Several studies have shown that the receptor present on vascular endothelium responsible for the release of nitric oxide (termed ET_{B1}) has a unique pharmacological profile compared to the ET_B receptor that mediates vasoconstriction, termed ET_{B2} *(14,15)*. In isolated smooth-muscle preparations, Warner et al. *(14)* observed that the "non-selective" antagonist, PD 142893, blocks ET_A-induced contractions and ET_B-induced relaxations, but has no effect on non-ET_A contractions. Interestingly, the ET_{B1} and ET_{B2} subclassification is consistent with that identified by Sokolovsky et al. *(16)*, who identified ET_{B1} and ET_{B2} binding sites using membrane preparations from different brain regions. These authors distinguished the ET_{B1} and ET_{B2} subtypes by differences in affinity for ET peptides being "super-high" and "high," respectively. Additional evidence that the ET_{B2} receptor on vascular smooth muscle has a lower affinity for ET-1 compared to the ET_{B1} or ET_A receptor comes from the observation that ET_A receptor blockade completely prevents ET-1-induced decreases in renal-blood flow at low doses of the peptide, but has no effect on higher doses of ET-1 *(9,17)*. These results cannot be explained by insufficient blockade of ET_A receptors because the pressor response was completely prevented at both high and low doses of ET-1 and higher doses of ET_A antagonist yielded the same results.

At present, there is no clear biochemical or molecular evidence for ET_{B1} and ET_{B2} receptor subtypes. In fact, RT-PCR and *in situ* hybridization experiments have revealed the presence of mRNA encoding both ET_A and ET_B receptors (the latter using cDNA from the endothelial ET_B receptor) in human vascular smooth muscle *(18)*. These data suggest that differences between the endothelium ET_B receptor, ET_{B1}, and the smooth muscle ET_B receptor, ET_{B2}, are either extremely minor or may be posttranslational in nature. There is some limited molecular evidence for variants of the ET_B receptor in human tissues. Shyamala et al. *(19)* recently published a study that described two distinct human ET_B receptors generated by alternative splicing from a single gene located within human brain, placenta, lung, and heart. Similarly, Cheng et al. *(20)* discovered a novel cDNA encoding a nonselective ET receptor found in rat brain and possibly other tissues as well. It has yet to be determined whether these findings could help explain some of the pharmacological characterization studies.

2.3. ET_A Receptor Subtypes

There have been several reports of novel ET receptors and receptor subtypes of the ET_A variety. Sudjarwo et al. *(21)* suggested the existence of a BQ-123-insensitive ET_A receptor present in rabbit saphenous vein. These authors proposed further subtyping of the ET_A receptor into ET_{A1} (BQ-123 sensitive) and ET_{A2} (BQ-123 insensitive). However, studies from three laboratories have each come to different conclusions regarding the exact receptor population in this tissue *(21–23)*. Other investigators have reported novel subtypes, possibly of the ET_A variety, in rat and human coronary artery *(24,25)*, calf zona glomerulosa *(26)*, rat pituitary *(27)*, and rat mesangial cells *(28)*.

2.4. ET_C Receptors

Because the initial receptor classification was based on isopeptide selectivity, it was postulated that another receptor subtype, named ET_C, would exist as a selective receptor for ET-3. In fact, there has been considerable evidence that all ET receptors cannot fit simply into the ET_A and ET_B classification. There is some indirect or pharmacological evidence for an ET-3-selective receptor located in a variety of tissues and species. Membrane-binding studies have suggested the presence of an ET-3-preferring receptor in chick cardiac membranes *(29)*, bovine and rat atria *(16,30)*, and rat brain and cerebellum *(31,32)*. Functional responses indicating greater potency of ET-3 or sarafotoxin 6c compared to ET-1 have been observed in bovine endothelial cells *(33,34)*, rat renal papilla *(35)*, rat pituitary *(36)*, and rat PC12 pheochromocytoma cells *(37)*. More recently, Douglas et al. *(22)* reported pharmacological evidence for the presence of three distinct receptor subtypes in the rabbit saphenous vein. They used ET-1, ET-3, and sarafotoxin 6c along with a combination of newly developed receptor antagonists to distinguish between ET_{B2}- and ET_C-mediated vasoconstriction as well as ET_{B1} receptors on the vascular endothelium of this tissue. In contrast, Gray et al. *(15)* observed that a significant portion of the vasoconstrictor response to ET-1 was inhibited by BQ-123, suggesting the existence of ET_A-mediated vasoconstriction in the rabbit saphenous vein. The reason for these conflicting results are not known. Finally, there have been several reports of an ET-3-specific receptor that is sensitive to BQ-123 *(38,39)*.

At present, however, the ET_C receptor still represents only a pharmacological phenomenon because there is yet no molecular confirmation of a third ET receptor in mammalian tissue. Karne et al. *(40)*

cloned a unique receptor with slightly higher affinity for ET-3 vs ET-1 from *Xenopus laevis* dermal melanophores, but it is not known whether this or a related receptor exists in mammalian tissues.

Although there is considerable evidence for pharmacologically distinct receptor subtypes beyond the ET_A /ET_B classification, no clear picture has emerged. Some of the lack of clarity in pharmacological studies of ET receptors may be owing to differences in glycosylation or other posttranslational modifications of ET receptors within various tissues and among species *(41)*. Progress in developing receptor ligands with higher specificity as well as localization and molecular studies will facilitate resolution of the receptor subtype questions.

3. Receptor Subtypes and Signal Transduction

Very little information is known about ET receptor subtype-specific signal transduction pathways. The most common feature of activation of each receptor subtype characterized thus far is an increase in cytosolic calcium (Ca^{2+}; *42*). Endothelin-induced vasoconstriction after binding to ET_A receptors occurs via a G protein-dependent signal-transduction pathway of phospholipase C (PLC) activation and inositol triphosphate (IP_3) generation. Multiple G proteins may be activated to stimulate a variety of other effector systems, such as phospholipase A_2 or ion-specific membrane channels, including the Na^+/H^+ antiporter. Although a number of mediators have been identified for their involvement in the Ca^{2+} mobilization response to ET, the precise function and coordination of these messengers is not fully resolved. In the vasculature, the assumption that the ET_A receptor is the predominant subtype underlies a number of studies investigating the nature of the vasoconstricting actions of ET. However, there has been little verification of receptor subtypes in these studies. Thus, the extent to which the signal transduction mechanisms may be receptor subtype-specific is unknown.

The focus of most research on ET-activated cellular events has clearly been on those occurring with activation of the ET_A receptor. It should be noted, however, that investigation of signaling mechanisms mediated by other ET-receptor subtypes is an evolving research area. A number of questions regarding the specificity of responses in various tissues must be addressed, such as the signal-transduction pathways for ET_{B2}-induced constriction. Furthermore, subtype-specific coupling may vary according to the type of cell or species involved. For example, Aramori and Nakanishi *(43)* observed that ET_A receptor activation produced an increase in cAMP accumulation whereas activation of the ET_B receptor had opposite effects in cells transfected with either ET_A or ET_B receptors. Because activation of both receptors also stimulated phosphatidylinositol hydrolysis and arachidonic-acid release, these results suggest that the two receptor subtypes have both common and distinct signal-transduction pathways mediated through different G proteins. Alternatively, it is possible that these mechanisms may be unique to transfected cells. In cultured smooth muscle cells of the bovine pulmonary artery, both ET_A and ET_B receptor subtypes are present, but stimulate distinct signals of IP_3 formation and inhibition of adenylate cyclase, respectively *(44)*. In rabbit saphenous vein, both ET_A and ET_B receptors produce vasoconstriction, but by PKC-dependent and -independent mechanisms, respectively. In terms of the ET-induced vasodilation, the ET_{B1} receptor activates a pertussis toxin-sensitive G protein and increases IP_3 production and cytosolic Ca^{2+} *(33)*. Subsequent release of nitric oxide then induces the underlying vascular smooth muscle to relax.

4. Termination of ET Signaling

A rather unique property of the ET ligand-receptor complex is the slow rate of dissociation and the near irreversibility of binding *(45)*. This property helps to explain the prolonged vasoconstriction of ET given its extremely short half-life within the circulation *(46)*. This finding also highlights the importance of understanding how the ET signal is terminated, yet it is a topic that has received relatively little scrutiny. The different ET isoforms display different rates and extents of dissociation *(47,48)*. Furthermore, dissociation rates vary among membrane preparations from different tissues or species *(49)*. These characteristics could be explained by different mechanisms involved in turning off the ET signal and/or dissociating the ligand-receptor complex.

It is doubtful that fast-acting mediators are involved in termination of ET signaling because of the prolonged vasoconstriction induced by ET. Researchers who believe that L-type Ca^{2+} channels have an exclusive role in facilitating Ca^{2+} entry would support the idea that membrane repolarization and channel inactivation would be responsible for terminating the signal. However, proponents of PKC-mediated constriction believe that metabolism of DAG leads to inactivation of PKC and subsequent termination of the response. Although the actual mechanism probably involves both of these actions, it is possible that an alternative pathway is involved. Goligorsky et al. *(50)* have recently proposed a novel mechanism by which nitric oxide (NO) may mediate the termination of the signal. When Chinese hamster ovary (CHO) cells were transfected with ET_A receptors and stimulated with ET, NO displaced ET from its receptor at the cell membrane, thus terminating the stimulation. Furthermore it was shown that NO interfered with the calcium-mobilization process during the cellular transduction of the ET signal. Another study conducted by Edano and colleagues *(51)* suggests that ET-1 is digested by a membrane-bound enzyme similar to enkephalinase. Homologous desensitization of the ligand-receptor complex is prevented because the degradation occurs while ET is still bound to its receptor. Thus, the proposed mechanism of termination involves desensitization of the ET receptor as well as downregulation of ET-induced second messengers. Termination of ET signaling is an area that needs more investigation in order to obtain a more complete understanding of the process of ET-induced activation and inactivation of the smooth-muscle contractile apparatus.

5. Tissue Distribution of ET and Its Receptors

Consistent with its putative role as an autocrine and paracrine factor, circulating levels of ET may represent spillover from the local environment between the endothelium and vascular smooth muscle. Several general observations support this conclusion. Endothelin concentrations in plasma are below the concentrations thought to be necessary to activate ET receptors (< 5 pM). Plasma ET is also degraded and cleared rapidly, with a half-life on the order of approx 1 min *(46)*. Furthermore, ET-neutralizing antibodies have no hemodynamic effects. Therefore, plasma ET concentrations, at least at normal to low levels, are poor predictors of the biological activity of ET. Tissue concentrations and mRNA expression measurements of ET and especially its receptors are perhaps a more reliable means of studying ET activity.

Endothelin-binding studies have revealed widespread distribution of ET receptors within virtually every organ system by virtue of ET's presence within the vascular endothelium. Much of the complexity surrounding the study of ET function is related to the fact that there is considerable variability in the distribution of receptor subtypes between different vascular beds and among species. In general, but not always, ET-1-induced vasoconstriction is produced via ET_A receptors on arterial vessels whereas ET_B receptors predominate on the low-pressure side of the circulation *(52,53)*. Endothelin receptors of both the ET_A and especially the ET_B classification are found on many other cell types aside from vascular endothelium and smooth muscle, including nonvascular structures within the heart, kidney, lung, and nervous system (Table 1).

5.1. Heart

Endothelin can influence cardiac function in a wide variety of ways including vasoconstriction, mitogenesis, release of atrial natriuretic peptide, and inotropic effects. Vascular endothelium, the conducting system, and cardiomyocytes themselves are all potential sources of ET. The initial work of MacCumber et al. *(54)* using Northern blot analysis of tissue extracts and *in situ* hybridization suggested very little ET present within normal cardiac tissue of the rat although Nunez et al. *(55)* observed notable expression of preproET mRNA when applying reverse transcription (RT) and the polymerase chain reaction (PCR) technique. These results would indicate that the heart normally synthesizes only small quantities of ET. Plumpton et al. *(56)* further showed that human myocardium expresses all three ET isoforms, ET-1, ET-2, and ET-3, based on RT-PCR, immunoreactivity, and chromatography of tissue extracts. Several laboratories demonstrated that cultured rat cardiomyocytes and endocardial cells synthesize and release ET-1 *(57–60)*, although very little information is yet available in regard to specific localized production in intact tissue.

Both ET_A and ET_B receptor subtypes have been identified within cardiac tissue of several species as determined in differential binding studies. In general, there appear to be a greater number of binding sites in the atria relative to ventricle and, in particular, the right atrium *(61–63)*. In fact, ET stimulates atrial-natriuretic peptide release probably through ET_A receptors located in the atrial myocardium *(64,65)*. Molenaar and colleagues *(66)* studied human receptor subtypes using radioligand binding, RT-PCR, and *in situ* hybridization techniques and identified both ET_A and ET_B receptors in atrial and ventricular myocardium, the atrioventricular conducting system, and endocardial cells.

Identification of receptor subtypes within the coronary circulation has been facilitated primarily by pharmacological ex vivo studies. Both receptor subtypes have been identified as mediating

Table 1
Distribution of ET_A and ET_B Receptor Subtypes in Human Tissue[a]

Heart	
Coronary artery	ET_A/ET_B
Tunica media	ET_A
Neointima	ET_B
Distal artery	ET_A
Proximal artery	ET_B
Coronary vein	ET_A
Left ventricle	$ET_A \gg ET_B$
Right atrium	ET_A
Atrioventricular conducting system	ET_A / ET_B
Pericardium	ET_A / ET_B
Girardi heart cells	ET_B
Embryonic carcinoma — cardiomyocyte origin	ET_A
Aorta	
Endothelium	ET_B
Vascular smooth muscle	$ET_A \gg ET_B$
Brachial artery	ET_A
Saphenous vein	$ET_B > ET_A$
Lung	
Pulmonary artery	ET_A
Airway smooth muscle	$ET_B > ET_A$
Alveoli	$ET_B > ET_A$
Kidney	
Collecting tubules	ET_B
Renal artery and vein	$ET_A > ET_B$
Vasa recta bundles	ET_A
Nervous system	
Cerebral cortex	ET_B
Glia, epithelial ependymal cells	ET_B
Astrocytoma	ET_B
Neuroblastoma	ET_A
Meningioma	ET_A
Embryonic carcinomal — neural origin	ET_B
Cerebral microvascular endothelium	ET_A
Cerebral, meningial, and temporal artery	ET_A
Glioblastoma capillaries	ET_A
Bone	
Osteoblasts	ET_A / ET_B
Osteogenic cells (embryonic mandibular process)	ET_A / ET_B
Synovial blood vessels	ET_A
Skin	
Subcutaneous resistance arteries	$ET_A > ET_B$
Dermal fibroblasts	ET_A

Table 1 *(continued)*

Keratinocytes	ET_A / ET_B
Platelets	ET_A (maybe ET_B)
Female reproductive system	
Endometrium	
Proliferative phase	ET_A
Secretory, menstrual phase	ET_B
Myometrium	$ET_A \gg ET_B$
Small placental arteries	ET_A
Placental vein	ET_B
Umbilical artery	ET_A / ET_B?
Human umbilical vein endothelial cells	ET_B
Decidua	ET_B
Mammary artery	$ET_A > ET_B$
Mammary vein	$ET_B > ET_A$
Prostate	
Stroma	ET_A
Glandular epithelium	ET_B
Liver	
Myofibroblastic Ito cells	$ET_B > ET_A$
Gastrointestinal tract	
Enteric ganglia	ET_B
Omental arteries	ET_A
Eye	
Retinal and choroidal blood vessels	ET_A
Neural and glial substance	ET_B
Adrenal gland	
Zona glomerulosa	$ET_A > ET_B$
Aldosterone-producing adenoma	ET_A / ET_B

[a]This table is a best representation of available binding and mRNA expression data obtained exclusively from human tissues or cell lines of human origin. Refer to text for selected references. Unless indicated, relative amounts in tissues expressing both subtypes are unknown.

ET-1-induced contraction in the coronary circulation although a high degree of species variability appears to exist. In porcine coronary vessels, ET_{B2} but not ET_{B1} receptors have been pharmacologically identified *(67)* whereas canine coronary arteries possess both ET_{B1} and ET_{B2} *(68)*. In human coronary artery, however, a clear picture has not emerged because several investigators have indicated the presence of non-ET_A-induced vasoconstriction *(69,70)*, whereas others suggest that ET-1-induced constriction is predominantly mediated by the ET_A subtype *(71,72)*. Both ET_A and ET_B receptors have been identified on smooth muscle from human coronary vessels using RT-PCR, *in situ* hybridization, and membrane-binding techniques *(18,73)*. However, the functional response attributed to non-ET_A receptors may be relatively weak compared to the degree of ET_A-mediated constrictor effects *(72,73)*.

5.2. Kidney

In addition to vascular endothelium, cells of renal tubular, mesangial and interstitial origin have been shown to synthesize and release ET in culture. Immunohistochemical analysis has consistently demonstrated higher amounts of ET-1-like immunoreactivity in the renal medulla compared to the cortex in a variety of species, including human *(74–77)*. In the rat kidney, Wilkes et al. *(77)* reported that immunostaining density was greatest in vasa recta whereas lesser staining was observed within the cytosol of collecting duct cells in the papilla. Within the renal cortex, ET-like immunoreactivity was predominantly localized to endothelial cells of arcuate arteries, arterioles, peritubular capillaries, and veins. Lesser amounts of staining appeared in both glomerular capillaries and mesangial cells along with the early proximal tubule.

Studies examining ET-gene expression confirm that higher amounts of the peptide are produced within the medullary regions of the kidney *(78,79)*. Specific cellular localization using microdissection and RT-PCR or RNase protection reveal that in both rat and human, the inner medulla (specifically, inner medullary collecting duct cells) is the site of the highest amount of ET-1 gene expression *(80,81)*. *In situ* hybridization studies identified ET-1 mRNA expression within the vasa recta *(79)*. Glomerular expression of ET-1 mRNA has been reported in the rat *(80)* but not the human, although technical differences may not have allowed detection of a low-expression level in human glomeruli *(81)*.

Autoradiographic-binding studies have shown a pattern of ET-receptor localization consistent with its role as a paracrine factor; that is, the receptors are present at sites where ET synthesis occurs. Within the kidney, a particularly high density of binding sites have been identified in the inner medulla, inner stripe of the outer medulla, and glomeruli, with moderate to low levels of binding distributed throughout the outer cortex *(82,83)*. In terms of receptor subtypes, kidneys from all species, including human, contain both ET_A and ET_B receptors, although the role of each of these receptors in producing vasoconstriction are species dependent. In the rat, both ET_A and ET_B receptor activation produces vasoconstriction in the kidney *(9,17)*. In the dog, ET_B agonists or low doses of ET-3 will produce renal vasodilation although they have no effect in the rabbit kidney *(84,85)*. Binding studies suggest a mixed population of both ET_A and ET_B receptors in kidneys of all species tested thus far, although the relative quantities of each subtype are not correlated to functional responses *(9,17,84,85,87,88)*. The vascular response to ET-1 appears to be ET_A-dependent in the human kidney, even though the tissue contains a majority of ET_B receptors *(74)*. Specific cellular localization has not been completely elucidated. In vitro radioligand binding indicates the presence of receptors in the renal vascular smooth muscle, mesangial cells, and cultured tubular cells *(82,83,89)*. Intravenous injection of ^{125}I-labeled ET-1 in the rat indicates specific binding localized to endothelial cells of glomeruli and peritubular capillaries of the cortex *(90)*.

The function of ET within the renal medulla appears to involve inhibition of ADH-induced changes in water permeability *(91,92)* that occurs via interaction with ET_B receptors located on inner-medullary collecting-duct cells *(93,94)*. However, ET_A receptors present on medullary-interstitial cells may also influence water excretion by regulating medullary hemodynamics *(95)*. Synthesis and release of ET has been demonstrated in cultured collecting-duct cells and cells originating from the proximal tubule *(96)*. Several studies have provided evidence that ET-1 may regulate proximal tubular-transport mechanisms, including Na^+-K^+-ATPase, Na^+/H^+ exchange, Na^+-HCO_3^- cotransport, and Na^+-P_i cotransport *(97–99)*.

5.3. Lung

Pulmonary tissue contains some of the highest concentrations of ET-1 of any organ *(100)*. Rozengurt et al. *(101)* observed in rats and mice that ET-like immunoreactivity is found primarily in airway epithelium. ET-1 is also released in vitro from tracheal and bronchial epithelial cells in addition to the pulmonary vascular endothelial cells. Marciniak and coworkers *(102)* identified significant ET-like immunoreactivity in human-lung parenchyma, airway smooth muscle, and airway epithelia. Similarly, Giaid et al. *(103)* identified high proportions ET-1 in human-lung parenchyma using immunocytochemistry and *in situ* hybridization with lesser amounts being found in airway epithelium and vascular endothelium.

Both ET_A and ET_B receptors have also been found throughout the pulmonary vasculature, airways, and alveoli. Similar to other organs, specific receptor distribution differs among species. In the pulmonary circulation of the guinea pig, ET_A receptors appear to mediate ET-1-induced contractions as demonstrated in vitro and in vivo *(104–106)*. ET-1 can contract isolated airway tissues via both ET_A and ET_B receptor subtypes *(104,107–110)*. In the anesthetized, ventilated guinea pig, iv injection of ET-1 results in a potent pressor response along with an increase in airway resistance *(111,112)*. Intravenous infusion of an ET_A receptor antagonist inhibited the pressor response to ET-1, but had little effect on bronchoconstriction, suggesting that non-ET_A receptors are functional in bronchial smooth muscle *(106)*. Using autoradiography and isolated tracheal strips from the rat, Henry *(110)* reported that ET_A and ET_B receptors may coexist in tracheal smooth muscle. Inui et al. *(113)* have also localized both ET_A and ET_B receptors on single smooth-muscle cells of the guinea-pig trachea both of which appear to be linked to a contractile mechanism. Nakamichi et al. *(114)* have shown in porcine pulmonary tissues that blood vessels and bronchi are rich in ET_A receptors and the lung parenchyma is rich in ET_B receptors, which is consistent with the results of Abraham et al. *(115)* in sheep. In contrast, Hay et al. *(105)* have reported the opposite results in guinea pigs. Similar to the porcine species, human pulmonary vessels contain primarily ET_A receptors, whereas there is a high proportion of ET_B receptors in the rabbit pulmonary artery *(88,114,116)*. In the human pulmonary artery, functional data confirms binding studies because the selective ET_A receptor antagonist, BQ-123, inhibited ET-1-induced contraction and the ET_B agonist, sarafotoxin 6c, caused no contraction *(117)*. In human airways, Knott et al. *(118)* reported the presence of both ET_A and ET_B receptor sites in airway smooth muscle and alveoli; the great majority within airway smooth muscle were of the ET_B subtype. In other species, ET_B receptors present on endothelial cells within the pulmonary vasculature produce vasodilation via release of NO. Regardless of species, ET-1 appears to be a more potent constrictor of pulmonary veins than arteries *(119–121)*.

Seldeslagh and Lauweryns *(122)* identified significant amounts of ET-3 in neuroepithelial bodies in the intrapulmonary airways and alveolar parenchyma. Furthermore, ET-3 colocalized to areas rich in serotonin and/or calcitonin gene-related peptide. Interestingly, ET_B receptors, for which ET-3 has the highest affinity, are found in highest concentrations in parenchyma, parasympathetic ganglia, pulmonary and submucosal plexuses *(123)*.

5.4. Central and Peripheral Nervous System

Components of the ET system have been identified throughout the central and peripheral nervous system, although there is still much that remains unknown about the role of ET in neural function. *In situ* hybridization and immunohistochemistry have identified ET peptides in a variety of structures, including the paraventricular and supraoptic nuclei of the hypothalamus *(124,125)*, both glia and neurons of the cerebellum *(126)*, the hippocampus, granular cerebellum, motor neurons in the spinal cord *(127)*, and peripheral ganglia *(123)*. The predominant ET isoform within the brain is thought by many to be ET-3, particularly within the hypothalamus and cerebellum *(100,125)*, which could explain why the ET_B receptor is the predominant subtype found within such areas as the cerebellum *(128)*.

A unique finding with regard to ET receptors is the observation that receptors of the ET_A variety have been identified on rat and human endothelial cells derived from the cerebral microcirculation *(129,130)*. The function of these receptors has not been elucidated. As expected, ET_A receptors have also been identified on smooth muscle within this vascular bed *(131,132)*.

The functional role of ET within the brain has yet to be clearly elucidated, although there is a fair amount of evidence that it is important in central control of fluid-volume status and blood pressure. One line of evidence to support this idea is simply the localization of portions of the ET system within the regions of the brain known to be involved in regulation of circulatory and renal function, i.e., the hypothalamus and pituitary gland *(see* Section 5.5.). Endothelin may also play a role as a neuromodulator within the central nervous system (CNS) because intraventicular infusion of ET results in an increase in mean arterial pressure and heart rate *(133,134)*.

5.5. Endocrine Organs

Endothelin modulates the activity of many endocrine systems and is the subject of two recent reviews *(135,136)*. It seems certain that in addition to its direct cardiovascular effects, ET has a neuroendocrine function based on localization experiments (that have identified ET immunoreactivity and mRNA in hypothalamus, pituitary, and adrenal glands) as well as numerous functional studies. In addition, there is considerable evidence that ET and atrial natriuretic peptide have an interactive role *(see* Section 5.1.).

The observation that ET-like immunoreactivity is localized within the neurohypophysis suggests an autocrine role for ET in regulating antidiuretic hormone release *(125)*. Both in vitro and in vivo studies have demonstrated that exogenous ET-1 and/or ET-3 stimulates the release of ADH *(137–139)*. These actions most likely involve ET_A receptor activation *(140)*. There is evidence that both ET_A and ET_B receptors are expressed in the anterior pituitary, although ET_A receptors appear to mediate the actions of ET in terms of gonadotrophin release *(27,141,142)*. However, the anterior pituitary is one of the few tissues where the concentration of ET-3 is found in great abundance *(100)*.

Many investigators have demonstrated that ET-1 can stimulate the release of aldosterone. The adrenal gland expresses ET-1 mRNA and contains a large amount of ET-1 immunoreactivity *(126)*. It is not clear which receptor subtype mediates the stimulatory effect of ET-1 on aldosterone release. A preliminary report by Naruse et al. *(143)* indicated that the ET_A receptor antagonist, BQ-123, can inhibit ET-1-induced aldosterone release. However, Imai et al. *(144)* used mRNA expression studies to show that the major subtype present within the zona glomerulosa is of the ET_B variety, although Rossi et al. *(145)* found an equal amount of ET_A and ET_B receptors within this cell type. It is possible that the ET_B receptor functions to mediate indirect actions of ET-1 by potentiating angiotensin II-induced aldosterone release. As suggested by Cozza et al. *(146)*, this mechanism would be separate from direct ET_A-mediated stimulation.

5.6. Reproductive Organs

Endothelin may have a role in various aspects of the female reproductive system. ET-1 is a potent contractor of uterine smooth muscle and can reduce uterine and placental blood flow through its vasoconstrictive properties. Immunoreactive ET-1 and ET-1 mRNA have been identified within the endometrium of several species with limited detection in myometrium *(147,48)*. Human amnionic fluid also contains ET-1, which probably originates from amnion cells *(149)*. ET-1 in the human placenta is thought to be synthesized in a developmentally regulated manner and may be important in regulating growth of placental mesenchymal cells, in addition to controlling placental blood flow.

Both ET_A and ET_B receptors are expressed in normal human myometrium as well as placenta, with ET_B receptors predominating in the latter tissue *(150,151)*. The ET_A receptor is responsible for

ET-1-induced uterine contraction whereas the role of the ET_B receptor has yet to be defined *(152,153)*.

Within the male reproductive system, Ergul et al. *(154)* demonstrated that ET-1 can be synthesized and secreted by rat testicular Sertoli cells, whereas specific binding sites were found on rat testicular Leydig cells. In the human prostate, ET_A receptors appear to be localized in the stroma and ET_B in the epithelium *(155)*. However, both ET-1 and an ET_B-selective agonist, sarafotoxin 6c, contract isolated prostatic tissue and are not inhibited by ET_A receptor blockade *(156)*.

5.7. Gastrointestinal System

In addition to the vascular endothelium, ET-1 and its receptors have been localized within the mucosal layer of the rat colon, intestine, and stomach by Takahashi et al. *(157)* using autoradiographic and mRNA-expression techniques. A role for ET in the control of ion transport in the gut may be mediated by ET_A receptors and may involve submucosal cholinergic nerves *(158)*. ET-2, also known as vasoactive intestinal contractor (VIC), is found in high concentrations within the gastrointestinal (GI) tract and is a potent contractor of GI smooth muscle. Pharmacological studies with receptor agonists and antagonists suggest that intestinal smooth muscle contains both ET_A and ET_{B2} constrictor elements as well as ET_{B1}-mediated relaxation *(159–161)*. Both ET-1 and VIC have also been identified in enteric and myenteric neurons *(162–164)*. Puffenberger et al. *(165)* have reported that patients with Hirschsprung's disease, characterized by an absence of enteric ganglia in the distal colon, have a missense mutation of the ET_B receptor gene, which suggests a role for ET in ganglion formation.

6. Summary

Considerable progress has been made in our efforts to localize the various components of the ET system in the short time since its discovery. However, there remains much to be learned about many aspects of ET physiology and pathophysiology. The family of ET peptides are synthesized by not only the vascular endothelium, but also by a wide variety of nonendothelial cell types. Although we are confident that synthesis of ET involves the activity of a unique ET-converting enzyme, we know very little about this enzyme, especially in regard to specific localization. Two receptor subtypes have been cloned, but there is a large and growing body of evidence that the two receptor model is incomplete. Investigation in this area is made difficult by the complexity of the system, but perhaps even more so because ET is an autocrine and/or paracrine factor. Further progress will depend on a proper blend of molecular biology and cell biology, with both in vitro and in vivo approaches. It is certain that over the coming years we will slowly unlock the secrets behind this sometimes mysterious family of peptides.

References

1. Hickey, K. A., Rubanyi, G. M., Paul, R. J., and Highsmith, R. F. (1985) Characterization of a coronary vasoconstrictor produced by cultured endothelial cells. *Am. J. Physiol.* **248:**C550–C556.
2. Yanagisawa, M., Kurihara, H., Kimura, S., Tomobe, Y., Kobayashi, M., Mitsui, Y., Yazaki, K., Goto, Y., and Masaki, T. (1988) A novel potent vasoconstrictor peptide produced by vascular endothelial cells. *Nature* **332:**411–415.
3. Inoue, A., Yanagisawa, M., Takuwa, Y., Kobayashi, M., and Masaki, T. (1989) The human endothelin family: three structurally and pharmacologically distinct isopeptides predicted by three separate genes. *Proc. Natl. Acad. Sci. USA* **86:**2863–2867.
4. Warner, T. D., Mitchell, J. A., de Nucci, G., and Vane, J. R. (1989) Endothelin-1 and endothelin-3 release EDRF from isolated perfused arterial vessels of the rat and rabbit. *J. Cardiovasc. Pharmacol.* **13:** S85–S88.
5. Gardiner, S. M., Compton, A. M., and Bennett, T. (1990) Effects of indomethacin on the regional haemodynamic responses to low doses of endothelins and sarafotoxin. *Br. J. Pharmacol.* **100:**158–162.
6. Arai, H., Nori, S., Aramori, I., Ohkubu, H., and Nakanishi, S. (1990) Cloning and expression of a cDNA encoding an endothelin receptor. *Nature* **348:**730–732.
7. Sakurai, T., Yanagisawa, M., Takuwa, Y., Miyazaki, H., Kimura, S., Goto, K., and Masaki, T. (1990) Cloning of a cDNA encoding a non-isopeptide-selective subtype of the endothelin receptor. *Nature* **348:**732–735.
8. Masaki, T., Vane, J. R., and Vanhoutte, P. M. (1994) V. International union of pharmacology nomenclature of endothelin receptors. *Pharmacol. Rev.* **46:**137–142.
9. Pollock, D. M. and Opgenorth, T. J. (1993) Evidence for endothelin-induced renal vasoconstriction independent of ET_A receptor activation. *Am. J. Physiol.* **264:**R222–R226.
10. Bigaud, M. and Pelton, J. T. (1992) Discrimination between ET_A- and ET_B-receptor-mediated effects of endothelin-1 and [Ala[1,3,11,15]]endothelin-1 by BQ-123 in the anesthetized rat. *Br. J. Pharmacol.* **107:**912–918.

11. Clozel, M., Gray, G. A., Breu, V., Löffler, B.-M., and Osterwalder, R. (1992) The endothelin ET_B receptor mediates both vasodilation and vasoconstriction in vivo. *Biochem. Biophys. Res. Comm.* **186**:867–873.

12. Cristol, J.-P., Warner, T. D., Thiemermann, C., and Vane, J. R. (1993) Mediation via different receptors of the vasoconstrictor effects of endothelins and sarafotoxins in the systemic circulation and renal vasculature of the anaesthetized rat. *Br. J. Pharmacol.* **108**:776–779.

14. Warner, T. D., Allcock, G. H., Corder, R., and Vane, J. R. (1993) Use of the endothelin antagonists BQ-123 and PD 142893 to reveal three endothelin receptors mediating smooth muscle contraction and the release of EDRF. *Br. J. Pharmacol.* **110**:777–782.

15. Gray, G. A. and Clozel, M. (1994) Three endothelin receptor subtypes suggested by the differential potency of bosentan, a novel endothelin receptor antagonist, in isolated tissues. *Br. J. Pharmacol.* **112**:U62.

16. Sokolovsky, M., Ambar, I., and Galdron, R. (1992) A novel subtype of endothelin receptors. *J. Biol. Chem.* **267**:20,551–20,554.

17. Pollock, D. M. and Opgenorth, T. J. (1994) ET_A receptor-mediated responses to endothelin-1 and big endothelin-1 in the rat kidney. *Br. J. Pharmacol.* **111**:729–732.

18. Davenport, A. P., O'Reilly, G., Molenaar, P., Maguire, J. J., Kuc, R. E., Sharkey, A., Bacon, C. R., and Ferro, A. (1993) Human endothelin receptors characterized using reverse transcriptase-polymerase chain reaction, in situ hybridization, and subtype-selective ligands BQ123 and BQ3020: evidence for expression of ET_B receptors in human vascular smooth muscle. *J. Cardiovasc. Pharmacol.* **22(Suppl. 8)**:S22–S25.

19. Shyamala, V., Moulthrop, T. H., Stratton-Thomas, J., and Tekamp-Olson, P. (1994) Two distinct human endothelin B receptors generated by alternative splicing from a single gene. *Cell. Mol. Biol. Res.* **40**:285–296.

20. Cheng, H. F., Su, Y. M., Yeh, J. R., and Chang, K. J. (1993) Alternative transcript of the nonselective-type endothelin receptor from rat brain. *Mol. Pharmacol.* **44**:533–538.

21. Sudjarwo, S. A., Hort, M., Tanaka, T., Matsuda, Y., Okada, T., and Karaki, H. (1994) Subtypes of endothelin ET_A and ET_B receptors mediating venous smooth muscle contraction. *Biochem. Biophys. Res. Comm.* **200**:627–633.

22. Douglas, S. A., Beck, G. R., Jr., Elliott, J. D., and Ohlstein, E. H. (1995) Pharmacological evidence for the presence of three distinct functional endothelin receptor subtypes in the rabbit lateral saphenous vein. *Br. J. Pharmacol.* **114**:1529–1540.

23. Gray, G. A., Löffler, B.-M., and Clozel, M. (1994) Characterization of endothelin receptors mediating contraction of rabbit saphenous vein. *Am. J. Physiol.* **266**:H959–H966.

24. Bax, W. A., Peterson, R. W. G., Inan, T., Bos, E., and Saxena, P. R. (1994) Heterogeneity of endothelin/sarafotoxin receptors mediating contractions of the human isolated coronary artery. *Br. J. Pharmacol.* **111**:15P.

25. Gulati, A. and Sharma, A. C. (1994) Evidence for the existence of a different type of endothelin (ET) receptor in the coronary blood vessels of rats. *Ped. Res.* **35**:35A.

26. Gomez-Sanchez, C. E., Cozza, E. N., Foecking, M., Chiou, F. S., and Ferris, M. W. (1990) Endothelin receptor subtypes and stimulation of aldosterone secretion. *Hypertension* **15**:744–747.

27. Kanyicska, B. and Freeman, M. E. (1993) Characterization of endothelin receptors in the anterior pituitary gland. *Am. J. Physiol.* **265**:E601–E608.

28. Simonson, M. S. and Rooney, A. (1994) Characterization of endothelin receptors in mesangial cells: evidence for two functionally distinct endothelin binding sites. *J. Pharmacol. Exp. Therap.* **46**:41–50.

29. Watanabe, H., Miyazaki, H., Kondoh, M., Masuda, Y., Kimura, S., Yanagisawa, M., Masaki, T., and Murakami, K. (1989) Two distinct types of endothelin receptors are present on chick cardiac membranes. *Biochem. Biophys. Res. Comm.* **161**:1252–1259.

30. Schvartz, I., Ittoop, O., and Hazum, E. (1991) Direct evidence for multiple endothelin receptors. *Biochemistry* **30**:5325–5327.

31. Nambi, P., Pullen, M., and Feuerstein, G. (1990) Identification of endothelin receptors in various regions of the rat brain. *Neuropeptides* **16**:195–199.

32. Kloog, Y., Bousso-Mittler, D., Bdolah, A., and Sokolovsky, M. (1989) Three apparent receptor subtypes for the endothelin/sarafotoxin family. *FEBS Lett.* **253**:199–202.

33. Emori, T., Hirata, Y., and Marumo, F. (1990) Specific receptors for endothelin-3 in cultured bovine endothelial cells and its cellular mechanism of action. *FEBS Lett.* **263**:261–264.

34. Warner, T. D., Schmidt, H. H. H. W., and Murad, F. (1992) Interactions of endothelins and EDRF in bovine native endothelial cells: selective effects of endothelin-3. *Am. J. Physiol.* **262**:H1600–H1605.

35. Woodcock, E. A. and Land, S. (1991) Endothelin receptors in rat renal papilla with a high affinity for endothelin-3. *Eur. J. Pharmacol.* **208**:255–260.

36. Samson, W. K., Skala, K. D., Alexander, B. D., and Huang, F. L. (1990) Pituitary site of action of endothelin: selective inhibition of prolactin release in vitro. *Biochem. Biophys. Res. Comm.* **169**:737–743.

37. Martin, E. R., Brenner, B. M., and Ballermann, B. J. (1990) Heterogeneity of cell surface endothelin receptors. *J. Biol. Chem.* **265**:14,044–14,049.

38. Battistini, B., O'Donnell, L. J. D., Warner, T. D., Fournier, A., Farthing, M. J. G., and Vane, J. R. (1994) Characterization of endothelin (ET) receptors in the isolated gall bladder of the guinea pig: evidence for an additional ET receptor subtype. *Br. J. Pharmacol.* **112**:1244–1250.

39. Sedo, A., Rovero, P., Revoltella, R. P., di Bartolo, V., Beffy, P., and Mizrahi, J. (1993) BQ-123 inhibits both endothelin 1 and endothelin 3 mediated C6 rat glioma cell proliferation suggesting an atypical endothelin receptor. *J. Biol. Regul. Homeostat. Agents* **7**:95–98.

40. Karne, S., Jayawickreme, C. K., and Lerner, M. R. (1993) Cloning and characterization of an endothelin-3 specific receptor (ET_C) receptor from Xenopus laevis dermal melanophores. *J. Biol. Chem.* **268**:19,126–19,133.

41. Bousso-Mittler, D., Galron, R., and Sokolovsky, M. (1991) Endothelin/ sarafotoxin receptor heterogeneity: evidence for different glycosylation in receptors from different tissues. *Biochem. Biophys. Res. Comm.* **178:**921–926.

42. Pollock, D. M., Keith, T. L., and Highsmith, R. F. (1995) Endothelin receptors and calcium signaling. *FASEB J.* **9:**1196–1204.

43. Aramori, I. and Nakanishi, S. (1992) Coupling of two endothelin receptor subtypes to differing signal transduction in transfected Chinese hamster ovary cells. *J. Biol. Chem.* **267:**12,468–12,474.

44. Kent, A. and Keenan, A. K. (1994) Evidence for signaling by endothelin ET_A and ET_B receptors in bovine pulmonary artery smooth muscle cells. *Br. J. Pharmacol.* **122:**U62.

45. Hirata, Y., Yoshimi, H., Takaichi, S., Yanagisawa, M., and Masaki, T. (1988) Binding and receptor down-regulation of a novel vasoconstrictor endothelin in cultured rat vascular smooth muscle cells. *FEBS Lett.* **239:**13–17.

46. Anggard, E., Galton, S., Rae, G., Thomas, R., McLoughlin, L., De Nucci, G., and Vane, J. R. (1989) The fate of radioiodinated endothelin-1 and endothelin-3 in the rat. *J. Cardiovasc. Pharmacol.* **13(Suppl. 5):**S46–S49.

47. Galdron, R., Kloog, Y., Bdolah, A., and Sokolovsky, M. (1989) Functional endothelin/sarafotoxin receptors in rat heart myocytes: structure-activity relationships and receptor subtypes. *Biochem Biophys. Res. Comm.* **163:**936–943.

48. Devesly, P., Phillips, P. E., Johns, A., Rubanyi, G., and Parker-Botelho, L. H. (1990) Receptor kinetics differ for endothelin-1 and endothelin-2 binding to Swiss 3T3 fibroblasts. *Biochem. Biophys. Res. Comm.* **172:**126–134.

49. Galdron, R., Bdolah, A., Kochva, A., Wollberg, Z., Kloog, Y., and Sokolovsky, M. (1991) Kinetic and cross-linking studies indicate different receptors for endothelins and sarafotoxins in ileum and cerebellum. *FEBS Lett.* **238:**11–14.

50. Goligorsky, M., Tsukhara, H., Magazine, H., Anderson, T., Malik, A., and Bahou, W. (1994) Termination of endothelin signaling: role of nitric oxide. *J. Cell. Physiol.* **158:**485–494.

51. Edano, T., Arai, K., Koshi, T., Torii, T., Ohshima, T., Hirata, M., Ohkuchi, M., and Okabe, T. (1994) Digestion of endothelin-1 on cultured vascular smooth muscle cells. *Biol. Pharm. Bull.* **17:**376–378.

52. Miller, V. M., Komori, K., Burnett, J. C., Jr., and Vanhoutte, P. M. (1989) Differential sensitivity to endothelin in canine arteries and veins. *Am. J. Physiol.* **257:**H1127–H1131.

53. Moreland, S., McMullen, D., Abboa-Offei, B., and Seymour, A. (1994) Evidence for a different location of vasoconstrictor endothelin receptors in the vasculature. *Br. J. Pharmacol.* **112:**704–708.

54. MacCumber, M. W., Ross, C. A., Glaser, B. M., and Snyder, S. H. (1989) Endothelin: visualization of mRNAs by in situ hybridization provides evidence for local action. *Proc. Natl. Acad. Sci. USA* **86:**7285–7289.

55. Nunez, D. J. R., Brown, M. J., Davenport, A. P., Neylon, C. B., Schofield, J. P., and Wyse, R. K. (1990) Endothelin-1 mRNA is widely expressed in porcine and human tissues. *J. Clin. Invest.* **85:**1537–1541.

56. Plumpton, C., Champeney, R., Ashby, M. J., Kuc, R. E., and Davenport, A. P. (1993) Characterization of endothelin isoforms in human heart: endothelin-2 demonstrated. *J. Cardiovasc. Pharmacol.* **22(Suppl. 8):** S26–S28.

57. Suzki, T., Jumazaki, T., and Mitsui, Y. (1993) Endothelin-1 is produced and secreted by neonatal rat cardiac myocytes in vitro. *Biochem. Biophys. Res. Comm.* **191:**823–830.

58. Ito, H., Hirata, Y., Adachi, S., Tanaka, M., Tsujino, M., Koike, A., Nogami, A., Marumo, F., and Hiroe, M. (1993) Endothelin-1 is an autocrine/paracrine factor in the mechanism of angiotensin II-induced hypertrophy in cultured rat cardiomyocytes. *J. Clin. Invest.* **92:**398–403.

59. Eid, H., de Bold, M. L., Chen, J. H., and de Bold, A. J. (1994) Epicardial mesothelial cells synthesize and release endothelin. *J. Cardiovasc. Pharmacol.* **24:**715–720.

60. Evans, H. G., Lewis, M. J., and Shah, A. M. (1994) Modulation of myocardial relaxation by basal release of endothelin from endocardial endothelium. *Cardiovasc. Res.* **28:**1694–1699.

61. Bax, W. A., Bruinvels, A. T., van Suylen, R.-J., Saxena, P. R., and Hoyer, D. (1993) Endothelin receptors in the human coronary artery, ventricle and atrium. A quantitative autoradiographic analysis. *Naunyn-Schmeid. Arch. Pharmacol.* **348:**403–410.

62. Davenport, A. P., Morton, A. J., and Brown, M. J. (1991) Localization of endothelin-1 (ET-1), ET-2, and ET-3, mouse VIC, and sarafotoxin S6b binding sites in mammalian heart and kidney. *J. Cardiovasc. Pharmacol.* **17(Suppl. 7):**S152–S155.

63. Hemsen, A., Franco-Cereceda, A., Matran, R., Rudehill, A., and Lundberg, J. M. (1990) Occurrence, specific binding sites and functional effects of endothelin in human cardiopulmonary tissue. *Eur. J. Pharmacol.* **191:**319–328.

64. Thibault, G., Doubell, A. F., Garcia, R., Lariviere, R., and Schiffrin, E. L. (1994) Endothelin-stimulated secretion of natriuretic peptides by rat atrial myocytes is mediated by endothelin A receptors. *Circ. Res.* **74:**460–470.

65. Williams, D. L., Jr., Jones, K. L., Pettibone, D. J., Lis, E. V., and Clineschmidt, B. V. (1991) Sarafotoxin S6c: an agonist which distinguishes between endothelin receptor subtypes. *Biochem. Biophys. Res. Comm.* **175:**556–561.

66. Molenaar, P., O'Reilly, G., Sharkey, A., Kuc, R. E., Harding, D. P., Plumpton, C., Gresham, G. A., and Davenport, A. P. (1993) Characterization and localization of endothelin receptor subtypes in the human atrioventricular conducting system and myocardium. *Circ. Res.* **72:**526–538.

67. Seo, B., Oemar, B. S., Siebenmann, R., von Segesser, L., and Luscher, T. F. (1994) Both ET_A and ET_B receptors mediate contraction to endothelin-1 in human blood vessels. *Circulation* **89:**1203–1208.

68. Teerlink, J. R., Breu, V., Sprecher, U., Clozel, M., and Clozel, J. P. (1994) Potent vasoconstriction mediated by endothelin ET_B receptors in canine coronary arteries. *Circ. Res.* **74**:105–114.

69. Bax, W. A., Aghai, Z., van Tricht, C. L. J., Wassenaar, C., and Saxena, P. R. (1994) Different endothelin receptors involved in endothelin-1- and sarafotoxin S6B-induced contractions of the human isolated coronary artery. *Br. J. Pharmacol.* **113**:1471–1479.

70. Godfraind, T. (1993) Evidence for heterogeneity of endothelin receptor distribution in human coronary artery. *Br. J. Pharmacol.* **110**:1201–1205.

71. Opgaard, O. S., Adner, M., Gulbenkian, S., and Edvinsson, L. (1994) Localization of endothelin immunoreactivity and demonstration of constrictory endothelin-A receptors in human coronary arteries and veins. *J. Cardiovasc. Pharmacol.* **23**:576–583.

72. Davenport, A. P. and Maguire, J. J. (1994) Is endothelin-induced vaso-constriction mediated only by ET_A receptors in humans? *Trends Pharmacol. Sci.* **15**:9–11.

73. Davenport, A. P., O'Reilly, G., and Kuc, R. E. (1995) Endothelin ET_A and ET_B mRNA and receptors expressed by smooth muscle in the human vas-culature: majority of the ET_A subtype. *Br. J. Pharmacol.* **114**:1110–1116.

74. Karet, F. E., Kuc, R. E., and Davenport, A. P. (1993) Novel ligands BQ123 and BQ3020 characterize endothelin receptor subtypes ET_A and ET_B in human kidney. *Kidney Int.* **44**:36–42.

75. Kitamura, K., Tanaka, T., Kato, J., Ogawa, T., Eto, T., and Tanaka, K. (1989) Immunoreactive endothelin in rat kidney inner medulla: marked decrease in spontaneously hypertensive rats. *Biochem. Biophys. Res. Comm.* **162**:38–44.

76. Morita, S., Kitamura, K., Yamamoto, Y., Eto, T., Osada, Y., Sumiyoshi, A., Koono, M., and Tanaka, K. (1991) Immunoreactive endothelin in human kidney. *Ann. Clin. Biochem.* **28**:267–271.

77. Wilkes, B. M., Susin, M., Mento, P. F., Macica, C. M., Girardi, E. P., Boss, E., and Nord, E. P. (1991) Localization of endothelin-like immu-noreactivity in rat kidneys. *Am. J. Physiol.* **260**:F913–F920.

78. Firth, J. D. and Ratcliffe, P. J. (1992) Organ distribution of the three rat endothelin messenger RNAs and the effects of ischemia on renal gene expression. *J. Clin. Invest.* **90**:1023–1031.

79. Nunez, D. J. R., Taylor, E. A., Oh, V. M. S., Schofield, J. P., and Brown, M. J. (1991) Endothelin-1 mRNA expression in the rat kidney. *Biochem. J.* **275**:817–819.

80. Chen, M., Todd-Turla, K., Wang, W. H., Cao, X., Smart, A., Brosius, F. C., Killen, P. D., Keiser, J. A., Briggs, J. P., and Schnermann, J. (1993) Endothelin-1 mRNA in glomerular and epithelial cells of kidney. *Am. J. Physiol.* **265**:F542–F550.

81. Pupilla, C., Brunori, M., Misciglia, N., Selli, C., Ianni, L., Yanagisawa, M., Mannelli, M., and Serio, M. (1994) Presence and distribution of endothelin-1 gene expression in human kidney. *Am. J. Physiol.* **267**: F679–F687.

82. Jones, C. R., Hiley, C. R., Pelton, J. T., and Miller, R. C. (1989) Autoradiographic localization of endothelin binding sites in kidney. *Eur. J. Pharmacol.* **163**:379–382.

83. Kohzuki, M., Johnson, C. I., Chai, S. Y., Casley, D. J., and Mendelsohn, F. A. O. (1989) Localization of endothelin receptors in rat kidney. *Eur. J. Pharmacol.* **160**:193,194.

84. Télémaque, S., Gratton, J.-P., Claing, A., and D'Orléans-Juste, P. (1993) Endothelin-1 induces vasoconstriction and prostacyclin release via the activation of endothelin ET_A receptors in the perfused rabbit kidney. *Eur. J. Pharmacol.* **237**:275–281.

85. Yamashita, Y., Yukimura, T., Miura, K., Okumura, M., and Yamamoto, K. (1991) Effects of endothelin-3 on renal functions. *J. Pharmacol. Exp. Ther.* **259**:1256–1260.

86. Brooks, D. P., DePalma, P. D., Pullen, M., and Nambi, P. (1994) Characterization of canine renal endothelin receptor subtypes and their function. *J. Pharmacol. Exp. Ther.* **268**:1091–1097.

87. Nambi, P., Pullen, M., and Spielman, W. (1994) Species differences in the binding characteristics of [^{125}I]IRL-1620, a potent agonist specific for endothelin-B receptors. *J. Pharmacol. Exp. Ther.* **268**:202–207.

88. Fukuroda, T., Kobayashi, M., Ozaki, S., Yano, M., Miyauchi, T., Onizuka, M., Sugishita, Y., Goto, K., and Nishikibe, M. (1994) Endothelin receptor subtypes in human versus rabbit pulmonary arteries. *J. Appl. Physiol.* **76**:1976–1982.

89. Neuser, D., Zaiss, S., and Stasch, J. P. (1990) Endothelin receptors in cultured renal epithelial cells. *Eur. J. Pharmacol.* **176**:241–243.

90. Dean, R., Zhuo, J., Alcorn, D., Casley, D., and Mendelsohn, F. A. O. (1994) Cellular distribution of ^{125}I-endothelin-1 binding in rat kidney following in vivo labeling. *Am. J. Physiol.* **267**:F845–F852.

91. Oishi, R., Nonoguchi, H., Tomita, K., and Marumo, F. (1991) Endothelin-1 inhibits AVP-stimulated osmotic water permeability in rat inner medullary collecting duct. *Am. J. Physiol.* **261**:F951–F956.

92. Schnermann, J., Lorenz, J. N., Briggs, J. P., and Keiser, J. A. (1992) Induction of water diuresis by endothelin in rats. *Am. J. Physiol.* **263**:F516–F526.

93. Kohan, D. E., Padilla, E., and Hughes, A. K. (1993) Endothelin B receptor mediates ET-1 effects on cAMP and PGE2 accumulation in rat IMCD. *Am. J. Physiol.* **265**:F670–F676.

94. Edwards, R. M., Stack, E. J., Pullen, M., and Nambi, P. (1993) Endothelin inhibits vasopressin action in rat inner medullary collecting duct via the ET_B receptor. *J. Pharmacol. Exp Ther.* **267**:1028–1033.

95. Wilkes, B. M., Ruston, A. S., Mento, P., Girardi, E., Hart, D., Vander Molen, M., Barnett, R., and Nord, E. P. (1991) Characterization of endothelin 1 receptor and signal transduction mechanisms in rat medullary interstitial cells. *Am. J. Physiol.* **260**:F576–F589.

96. Kohan, D. E. (1991) Endothelin synthesis by rabbit renal tubule cells. *Am. J. Physiol.* **261**:F221–F226.

97. Garvin, J. and Sanders, K. (1991) Endothelin inhibits fluid and bicarbonate transport in part by reducing the Na^+/K^+-ATPase activity in the rat proximal straight tubule. *J. Am. Soc. Nephrol.* **2**:976–982.

98. Eiam-ong, S., Hildew, S. A., King, A. J., Johns, C. A., and Madias, N. E. (1992) Endothelin-1 stimulates the Na^+/H^+ and Na^+/HCO_3^- transporters in rabbit renal cortex. *Kidney Int.* **42**:18–24.

99. Guntupalli, J. and DuBose, T. D., Jr. (1994) Effects of endothelin on rat renal proximal tubule $Na+-P_i$ cotransport and Na^+/H^+ exchange. *Am. J. Physiol.* **266**:F658–F666.

100. Matsumoto, H., Suzuki, N., Onda, H., and Fujno, M. (1989) Abundance of endothelin-3 in rat intestine, pituitary gland, and brain. *Biochem. Biophys. Res. Comm.* **164**, 74-80.

101. Rosengurt, N., Springall, D., and Polak, J. (1990) Localization of endothelin-like immunoreactivity in airway epithelia of rats and mice. *J. Pathol.* **160**:5–8.

102. Marciniak, S. J., Plumpton, C., Barker, P. J., Huskisson, N. S., and Davenport, A. P. (1992) Localization of immunoreactive endothelin and proendothelin in the human lung. *Pulm. Pharmacol.* **5**:175–182.

103. Giaid, A., Polak, J. M., Gaitonde, V., Hamid, Q. A., Moscoso, G., Legon, S., Uwanogho, D., Roncalli, M., Shinmi, O., Sawamura, T., Kimura, S., Yanagisawa, M., Masaki, T., and Springall, D. R. (1991) Distribution of endothelin-like immunoreactivity and mRNA in the developing and adult human lung. *Am. J. Respir. Cell. Mol. Biol.* **4**:50–58.

104. Cardell, L. O., Uddman, R., and Edvinsson, L. (1993) A novel ET_A-receptor antagonist, FR 139317, inhibits endothelin-induced contractions of guinea-pig pulmonary arteries, but not trachea. *Br. J. Pharmacol.* **108**:448–452.

105. Hay, D. W. P., Luttmann, M. A., Hubbard, W. C., and Undem, B. J. (1993) Endothelin receptor subtypes in human and guinea pig pulmonary tissues. *Br. J. Pharmacol.* **110**:1175–1183.

106. Noguchi, K., Noguchi, Y., Hirose, H., Nishikibe, M., Ihara, M., Ishikawa, K., and Yano, M. (1993) Role of endothelin ET_B receptors in bronchoconstrictor and vasoconstrictor responses in guinea pigs. *Eur. J. Pharmacol.* **223**:47–51.

107. Battistini, B., Warner, T. D., Fournier, A., and Vane, J. R. (1994) Comparison of PD 145065 and Ro 46-2005 as antagonists of contractions of guinea pig airways induced by endothelin-1 or IRL 1620. *Eur. J. Pharmacol.* **252**:341–345.

108. Battistini, B., Warner, T. D., Fournier, A., and Vane, J. R. (1994) Characterization of ET_B receptors mediating contractions induced by endothelin-1 or IRL 1620 in guinea pig isolated airways: effects of BQ-123, FR139317 or PD 145065. *Br. J. Pharmacol.* **111**:1009–1016.

109. Cardell, L. O., Uddman, R., and Edvinsson, L. (1992) Evidence for multiple endothelin receptors in the guinea-pig pulmonary artery and trachea. *Br. J. Pharmacol.* **105**:376–380.

110. Henry, P. J. (1993) Endothelin-1 (ET-1)-induced contraction in rat isolated trachea: involvement of ET_A and ET_B receptors and multiple signal transduction systems. *Br. J. Pharmacol.* **110:**435–441.

111. Macquin-Mavier, I., Levame, M., Istin, N., and Harf, A. (1989) Mechanism of endothelin-mediated bronchoconstriction in the guinea pig. *J. Pharmacol. Exp. Ther.* **250:**740–745.

112. Touvay, C., Vilian, B., Pons, F., Chabrier, P. E., Mencia-Huerta, J. M., and Braquet, P. (1990) Bronchopulmonary and vascular effect of endothelin in the guinea pig. *Eur. J. Pharmacol.* **176:**23–33.

113. Inui, T., James, A. F., Fujitani, Y., Takimoto, M., Okada, T., Yamamura, T., and Urade, Y. (1994) ET_A and ET_B receptors on single smooth muscle cells cooperate in mediating guinea pig tracheal contraction. *Am. J. Physiol.* **266:**L113–L124.

114. Nakamichi, K., Ihara, M., Kobayashi, M., Saeki, T., Ishikawa, K., and Yano, M. (1992) Different distribution of endothelin receptor subtypes in pulmonary tissues revealed by the novel selective ligands BQ-123 and [Ala^{1,3,11,15}]ET-1. *Biochem. Biophys. Res. Comm.* **182:**144–150.

115. Abraham, W. M., Ahmed, A., Cortes, A., Spinella, M. J., Malik, A. B., and Andersen, T. T. (1993). A specific endothelin-1 antagonist blocks inhaled endothelin-1-induced bronchoconstriction in sheep. *J. Appl. Physiol.* **74:**2537–2542.

116. Panek, R. L., Major, T. C., Hingorani, G. P., Doherty, A. M., Taylor, D. G., and Rapundalo, S. T. (1992) Endothelin and structurally related analogs distinguish between endothelin receptor subtypes. *Biochem. Biophys. Res. Comm.* **183:**1566–1571.

117. Buchan, K. W., Magnusson, H., Rabe, K. F., Sumner, M. H., and Watts, I. S. (1994) Characterisation of the endothelin receptor mediating contraction of human pulmonary artery using BQ123 and Ro 46-2005. *Eur. J. Pharmacol.* **260:**221–225.

118. Knott, P. G., D'Aprile, A. C., Henry, P. J., Hay, D. W. P., and Goldie, R. G. (1995) Receptors for endothelin-1 in asthmatic human peripheral lung. *Br. J. Pharmacol.* **114:**1–3.

119. Horgan, M. J., Pinheiro, J. M. B., and Malik, A. B. (1991) Mechanism of endothelin-1-induced pulmonary vasoconstriction. *Circ. Res.* **69:**157–164.

120. Brink, C., Gillard, V., Roubert, P., Mencia-Huerta, J. M., Chabrier, P. E., Braquet, P., and Verley, J. (1991) Effects of specific binding sites of endothelin in human lung preparations. *Pulm. Pharmacol.* **4:**54–59.

121. Toga, H., Ibe, B. O., and Raj, J. U. (1992) In vitro responses of ovine intrapulmonary arteries and veins to endothelin-1. *Am. J. Physiol.* **263:**L15–L21.

122. Seldeslagh, K. A. and Lauweryns, J. M. (1993) Sarafotoxin expression in the bronchopulmonary tract: immunohistochemical occurrence and colocalization with endothelins. *Histochemistry* **100:**257–263.

123. Kobayashi, M., Ihara, M., Sato, N., Saeki, T., Ozaki, S., Ikemoto, F., and Yano, M. (1993) A novel ligand, [^{125}I]BQ-3020, reveals the localization of endothelin ET_B receptors. *Eur. J. Pharmacol.* **235:**95–100.

124. Lee, M. E., de la Monte, S. M., Ng, S.-C., Bloch, K. D., and Quertermous, T. (1990) Expression of the potent vasoconstrictor endothelin in human central nervous system. *J. Clin. Invest.* **86:**141–147.

125. Yoshizawa, T., Shinmi, O., Giaid, A., Yanagisawa, M., Gibson, S. J., Kimura, S., Uchiyama, Y., Polak, J. M., Masaki, T., and Kanazawa, I. (1990) Endothelin: a novel peptide in posterior pituitary system. *Science* **247:**462–464.

126. MacCumber, M. W., Ross, C. A., and Snyder, S. H. (1990) Endothelin in brain: receptors, mitogenesis, and biosynthesis in glial cells. *Proc. Natl. Acad. Sci. USA* **87:**2359–2363.

127. Giaid, A., Bibson, S. J., Ibrahim, B. N., Legon, S., Bloom, S. R., Yanagisawa, M., Masaki, T., Varndell, I. M., and Polak, J. M. (1989) Endothelin 1, an endothelium derived peptide, is expressed in neurons of the human spinal cord and dorsal root ganglia. *Proc. Natl. Acad. Sci. USA* **86:**7634–7638.

128. Elshourbagy, M. A., Lee, J. A., Korman, D. R., Nuthalaganti, P., Sylvester, D. R., Dilella, A. G., Sutiphong, J. A., and Kumar, C. S. (1992) Molecular cloning and characterization of the major endothelin receptor subtype in porcine cerebellum. *Mol. Pharmacol.* **41:**465–473.

129. Vigne, P., Breittmayer, J. P., and Felin, C. (1993) Competitive and noncompetitive interactions of BQ-123 with endothelin ET_A receptors. *Eur. J. Pharmacol.* **245:**229–232.

130. Stanimirovic, D. B., Yamamoto, T., Uematsu, S., and Spatz, M. (1994) Endothelin-1 receptor binding and cellular signal transduction in cultured human brain endothelial cells. *J. Neurochem.* **62:**592–601.

131. De Olivera, A. M., Viswanathan, M., Capsoni, S., Heemskerk, F. M., Correa, F. M., and Saavedra, J. M. (1995) Characterization of endothelin A receptors in cerebral and peripheral arteries of the rat. *Peptides* **16:**139–144.

132. Sagher, O., Jim, Y., Thai, Q. A., Fergus, A., Kassell, N. F., and Lee, K. S. (1994) Cerebral microvascular responses to endothelins: the role of ET_A receptors. *Brain Res.* **658:**179–184.

133. Mosqueda-Garcia, R., Inagami, T., Appalsamy, M., Sugiura, M., and Robertson, R. M. (1992) Endothelin as a neuropeptide. Cardiovascular effects in the brainstem of normotensive rats. *Circ. Res.* **72:**20–35.

134. Ouchi, Y., Kim, S., Souza, A.C., Iijima, S., Hattori, A., Orimo, H., Yoshizumi, M., Kurihara, H., and Yazaki, Y. (1989) Central effect of endothelin on blood pressure in conscious rats. *Am. J. Physiol.* **256:** H1747–H1751.

135. Takuwa, Y. (1993) Endothelin in vascular and endocrine systems: biological activities and its mechanisms of action. *Endocrine J.* **40:**489–506.

136. Naruse, M., Naruse, K., and Demura, H. (1994) Recent advances in endothelin research on cardiovascular and endocrine systems. *Endocrine J.* **41:**491–507.

137. Samson, W. K., Skala, K. D., Alexander, B. D., and Huang, F. L. (1991) Hypothalamic endothelin: presence and effects related to fluid and electrolyte homeostasis. *J. Cardiovasc. Pharmacol.* **17(Suppl. 7):**S346–S349.

138. Shichiri, M., Hirata, Y., Kanno, K., Ohta, K., Emori, T., and Marumo, F. (1989) Effect of endothelin-1 on release of arginine-vasopressin from perfused rat hypothalamus. *Biochem. Biophys. Res. Comm.* **163:**1332–1337.

139. Makino, S., Hashimoto, K., Hirasawa, R., Hattori, T., and Ota, Z. (1992) Central interaction between endothelin and brain natriuretic peptide on vasopressin secretion. *J. Hypertens.* **10:**25–28.

140. Ritz, M. F., Stuenkel, E. L., Dayanithi, G., Jones, R., and Nordmann, J. J. (1992) Endothelin regulation of neuropeptide release from nerve endings of the posterior pituitary. *Proc. Natl. Acad. Sci.* **89:**8371–8375.

141. Samson, W. K. (1992) The endothelin-A receptor subtype transduces the effects of the endothelins in the anterior pituitary gland. *Biochem. Biophys. Res. Comm.* **187:**590–595.

142. Stojilkovic, S. S., Balla, T., Fukuda, S., Cesnjaj, M., Merelli, F., Krsmanovic, L. Z., and Catt, K. J. (1992) Endothelin ET_A receptors mediate the signaling and secretory actions of endothelins in pituitary gonadotrophs. *Endocrinology* **130:**465–474.

143. Naruse, M., Naruse, K., Kawai, M., Yoshimoto, Y., Tanabe, A., Tanaka, M., and Demura, H. (1994) Endothelin as a local regulator of aldosterone secretion from bovine adrenocortical cells. *Am. J. Hyper.* **7:**74A.

144. Imai, T., Hirata, Y., Eguchi, S., Kanno, K., Ohta, K., Emori, T., Sakamoto, A., Yanagisawa, M., and Masaki, T. (1992) Concomitant expression of receptor subtype and isopeptide of endothelin by human adrenal gland. *Biochem. Biophys. Res. Comm.* **182:**1115–1121.

145. Rossi, G., Albertin, G., Belloni, A., Zanin, L., Biasolo, M. A., Prayer-Galetti, T., Bader, M., Nussdorfer, G. G., Palu, G., and Pessina, A. C. (1994) Gene expression, localization, and characterization of endothelin A and B receptors in the human adrenal cortex. *J. Clin Invest.* **94:**1226–1234.

146. Cozza, E. N., Chiou, S., and Gomez-Sanchez, C. E. (1992) Endothelin-1 potentiation of angiotensin II stimulation of aldosterone production. *Am. J. Physiol.* **262:**R85–R89.

147. Malassine, A., Cronier, L., Mondon, F., Mignot, T. M., and Ferre, F. (1993) Localization and production of immunoreactive endothelin-1 in the trophoblast of human placenta. *Cell Tissue Res.* **271:**491–497.

148. O'Reilly, G., Charnock-Jones, D. S., Davenport, A. P., Cameron, I. T., and Smith, S. K. (1992) Presence of messenger ribonucleic acid for endothelin 1, endothelin 2, and endothelin 3 in human endometrium and a change in the ratio of ET_A and ET_B receptor subtype across the menstrual cycle. *J. Clin. Endocrinol. Metab.* **75:**1545–1549.

149. Sagawa, N., Hasegawa, M., Itoh, H., Nanno, H., Mori, T., Yano, J., Yoshimasa, T., and Nakao, K. (1994) Current topic: the role of amnionic endothelin in human preganancy. *Placenta* **15:**565–575.

150. Buchan, K. W., Sumner, M. J., and Watts, I. S. (1993) Human placental membranes contain predominantly ET_B receptors. *J. Cardiovasc. Pharmacol.* **22(Suppl. 8):**S136–S139.

151. Kilpatrick, S. J., Roberts, J. M., Lykins, D. L., and Taylor, R. N. (1993) Characterization and ontogeny of endothelin receptors in human placenta. *Am. J. Physiol.* **264:**E367–E372.

152. Rae, G. A., Calixto, J. B., and D'Orleans-Juste, P. (1993) Big endothelin-1 contracts isolated uterus via a phosphoramidon-sensistive endothelin ET_A receptor mediated mechanism. *Eur. J. Pharmacol.* **240:**113–119.

153. Tsunoda, H., Miyauchi, T., Fujita, K., Kubu, T., and Goto, K. (1993) Mechanism of rat uterine smooth muscle contraction induced by endothelin-1. *Br. J. Pharmacol.* **110:**1437–1446.

154. Ergul, A., Glassberg, M. K., Majercik, M. H., and Puett, D. (1993) Endothelin 1 promotes steroidogenesis and stimulates protooncogene expression in transformed murine Leydig cells. *Endocrinology* **132:**598–603.

155. Kobayashi, S., Tang, R., Wang, B., Opgenorth, T., Stein, E., Shapiro, E., and Lepor, H. (1994) Localization of endothelin receptors in the human prostate. *J. Urol.* **151:**763–766.

156. Kobayashi, S., Tang, R., Wang, B., Opgenorth, T., Langenstroer, P., Shapiro, E., and Lepor, H. (1994) Binding and functional properties of endothelin receptor subtypes in the human prostate. *J. Pharmacol. Exp. Ther.* **45:**306–311.

157. Takahashi, K., Jones, P. M., Kanse, S. M., Lam, H. C., Spokes, R. A., Ghatei, M. A., and Bloom, S. R. (1990) Endothelin in the gastrointestinal tract. Presence of endothelin like immunoreactivity, endothelin-1 messenger RNA, endothelin receptors, and pharmacological effect. *Gastroenterology* **99:**1660–1667.

158. Kiyohara, T., Okuno, M., Nakanishi, T., Shinomura, Y., and Matsuzawa, Y. (1993) Effect of endothelin 1 on ion transport in isolated rat colon. *Gasteroenterology* **104:**1328–1336.

159. Lin, W. W. and Lee, C. Y. (1992) Intestinal relaxation by endothelin isopeptides: involvement of Ca^{2+} activated K^+ channels. *Eur. J. Pharmacol.* **219:**355–360.

160. Douglas, S. A. and Hiley, C. R. (1991) Endothelium-dependent mesenteric vasorelaxant effects and systemic actions of endothelin (16–21) and other endothelin-related peptides in the rat. *Br. J. Pharmacol.* **104:**311–320.

161. Yoshinaga, M., Chijiiwa, Y., Misawa, T., Harada, N., and Nawata, H. (1992) Endothelin B receptor on guinea pig small intestinal smooth muscle cells. *Am. J. Physiol.* **262:**G308–G311.

162. Inagaki, H., Bishop, A. E., Yura, J., and Polak, J. M. (1991) Localization of endothelin-1 and its binding sites to the nervous system of the human colon. *J. Cardovasc. Pharmacol.* **17(Suppl. 7):**S455–S471.

163. Eaker, E., Sallusito, J., Kohler, J., and Visner, G. (1995) Endothelin-1 expression in myenteric neurons cultured from rat small intestine. *Regulatory Pep.* **55:**167–177.

164. Fang, S., Ledlow, A., Murray, J. A., Christensen, J., and Conklin, J. L. (1994) Vasoactive intestinal contractor: localization in the opossum esophagus and effects on motor functions. *Gastroenterology* **107:**1621–1626.

165. Puffenberger, E. G., Hosoda, K., Washington, S. S., Nakao, K., deWit, D., Yanagisawa, M., and Chakravarti, A. (1994) A missense mutation of the endothelin-B receptor gene in multigenic Hirschsprung's disease. *Cell* **79:**1257–1266.

Chapter 2

Molecular Biology of the Endothelin Receptors

Jonathan A. Lee, Eliot H. Ohlstein, Catherine E. Peishoff, and John D. Elliott

1. Introduction

Since the initial discovery of the endothelium-derived constricting factor, endothelin-1 (ET-1) *(1)* and determination of its peptidic nature *(2)*, elucidation of the molecular details of the endothelin (ET) system has progressed rapidly via a multidisciplinary approach using the tools of biochemistry, chemistry, pharmacology, and molecular biology. Milestones in the development of this area include the isolation *(3)* and three-dimensional structure determination *(4,5)* of ET-1 and related peptides, the pharmacological characterization and molecular cloning of ET-receptor subtypes *(6,7)* which was followed by the development of potent peptide and nonpeptide antagonists *(8–13)*, and, more recently, the disruption of the genes encoding ET-1, ET-3, and the ET_B receptor subtype *(14–16)*. Thus elucidation of the intricacies of the endothelin system has been the product of a truly molecular approach to pharmacology.

The endothelins, ET-1, -2, and -3, are known to elicit their biological effects through activation of receptors belonging to the G protein-coupled receptor superfamily. Structurally, this receptor family is characterized by an amino-terminal region located on the extracellular surface of the plasma membrane, an integral-membrane region consisting of seven helical transmembrane domains (TMs 1–7) connected by hydrophilic loops alternately on the cytoplasmic and

From: *Endothelin: Molecular Biology, Physiology, and Pathology*
Edited by R. F. Highsmith © Humana Press Inc., Totowa, NJ

extracellular surfaces of the plasma membrane, and a carboxyl terminal region in the cytoplasm *(17)*. There are two fully characterized ET receptor subtypes, ET_A, which binds the ET peptides in the order ET-1 ~ ET-2 (K_i ~ 20–60 pM) > ET-3 (6500 pM), and ET_B, which binds the ET peptides with equal and high affinity (K_i ~ 15 pM) *(18)*. Pharmacological evidence has been presented to support the existence of further subtypes of the ET_A and, in particular, the ET_B receptors although future progress in this area awaits the cloning and expression of these variants *(19)*. The ET receptors are also activated by the structurally similar snake-venom toxins, the sarafotoxins, of which the ET_B receptor selective-agonist sarafotoxin 6C has been extensively studied *(20)*. Linear analogs of these peptides, such as IRL-1620 and IRL-1736, have been found to be agonists-selective for the ET_B receptor *(21)*. Programs directed toward the discovery of antagonists of the ET receptors have provided both peptide (BQ 123) *(8)* and more recently, nonpeptide (SB 209670 *[10,11]*, Ro 47-0203 *[9,12]*, and BMS 182874 *[13]*) molecules. Thus, a number of structurally diverse ligands are available (*see* Fig. 1) for the ET receptors and these are being used to investigate receptor/ligand interactions as well as to establish the pharmacological significance of the ET system.

This chapter reviews the molecular biology of ET receptors, including their gene structure (*see* Section 2.), tissue localization of mRNA and alteration of mRNA levels in pathophysiology (*see* Section 3.), and cDNA cloning (*see* Section 4.). Sections 5. and 6. describe the implications of mutagenesis results on the ET receptors, Section 5. emphasizing the area of signal/transduction, whereas Section 6. reviews the effects of mutagenesis on ligand binding and concludes with a binding site model. Finally, Section 7. considers some of the likely future directions of the area.

2. Endothelin Receptor Genes

ET_A and ET_B receptor genes are represented as single copies in the human, bovine, porcine, and murine genomes *(22–25)*; in humans, the ET_A and ET_B receptor genes are located on chromosomes 4 and 13, respectively *(22,24)*. Human, bovine, porcine, and murine ET receptor genes are composed of multiple exons and introns. At the present time, a single transcriptional start has been observed for the ET_A receptor gene in these species *(24)*; however, alternate transcrip-

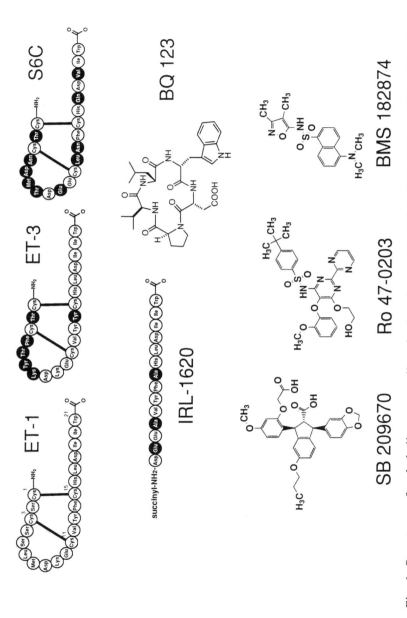

Fig. 1. Structures of endothelin-receptor ligands. Agonist peptides ET-1, ET-3, S6C, and IRL 1620: the positions of disulfide bonds and the amino acids that differ from ET-1 (reverse print) are indicated; BQ 123, a cyclic peptide ET_A-selective antagonist; nonpeptide endothelin-receptor antagonists SB 209670, Ro 47-0203, and BMS 182874.

33

tional initiation of the ET_B receptor gene has been observed in murine and bovine brain *(23,25)*. Furthermore, an ET_B receptor variant arising from alternative RNA splicing has been observed in human brain, placenta, lung, and heart *(26)*. The following section summarizes the current status of ET-receptor gene structure and regulation.

2.1. Promoter Elements

The 5'-flanking regions of the human ET_A and ET_B (hET_A, hET_B) receptor genes do not contain canonical TATA *(27)* or CCAAT *(28)* boxes *(22,24)* suggesting that transcriptional initiation of these genes may potentially originate at several sites. Recognition sites for Sp1 *(29)* are located within 80 bases of the major transcriptional start sites identified for hET_A and hET_B receptor genes, which are located at approx -230 bp *(22,24)*. Additional promoter motifs, the acute-phase reaction regulator element (APRRE) *(30)* and binding sites for MyoD-E2A *(31)* are located at nucleotides -1200 to -1360 within the hET_A receptor gene and -1220 to -850 within the hET_B receptor gene. These additional promoters may act as the transcriptional-initiation sites for the 5'-extended ET_B receptor mRNAs observed in bovine and murine brains *(23,25)*.

2.2. Exon–Intron Structure

Sequence comparisons between genomic DNA clones and the major mRNA species encoding hET_A and hET_B receptors have indicated that the hET_A receptor gene spans over 40 kb and contains 8 exons and 7 introns whereas the hET_B receptor gene spans over 24 kb and consists of 7 exons and 6 introns *(22,24)*. In the hET_A receptor gene, exon 1 corresponds to part of the 5' UTR of the mature mRNA and exons 2–8 encode the amino terminus (AT) through TM 2, TM 3, TM 4, TM 5, TM 6, TM 7, and the carboxyl terminal (CT) regions of the receptor, respectively (*see* Fig. 2). In the hET_B receptor gene, exon 1 corresponds to the 5' UTR through TM 2 whereas exons 2–7 encode TMs 3–7 and CT in a manner analogous to hET_A receptor exons 3–8 (Fig. 2).

For both the bovine and human ET_B receptor genes, however, transcription apparently can initiate at sites other than at the major transcriptional-start sites *(22,25)*. Recently, Cheng et al. *(23)* isolated a rat-brain cDNA representing an ET_B receptor mRNA transcribed from nucleotide -839, approx 600 bases upstream from the major tran-

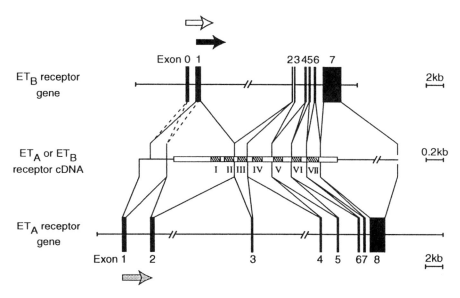

Fig. 2. Structural organization of ET-receptor genes. The ET_A and ET_B receptor genes are represented by solid lines with exons shown as black rectangles. Arrows indicate the transcriptional initiation sites for human ET_A gene (stippled arrow), the major transcriptional starts for bovine and human ET_B genes (solid arrow), and an alternative transcriptional start for murine ET_B gene (open arrow). The structure of the ET-receptor cDNAs derived ET_A and ET_B genes are indicated. The open reading frame is represented by a rectangle with putative TM regions indicated as hatched boxes. Exons in the genomic DNA and their corresponding regions in the cDNA are indicated. Upstream transcriptional initiation (open arrow) of murine ETB gene leads to an additional exon and intron not observed when transcription is initiated at the major start sites (solid arrow).

scription-start sites *(22,25)*. Comparison of this rat-brain cDNA with genomic DNA clones indicates the presence of an additional exon/intron (denoted exon 0; Fig. 2), containing consensus acceptor and donor splice sites, extending from nucleotide −51 to −638. Therefore, in rat brain, transcriptional activation from an alternative upstream promoter generates a 5' UTR-extended precursor RNA, which includes an additional exon/intron not detected when transcription initiates at the predominant start sites *(23)*. These data would indicate that the exon–intron structure of ET_A and ET_B receptor genes are more similar than previously recognized *(22,24,25,32)*, both containing 8 exons and 7 introns.

2.3. Deletion of Endothelin Receptor Genes

In a recent investigation, mice lacking ET_B receptor have been produced by means of targeted-gene disruption *(15)*. Homozygous ET_B receptor gene null mice displayed white spotting of the coat and gross distention of the intestine, anatomical features consistent with the diagnosis of aganglionic megacolon. Analysis of the ET_B receptor gene *(ednrb)* in Piebald mice, an animal-model system for hereditary aganglionic megacolon, and matings between Piebald-lethal and *ednrb*-deleted heterozygous mice indicate that *ednrb* is allelic to the Piebold locus *(15)*. Disruption of the ET-3 gene results in a similar phenotype of megacolon and coat-color spotting *(14)*. Taken together, these studies suggest that interaction of ET-3 with the ET_B receptor is required for normal development of two neural crest-derived cell lines, the enteric neurons, and epidermal melanocytes *(14,15)*. It is interesting to note that homozygous mice deleted in the ET-1 gene have various craniofacial abnormalities arising from organs derived principally from ectomesenchymal cells also originating from the neural crest *(16)*. A similar phenotype was reported for the deletion of the ET_A receptor gene more recently by Hosada et al. *(33)*. Therefore, disruption of the genes encoding ET-1 and ET-3 or their receptors has revealed the importance of ET receptor-mediated signaling to the normal development of cell lines derived from the neural crest. Although the vasoactive properties of the ET peptides have been well-documented pharmacologically, gene-deletion experiments have unexpectedly revealed the involvement of these peptides in embryonic development. These data generated in genetic models of human disease parallel recent findings that the hET_B receptor is a factor in the susceptibility of patients to aganglionic megacolon (Hirschsprung's Disease) *(34)*. It seems likely that future studies will lead to the further identification of human genetic disorders related to altered ET-signal transduction.

3. Endothelin Receptor mRNA

A multitude of techniques that include Northern analysis, reverse transcription-polymerase chain reaction (RT-PCR), *in situ* hybridization, autoradiography, and immunocytochemistry have been employed with traditional pharmacological studies to identify the tissue distribution of ET-receptor subtypes. Altered mRNA levels and, by implication, levels of the corresponding ET receptor, have been observed in a variety of pathophysiological conditions.

3.1. Tissue Localization of mRNA

ET_A and ET_B receptor mRNAs are widely distributed; however, the mRNA levels for the two receptor subtypes vary independently among different cells and tissues *(35,36)*. In humans, hET_A receptor mRNA is present at the highest levels in the aorta, with moderate to high levels found in other vascular and nonvascular tissues, with the exception of liver and cultured endothelial cells where it is not detected. In contrast, hET_B receptor mRNA is present at the highest levels in brain tissue, but also occurs to a moderate degree in all other tissues examined, including endothelial cells and blood vessels *(36,37)*.

Pharmacological evidence has been advanced to support the fact that the ET_A receptor represents the major subtype present in vascular smooth muscle cells, and that the ET_B receptor is the predominant subtype in vascular endothelial cells *(38–40)*. Thus, it appears that the ET_A receptor on vascular smooth muscle cells may mediate ET-1-induced vasoconstriction, whereas the ET_B receptor expressed on endothelial cells may mediate the release of endothelium-derived nitric oxide. In the rat kidney, Terada and colleagues *(41)* detected large signals for the ET_B receptor mRNA in the initial and terminal inner-medullary collecting duct and glomerulus, whereas lower levels were found in the cortical and outer medullary collecting ducts, vasa recta, and arcuate artery. ET_A receptor mRNA was only found in the glomerulus, vasa recta, and arcuate artery. Thus, there appears to be differential expression of the ET receptors along the nephron; however, some segments, such as the inner-medullary collecting duct, may possess both receptor subtypes *(42)*. It seems likely, therefore, that differential ET-receptor subtype expression in distinct cell types may result in profoundly disparate pharmacological effects of the ET peptides, the complexity of this situation being acutely demonstrated in the rat kidney.

3.2. Alterations of mRNA Levels in Pathophysiology

Although there have been many reports on the overexpression of ET-1 in a variety of pathophysiological processes, much less is known concerning the alterations of ET_A and ET_B receptor mRNA levels.

3.2.1. Cardiovascular Indications

Most of the reports on the regulation of ET-receptor expression have addressed cardiovascular-related diseases. Hasegawa et al. *(43)*

evaluated the expression of ET_A receptor genes in blood vessels of hypertensive patients where ET_A receptor mRNA was high in medial smooth-muscle cells, but low in intimal smooth-muscle cells. Thus, modulation of ET_A receptor-gene expression differs between the intima and media, which may be linked to the proliferative activity of these cells in patients with hypertension.

The temporal expression of mRNAs encoding ET-converting enzyme-1 (ECE-1), preproET-1, ET_A, and ET_B receptors has been examined by Wang et al. *(44)* in the rat carotid-artery balloon angioplasty model. A significant two-fold increase in ECE-1 and preproET-1 mRNA expression was observed 6–24 h and 3–7 d, respectively, following angioplasty. In contrast, both ET_A and ET_B receptor mRNAs are elevated by approx 30-fold, 3–7 and 1–3 d after angioplasty, respectively. Furthermore, there is a marked increase in ET-1 immunoreactivity in the neointimal lesions. These data suggest a possible role for endogenous ET-1, as well as involvement of both ET_A and ET_B receptors, in the pathogenesis of angioplasty-induced neointima formation.

Marmosets fed a high-cholesterol diet have been reported to possess elevated quantities of ET_B, but not ET_A receptor mRNA in a variety of tissues, suggesting that ET_B receptors may be involved in the pathogenesis of atherosclerosis *(45)*. In atherosclerotic human-coronary arteries, ET_A receptors have been localized in the medial smooth-muscle layer, whereas "non-ET_A" receptor(s) (presumably ET_B) are localized in the regions of neovascularization *(46)*.

ET_A and ET_B receptor mRNA increases in the heart chambers and the pulmonary vasculature following acute or chronic hypoxic exposure *(47,48)*. These studies are consistent with the hypothesis that increased ET-1 synthesis in the lungs contributes to hypoxia-induced hypertension.

3.2.2. Renal Indications

The expression of renal ET receptors is altered under some pathophysiological conditions and possibly contributes to disease processes. An upregulation of the expression of ET_B, but not ET_A, receptor mRNA has been observed in rat-mesangial cells following treatment with cyclosporine *(49)*. Nakamura et al. *(50)* reported increased expression of ET_B, but not ET_A, receptor mRNA as a result of puromycin-induced nephrotoxicity. In NZB/W F1 mice, a model system for the autoimmune disease lupus, a five- and threefold respective increase in renal ET_A and ET_B receptor mRNA expression occurred relative to control mice *(51)*. In both chemical and genetic-model systems of renal disease, methylprednisoline attenuated the increase in ET receptor mRNA levels *(50,51)*. A similar downregulation of ET_A receptor mRNA and receptor expression by dexamethasone has been previously noted in murine smooth-muscle cell lines *(52)*, suggesting that the glucocorticoid-mediated decrease in ET-receptor mRNA is not specific to inflammatory models and may represent a generic negative regulation of ET-receptor gene expression in diverse tissues.

Although the observation of tissue localization and altered expression of ET receptors provide a somewhat compelling argument for the importance of the ET system in pathophysiological conditions, definitive evidence will only come through human clinical trials with receptor-specific antagonists.

4. Molecular Cloning of Endothelin Receptor cDNAs

Shortly following the biochemical isolation and molecular cloning of ET-1, the cDNAs encoding the two principal ET-receptor subtypes, ET_A, and ET_B, were obtained by expression cloning *(6,7)*. These initial reports were followed by a plethora of studies reporting ET_A and ET_B cDNAs obtained from various mammalian species by cloning techniques based on functional expression *(53,54)*, hybridization of oligonucleotide probes based on tryptic fragments of bovine ET_B *(55)*, and cDNA homology between species *(35,56–59)*. Recently Kumar et al. *(60)* have cloned and characterized an ET_A receptor variant from *Xenopus laevis* heart which displays selectivity similar to ET_A receptor for binding agonist peptides, but has low affinity for the ET_A-selective antagonist BQ123. Finally, Karne et al. have identified and cloned an ET receptor endogenous to *Xenopus laevis* melanocytes. This receptor is selective for ET-3 over ET-1, thus implicating it as a putative ET_C subtype *(61)*.

Figure 3 shows the alignment of the derived amino-acid sequences of bovine, human, and rat ET_A and ET_B receptors; the porcine ET_B receptor; the *Xenopus* ET_A receptor; and the *Xenopus* ET_C (xET_C) receptor. Recent cDNA and genomic DNA-sequence data *(23)* revised the original murine ET_B receptor sequence *(7)*, such that substitution of "SSAP" for "FRT" occurs within the AT region of rET_B. This change is consistent with the regional sequence in mammalian ET_B receptors (Fig. 3). Comparison of mammalian ET_A sequences

```
     1                                                                                                   100
bETB  MQPLPSLQGR ALVALLIACG VAGIQAEERE FPPAGATQPL PGTGEMETP  TETSWPGRSN ASDPRSSATP QIPRGERNAG IPPR..TPPP CIGPIEIKET
pETB  MQPLRSLQGR ALVALIFACG VAGVQSEERG FPPAGATTPPA LRTGEVIAPP TKTFWPRGSN ASLPRSSSPP QMPKGERNAG PPARTLTPPP CEGPIEIKUT
hETB  MQPPPSLQGR ALVALVLACG LSRIWGEERG FPPDRAT.PL  LQTAEIMTPP TKTLWPKGSN ASLARSLAPA EVPKGDRDAG SPPRTISPPP CQGPIEIKET
rETB  MQSSASRCGR ALVALLLACG LLGWGEKRG  FPPAQATPSL  LGTKEVMTPP TKTSWTRGSN SSLMRGSGAFA EVTKGGERVAG VPPRSF.PPP CQRKIEINKT
bETA  ...METFWLR LSFWALVGG  VISDNPESYS TNLSIHVISV  ..........  ..ATFHGTEL SFVVTHQPT  NL.......A  LPSNGSMHNY CPQQTKITSA
hETA  ...METLCLR ASFWLALVGC VISDNPERYS TNLSNHVDDF  ..........  ..TTFRGTEL SFLVTTHQPT NL.......V  LPSNGSMHNY CPQQTKITSA
rETA  ...MGVLCFL ASFWLALVGG AIADNAERYS ANLSSHVEDF  ..........  ..TPFRGTEF DFLGTTLRPF NL.......A  LPSNGSMHGY CPQQTKITTA
xETA  ...MGGNTLR FTVLLVLAGI AVSSSFGEYY QNRTDASTDF  ..........  ..TMLNRSHT SPVRKGNRSA DL........  .......... CPEKTKINHV
xETC  ......NATV ILFVAWACL  MGVGCYQEFQ TQQNFPDISN  PSQELNQEPA HRIVQLLSIQ NNGALNMSTG NV........  .......... CLSRAKIRHA

   101                                                                                                   200
bETB  FKYINTVVSC LVFVLGIIGN STLLFIIYKN KCMRNGENIL IASLALAGDLL HIIIDIPINT YKLLAEDWPF  .....GEMC KLVPFIQKAS VGITVLSLCA
pETB  FKYINTVVSC LVFVLGIIGN STLLFIIYKN KCMRNGENIL IASLALAGDLL HIIIDIPINV YKLLAEDWPF  .....GEMC KLVPFIQKAS VGITVLSLCA
hETB  FKYINTVVSC LVFVLGIIGN STLLFIIYKN KCMRNGENIL IASLALAGDLL HIVIDIPINV YKLLAEDWPF  .....GEMC KLVPFIQKAS VGITVLSLCA
rETB  FKYINTIVSC LVFVLGIIGN STLLFIIYKN KCMRNGENIL IASLALAGDLL HIIIDIPINV YKLLAEDWPF  .....GEMC KLVPFIQKAS VGITVLSLCA
bETA  FKYINTVISC TIFTVGMGVN ATLLFIIYQN KCMRNGENAL IASLALAGDLI YVVIDLPINV FKLLAGRWPF  EQNDFGVFLC KLFPFLQKSS VGITVLNLCA
hETA  FKYINTVISC TIFTVGMGVN ATLLFIIYQN KCMRNGENAL IASLALAGDLI YVVIDLPINV FKLLAGRWPF  IHNDFGVFLC KLFPFLQKSS VGITVLNLCA
rETA  FKYINTVISC TIFIVGMGVN ATLLFIIYQN KCMRNGENAL IASLALAGDLI YVVIDLPINV FKLLAGRWPF  IHNDFGVFLC KLFPFLQKSS VGITVLNLCA
xETA  FKYINTILSC TIFIIGGMWGN STLLFIIYKN KCMRNGENVL IASLALAGDLF YILIDIPIIV IQSPVGAFLC KLVPFIQKAS VGITVLNLCA
xETC  FKVTTILSC  VIFLMGIVGN STLRIIIYKN KMRNGPNVL  IASLALGDLF YILIAIPIIS ISF.......  ..WLSTYGSE YIYQLVHLYRARVYSLSLCA

                                                              TM 1        TM 2                              TM 3

   201                                                                                                   300
bETB  LSIDRYRAVA SWSRIKGIGV PKWTAVEIVL IWVVSVVLAV PEAVGFDIIT SDHIGNKLRI CLLHPTQKTA FMQFYKTAKD WWLFSFYFCL PLAITAFFYT
pETB  LSIDRYRAVA SWSRIKGIGV PKWTAVEIVL IWVVSVVLAV PEALGFIMIT TUYKGNRLRI CLLHPTQKTA FMQFYKTAKD WWLFSFYFCL PLAITAFFYT
hETB  LSIDRYRAVA SWSRIKGIGV PKWTAVEIVL IWVVSVVLAV PEAIGFDIIT MYKGSYLRI  CLLHPVQKTA FMQFYKTAKD WWLFSFYFCL PLAITAFFYT
rETB  LSIDRYRAVA SWSRIKGIGV PKWTAVEIVL IWVVSVVLAV PEAIGFDVIT SDMKGKPLRV CMLNPFQKTA FMQFYKTAKD WWLFSFYFCL PLAITAFFYT
bETA  LSVDRYRAVA SWSRVQGIGI PLVTAIEIVS IWILSPILAI PEAIGFVMVP FEYKGBQHKT CMLNATSK.. ........... FMEFYQDVKD WWLFGFYFYM PLVCTAIFYT
hETA  LSVDRYRAVA SWSRVQGIGI PLVTAIEIVS IWILSFILAI PEAIGFVMVP FEYRGBQHKT CMLNATSK.. FMEFYQIVKD WWLFGFYFYM PLVCTAIFYT
rETA  LSVDRYRAVA SWSRVQGIGI PLITAIEIVS IWILSFILAI PEAIGFVMVP FEYKGBQHRT CMLNAATTK. FMEFYQIVKD WWLFGFYFYM PLVCTAIFYT
xETA  LSVDRYRAVP SWSRVQGSGI PLITAIEIIS IWILSFVLAI PEAIAFNLVE FEYRGBQFRT CMFHATSP.. FMMFYKNAKD WWLFGLYFYV PLACTGVFYT
xETC  LSIDRYRAVA SWNRFSIGI  PVRKAIEILT IWAVAIAVAV PEAIAFNLVE LDFRGYITLUV CMLPMEQTHD EMFEYEVKV WWLFGFYFCL PLACTGVFET

                           TM 4                                                                            TM 5
```

40

```
          301
bETB  LMTCEML.RK KGSEMQIALND HLKQRREVAK │TVFCLVLVFA LCMLPLHLSR│ IL..KLTLY DQ..HLPRR. CEFL......... SFLL.VLDY IGINMASLNS
pETB  LMTCEML.RK KGSEMQIALND HLKQRREVAK │TVFCLVLVFA LCMLPLHLSR│ IL..KLTLY DQ..NLDNR. CELL......... SFLL.VLDY IGINMASLNS
hETB  LMTCEML.RK KGSEMQIALND HLKQRREVAK │TVFCLVLVFA LCMLPLHLSR│ IL..KLTLY NQ..NDPNR. CELL......... SFLL.VLIY IGINMASLNS
rETB  LMTCEML.RK KGSEMQIALND HLKQRREVAK │TVFCLVLVFA LCMLPLHLSR│ IL..KLTLY DQ..GNFQR. CELL......... SFLL.VLDY IGINMASLNS
bETA  LMTEMLNRR  NGSLRIALSE HLKQRREVAK │TVFCLVVIFA LCWFPLHLSR│ IL..KKTVV DE..MTTNR. CELL......... SFLL.LMDY IGINLATMNS
hETA  LMTEMLNRR  NGSLRIALSE HLKQRREVAK │TVFCLVVIFA LCWFPLHLSR│ IL..KKTVY NE..MDKNR. CELL......... SFLL.LMDY IGINLATMNS
rETA  LMTEMLNRR  NGSLRIALSE HLKQRREVAK │TVFCLVVIFA LCTTFPLHLSR│ IL..KKTVT DE..MDKNR. CELL......... SFLL.LMDY IGINLATMNS
xETA  MMTEMLHQR  KGSLRIALSE HLKQRREVAK │TVFCLVVIFA LCWLPLHLSR│ IL..KKMIY NE..LDPSR. CELL......... SFLL.VMIF IGINLAALNS
xETC  LMSGEMLSIK N.GMRIALND HMKQRREVAK │TVFCLWVIFA LAWLPLHVSS│ IFVRLSATVK RACILRNKRS CTMAELCTGVNY QLIMVVNY TGINMASLNS
                                       └─────── TM 6 ───────┘                                                    400

          401                                                                          469
bETB  CINPIA│LYLV SKRFKNCFKS CLCCWC.QSF EEKQSLEEKQ SCLKFKANH GYD...NF.R SSNKYSSS
pETB  CINPIA│LYLV SKRFKNCFKS CLCCWC.QSF EEKQSLEEKQ SCLKFKANH GYD...NF.R SSNKYSSS
hETB  CINPIA│LYLV SKRFKNCFKS CLCCWC.QSF EEKQSLEEKQ SCLKFKANH GYD...NF.R SSNKYSSS
rETB  CINPIA│LYLV SKRFKNCFKS CLCCWC.QTF EEKQSLEEKQ SCLKFKANH GYD...NF.R SSNKYSSS
bETA  CINPIA│LYFV SKRFKNCFQS CLCCCYQSK  SLMTSVPMNG TSIQWKNHBQ NNH...NTER SSHKQSIN
hETA  CINPIA│LYFV SKRFKNCFQS CLCCCYQSK  SLMTSVPMNG TSIQWKNHQ NNH...NTDR SSHKQSMN
rETA  CINPIA│LYFV SKRFKNCFQS CLCCCHQSK  SLMTSVPMNG TSIQWKNQBQ .NH...NTER SSHKQSMN
xETA  CINPIA│LYFV SKRFKNCFQS CLCCCC.QSK THINTAPMNV TSIQWKNHDQ NYY...GADR SIHKQSIN
xETC  IG│PVALYFV SRKFKNCTQS CLQCWCHRPT LTTTPMEKG SGGKWKANH DLDLLRSSCR LCNKYSSS
      └──────┘
                                                                                       TM 7
```

Fig. 3. Alignment of mammalian and amphibian ET receptor sequences. The primary structures of ET_A receptor from bovine (6), human (35,56), rat (54), and *Xenopus* (60), ET_B receptor from bovine (55), porcine (53), human (36,57,59), and rat (7), and amphibian ET_C receptor (61) were simultaneously aligned with the PILEUP program in GCG version 8.0 (114). In two regions, slight adjustments to the alignment were made to restrict sequence gaps to putative interhelical loop regions. Seven putative-transmembrane domains are indicated. In the rat ET_B-receptor sequence, the original sequence (7) was corrected on the basis of recent cDNA and genomic DNA sequencing data (23) indicated as SSAP. In the xET_C sequence, residues that are conserved in all ET_A and ET_B receptor sequences are underlined; residues in xET_C that differ from the ET_A/ET_B consensus sequence are designated in bold print.

yields overall identity and similarity values of 91/95%, respectively. The sequence identity/similarity drops to 73/83% between mammalian and amphibian ET_As and is 50/71% between amphibian ET_A/xET_C (Table 1).

Sequence homology and hydropathic analysis of the ET receptor primary structures indicate that all currently known ET receptors belong to the rhodopsin class of G-protein coupled receptors (GPCRs) *(17)*. By analogy to the β2-adrenergic receptor where information concerning the membrane topology of the receptor is available *(62,63)*, ET receptors are composed of a 50–70-residue AT region, seven helical transmembrane domains (TMs 1–7) connected by hydrophilic loops (C1–3 facing the cytoplasm; E1–3 at the extracellular surface), and a CT region consisting of approx 60 residues. All ET receptors have multiple-cysteine residues located approx 10–15-residues following the end of TM7 (Fig. 3) that are conserved in a number of rhodopsin GPCRs *(17)* and can participate in a thioester linkage with palmitic acid to produce a fourth cytoplasmic loop (C4) *(64,65)*. The general ET-receptor topology is shown in Fig. 4.

Conserved residues or sequence motifs within the ET receptors in TM 1 (GN), TM 2 (LAXXD), TM 3 (D/ERY), TM 4 (W(X)9–10P), E2 (C), TM 6 (P), and TM 7 (P(X)2–3Y) are conserved in the majority of rhodopsin class GPCRs *(17)* (Fig. 4). In addition, residues at the interface of E1 and TM 3 (C) and in TM 7 (NP(X)2–3Y) which are found to occur in the majority of rhodopsin class receptors also occur in ET_A and ET_B, but differ in xET_C *(61;* Figs. 3 and 4).

Several features of xET_C distinguish it from other mammalian and amphibian ET receptors. The apparent affinity for ET-3, estimated by the EC_{50} of melanin dispersion in melanocytes or by [^{125}I]ET-3 competition binding to xET_C expressed in *Xenopus* melanocytes or HeLa cells, ranges from 24 to 45 n*M* *(61)*. These data indicate that xETC binds its preferred ET peptide, i.e., ET-3, with at least two orders of magnitude lower binding affinity than mammalian or amphibian ET_A or ET_B receptors bind ET-1 (and also ET-3 in the case of ET_B) *(6,7,60)*.

Many of the conserved residues and sequence motifs observed within mammalian ET receptors are also observed in xET_C. An obvious exception is noted in the TM 3 region of xET_C (Fig. 3). The average values for amino-acid identities/similarities within TM 3 between ET_A/ET_B (amphibian or mammalian) are 81 and 88%, respectively. However, the average corresponding values for TM 3 of ET_A and ET_B receptors compared to xET_C are 9 and 44%, respectively (Table 1). Thus, the TM 3 region of xET_C is quite distinct from that of other species.

Table 1

Sequence Comparisons Between Endothelin-Receptor Subtypes[a]

ET receptors	TM 1	TM 2	TM 3	TM 4	TM 5	TM 6	TM 7	Overall
hET$_A$/hET$_B$	65 (91)	78 (96)	71 (81)	63 (88)	76 (91)	86 (100)	78 (96)	58 (77)
hET$_A$/xET$_B$	87 (100)	87 (96)	86 (91)	88 (100)	76 (95)	100 (100)	78 (96)	73 (83)
hET$_B$/xET$_A$	61 (91)	83 (91)	86 (91)	75 (88)	71 (91)	86 (100)	78 (96)	61 (78)
hET$_A$/xET$_C$	65 (87)	55 (82)	6 (44)	50 (81)	76 (91)	86 (95)	57 (87)	49 (70)
xET$_A$/xET$_C$	70 (87)	68 (86)	11 (50)	44 (81)	86 (95)	86 (95)	57 (87)	50 (71)
hET$_B$/xET$_C$	61 (96)	59 (73)	11 (44)	63 (88)	76 (86)	81 (95)	70 (91)	52 (70)

[a]Sequence comparisons between mammalian and amphibian endothelin-receptor subtypes. The sequences of human ET$_A$ (hET$_A$), human ET$_B$ (hET$_B$), Xenopus ET$_A$ (xET$_A$), and Xenopus ET$_C$ (xET$_C$) were compared using the GAP program of the GCG package version 8.0. The percent sequence identity and (similarity) are shown for the overall sequence and receptor regions corresponding to putatuve-transmembrane domains (TMs 1–7). TM domains are defined as in Fig. 3.

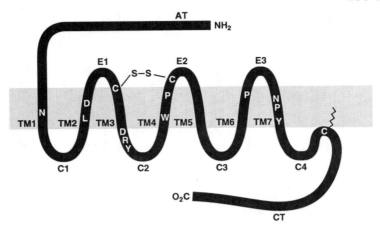

Fig. 4. Predicted membrane topology of endothelin receptors. The amino terminus (AT) and the carboxyl terminus (CT) are exposed to the extracellular and intracellular surfaces of the plasma membrane (stippled rectangle), respectively. Putative transmembrane helices (TMs 1–7), extracellular loops (E1–3), and intracellular loops (C1–4) are indicated. ET_A and ET_B receptor residues conserved in many rhodopsin class of G protein-coupled receptors are indicated. A potential disulfide bridge and site of cysteine palmitoylation is shown.

The large sequence variations within TM 3 of xET_C may explain the lower ligand-binding affinities observed in xET_C relative to the corresponding values in amphibian/mammalian ET_A or ET_B. In TM 3 of xET_C, a cysteine residue conserved through most of the rhodopsin class of GPCRs (Fig. 3) is missing. In hET_B receptor, replacement of this conserved cysteine, C174, results in an hET_B variant that has dramatically decreased binding affinity for ET-1 or is not expressed *(66)*. In addition, residues conserved within TM 3 of $ET_{A/B}$ and important for high affinity agonist peptide binding (Q165/181 and K166/182 within hET_A/hET_B, respectively, *vide infra*), are absent from the xET_C sequence (Fig. 3).

To date, no mammalian equivalent of xET_C has been identified. Further work will therefore be needed to determine whether mammalian homologs of xET_C exist and their relevance, if any, to mammalian physiology.

5. Endothelin Receptor Mutagenesis: Signal Transduction

Endothelin receptors mediate multiple signal-transduction processes in various tissues and cell lines. These processes include activation of phospholipases A2, C, and D, mobilization of both intra- and extracellularly calcium stores, activation of various protein kinase C isoforms with subsequent activation of mitogen-activated kinase, and activation of adenylate and guanylate cyclases (reviewed by Nambi et al., *67*). Although several of these events may not be directly mediated by G-proteins activated by ET receptors, it is clear that ET_A and ET_B receptors can directly couple to multiple, yet distinct signal transduction pathways. Currently, pharmacological evidence exists for further subtypes of the fully characterized ET_A and ET_B receptors *(19)*, however, these observations have not been confirmed at the molecular level. Relating pharmacological observations to molecular biology, therefore, should continue to be an active area of research.

5.1. G Protein Receptor Interactions

In addition to stimulating IP hydrolysis, each ET-receptor subtype can differentially alter cAMP metabolism in CHO cell lines; the ET_A receptor stimulates cAMP accumulation via $G\alpha s$ whereas the ET_B receptor inhibits forskolin-stimulated accumulation of cAMP via $G\alpha i$ *(68,69)*. The cytoplasmic loop regions of GPCRs appear to contribute significantly to G-protein/receptor binding (reviewed by Probst et. al., *17*) and receptor chimeras of hET_A and hET_B have been used to define the receptor regions that contribute to $G\alpha s$ and $G\alpha i$ activation in more detail *(69)*. An ET-receptor chimera in which TM 3-C3-TM 4 of hET_A is replaced by the corresponding hET_B sequence decreases forskolin-stimulated cAMP to levels comparable to wild-type hET_B. Thus C3 of the hET_B receptor appears to be sufficient for recognition and activation of $G\alpha i$ in CHO cell lines. In contrast, wild-type hET_A-like receptor activation of $G\alpha s$ requires the substitution of both C2 and C3 (with adjoining TMs) of hET_A receptor within an hET_B receptor framework. Substitution of the hET_A receptor C2 (with C1 and adjacent TMs) into the hET_B receptor generates a chimera that catalyzes $G\alpha s$-mediated cAMP accumulation with EC_{50} values that are comparable to wild-type hET_A receptor but with diminished maximal cAMP accumulation *(69)*. These results suggest that C2 and C3 regions of hET_A and hET_B, respectively, are major determinants of $G\alpha s/G\alpha i$ selectivity, and also suggest that amino-acid substitutions within these regions could subtly affect the activation of the various G protein pathways to which the ET receptors are coupled (Fig. 5).

Hashido et al. *(70)* have investigated the effects of amino-acid substitution by employing deletional and insertional mutagenesis tech-

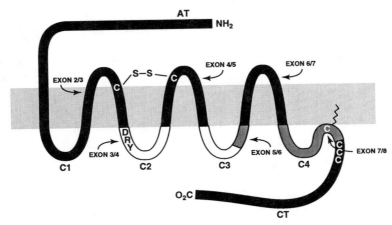

Fig. 5. Endothelin-receptor secondary-structure model: location of exon/ exon junctions and receptor regions implicated in signal transduction. Receptor regions designated according to the legend for Fig. 4. The C2 and C3 regions are important for G protein selectivity *(69)*. Receptor residues near the carboxyl end of C3 and C4 are important for signal transduction *(70)*. The location of the exon/exon boundaries that occur within the ET-receptor open reading frame are indicated.

niques in an effort to identify regions of hET_A receptor that are important to phospholipase C-mediated signal transduction. Deletion of residues 281–289 from the amino terminus of the C3 loop of hET_A does not affect receptor expression, ET-1 binding, or signal transduction. In contrast, perturbation of the carboxyl end of C3 by substitution of hET_A residues (296–305) with corresponding residues from the β2-adrenergic receptor or by deletion of residues (291–306) of the hET_A receptor, results in receptor variants with either impaired or undetectable calcium mobilization. These data suggest that the CT portion of C3 of hET_A is important for G-protein activation of phospholipase C (Fig. 5). Deletion of the CT region from N427 to C385 does not affect high-affinity ET-1 binding or calcium mobilization; however, further truncation of CT by a single residue (L384) results in an ET_A receptor variant with high-affinity ET-1 binding that is unable to mobilize intracellular calcium *(70)*. These data indicate that the majority of the CT region is not important for hET_A receptor expression, ET-1 binding, or signal transduction. However, the CT region proximal to the carboxy terminus of TM 7, containing conserved cysteine residues that may be palmitoylated (Fig. 5), is important for signal transduction, but not ligand binding. Taken together, the data available from chimeric ET receptors and site-directed ET-receptor mutants implicates the regions C2, C3, and part of C4 proximal to TM 7 as being influential to G protein-mediated signal transduction (Fig. 5).

5.2. Alternate RNA Splicing:
Potential Importance for Signal Diversification

At the present time, only one alternately spliced form of ET-receptor mRNA has been detected. Shyamala et al. *(26)* used PCR to identify an hET_B receptor splice variant (hET_{Bsv}) with a 10-amino acid in-frame insertion (SLKYNSIFIF) between R199 and Y200 of the highly conserved "DRY" sequence within the C2 loop of hET_B. hET_{Bsv} mRNA is found in brain, placenta, lung, and heart, but the inserted nucleotide sequence appears absent in bovine, rat and porcine genomic DNA. CHO cell lines expressing either hET_B or hET_{Bsv} receptor have identical ET-1 and ET-3 competition curves and display similar ET-1-mediated inhibition of forskolin-induced cAMP synthesis and stimulation of inositol phosphates *(26)*. Therefore, in the context of a CHO-recombinant cell line, the hET_{Bsv} receptor appears functionally identical to the hET_B receptor.

Despite the functional similarity between hET_B and hET_{Bsv} receptors *(26)*, the location of exon–exon boundaries within ET-receptor coding regions *(22,24,25)* suggests that undiscovered splice variants of ET receptors may have altered signal-transduction properties. Three exon–exon boundaries occur within ET_A and ET_B receptor coding sequences corresponding to regions of C2, C3, and C4 and have been demonstrated to be important for G protein coupling or selectivity *(69,70)* (Fig. 5). Specifically, exon 5/6 of the hET_A receptor is located within the carboxy terminus of C3 in the midst of the residues implicated as important for calcium mobilization and exon 7/8 in the hET_A receptor is located three residues upstream from the cysteine residue that is essential for G protein coupling *(70)*. Additionally, exon 3/4 interrupts the conserved DRY sequence demonstrated to be important for signal transduction in bioactive-amine receptors *(71,72)*.

It is noteworthy that altered signal transduction and/or G protein selectivities of various GPCRs arise from altered amino-acid sequences within the C1 *(73,74)*, C3 *(75,76)*, and C4 *(77–80)* receptor regions by alternate RNA splicing. Therefore, although speculative, alteration of ET-receptor primary structure in the C2, C3, or C4 regions may reasonably be expected to alter G protein coupling efficiencies and differentially affect various signaling pathways activated by an ET-receptor subtype. Future studies should investigate the role of alternate splicing as a potential molecular mechanism for the diversification of ET receptor-mediated signaling in tissues where physiological responses atypical of the fully characterized ET_A or ET_B receptors have been observed *(19,81)*.

6. Endothelin Receptor Mutagenesis: Ligand Binding

6.1. Receptor Chimeras

Owing to the high degree of sequence similarity between hET_A and hET_B receptors and the very large difference in binding affinity for subtype-selective peptides, ET-receptor chimera construction has been an effective way to gain insight into the receptor regions that contribute either directly or indirectly to ligand selectivity. Qualitatively, results from chimera studies *(82–86)* have identified receptor regions that contribute directly to the high-affinity binding of the ET_A receptor-selective antagonist BQ 123 (TMs 1–3 of hET_A) and indirectly to binding of the ET_B receptor-selective agonist peptide ET-3 (TMs 4–6 of hET_B).

Although experimental results cannot be directly compared across the chimeric-receptor studies, ligand affinity for chimeras can be expressed relative to that of the wild-type ET-receptor subtypes in order to characterize and compare their ligand-binding behavior. The ligand affinity of the chimeric receptor relative to its parent-receptor subtype ($K_{i\ chimera}/K_{i\ parent}$) is indicative of the degree to which the binding behavior of the chimera is similar to the parent subtype. Furthermore, the ligand affinity of the chimeric receptor relative to that of the nonparent receptor subtype ($K_{i\ chimera}/K_{i\ nonparent}$) is indicative of their similarity. These values are given in Table 2.

6.1.1. BQ 123 Affinity

Early studies implicated E1 (with adjoining parts of TM 3) of hET_A receptor as important for high affinity binding of BQ 123 *(87)*. Systematic studies using reciprocal ET chimeras indicated that replacement of AT and TM 1 of hET_A receptor with the corresponding sequence of hET_B receptor decreases BQ 123 affinity 5–20-fold (chimeras 1A1 and 1A2, Table 2) with further substitution of TM 2 and part of E1 decreasing BQ 123 affinity a total of 210-fold (chimera 3A, Table 2). These results highlight the importance of TM 1

Table 2

Endothelin Receptor Chimeras: Summary of BQ 123 Binding Affinities[a]

Code	Structure	Affinity change (fold)	K_i (chimera)/ K_i (wt chimera)	K_i (chimera)/ K_i (wt nonparent)	Reference/(chimera)
1A1		⇓4.8	4.8	0.004	86 (B(NI) A(IIC))
1A2		⇓19.7	19.7	0.04	84 (ETA-1)
2A		⇓145	145	0.3	84 (ETA-2)
3A		⇓208	208	0.017	86 (B(NII) A(IIIC))
4A		⇓2000	2000	1.6	86 (B(NIII) A(IVC))
5A		⇓>233	>233	1.0	85 (BAB)
1B1		⇑1.3	0.77	960	86 (A(NI) B(IIC))
1B2		⇓1.7	1.7	839	84 (ETB-2)
2B		⇓3.9	3.9	1870	84 (ETB-2)
3B		⇑3.5	0.29	356	86 (A(NII) B(IIIC))
4B		⇑155	0.007	8	86 (A(NIII) B(IVC))
5B		⇑>33	0.03	7.0	85 (ABA)

[a]Summary of BQ 123 binding-affinity changes observed with chimeras between ET_A and ET_B receptor subtypes. The approximate composition of each receptor chimera is indicated by its ET_A (dark-line) and ET_B (light-line) components. The change in BQ 123 binding affinity for ET-receptor chimeras is expressed as fold increases (up arrow) or decreases (down arrow) relative to the parental ET-receptor subtype. The change in BQ 123 affinity of an ET-receptor chimera relative to its parental ET-receptor subtype is expressed as a K_i of the receptor chimera/K_i of parent wild-type receptor. The similarity in binding-affinity relative to the opposite receptor subtype is expressed as K_i of the receptor chimera/K_i of nonparent wild-type receptor.

and TM 2 to BQ 123 binding because reciprocal exchange of the AT region between ET-receptor subtypes does not affect BQ 123 affinity *(86)*. Replacement of TM 2-E1-TM 3 of hET$_A$ receptor by the corresponding residues of hET$_B$ receptor decreased BQ 123 affinity 145-fold (chimera 2A, Table 2), suggesting that TM 3 also contributes to BQ 123 binding. This is consistent with the results from chimera 4A, where substitution of part of TM 3 from hET$_B$ to chimera 3A (containing TM 1 and TM 2 of hET$_B$; Table 2) further decreases BQ 123 affinity to 2000-fold overall (chimera 4A, Table 2). Therefore replacement of TM 1, TM 2-E1-TM 3 of hET$_A$ receptor by the corresponding regions of the hET$_B$ receptor results in chimeras (4A and 5A; Table 2) with BQ 123 affinities that are comparable to wild-type hET$_B$ receptor (Table 2).

In contrast, reciprocal constructs where AT-TM 1, TM2 -E1-TM 3, or AT-TM 1, TM 2 of hET$_B$ receptor are replaced by the corresponding sequence of hET$_A$ receptor do not significantly (less than fourfold) alter the BQ 123 affinities of the resulting chimeras (1B1, 1B2, 2B, and 3B; Table 2). Significantly, further substitution of TM 3 from the hET$_A$ receptor into chimera 3B (containing TM 1 and TM 2 of hET$_A$ receptor; Table 2) generates chimeras 4B and 5B which have significantly increased affinities for BQ 123 that are within 7–8-fold of wild-type hET$_A$ receptor affinity. Further sequential substitution of TM 4, E2-TM 5, and TM 6 to chimera 4B does not lead to an increase in BQ 123 affinity *(86)*. These data indicate that simultaneous inclusion of TM 1, TM 2-E1-TM 3 of hET$_A$ receptor can create a BQ 123 binding site within hET$_B$ receptor that has approx 10-fold lower affinity than that of wild-type hET$_A$ receptor. These results suggest a model whereby residues from TM 1, TM 2-E1, and TM 3 of hET$_A$ receptor are in three-dimensional proximity and form a binding site that directly engages BQ 123.

6.1.2. ET-3 Affinity

In contrast to the BQ 123 results, the results from chimeric studies aimed at elucidating the ET-3 binding site are not so straightforward to interpret. Reciprocal replacement of E2 with adjoining TMs 4 and 5 or E3 with adjoining TMs 6 and 7 of one ET-receptor subtype into the framework of the opposite receptor subtype alters the ET-3 affinity by 20–60-fold (chimeras 1A, 2A, 2B, and 3B; Table 3) *(86)*. Simultaneous substitution of TM 4-E2-TM 5, TM 6-E3 of hET$_B$ receptor into the hET$_A$ receptor framework results in a chimera with 500–900-fold higher ET-3 affinity than wild-type hET$_A$ receptor and

Table 3
Endothelin Receptor Chimeras: Summary of ET-3 Binding Affinities[a]

Code	Structure	Affinity change (fold)	K_i (chimera)/ K_i (wt chimera)	K_i (chimera)/ K_i (wt nonparent)	Reference/(chimera)
1A1		⇑15	0.07	333	82 (ET_A-C)
1A2		⇑39	0.03	6.6	84 (ET_A-3)
2A		⇑7.5	0.13	34	84 (ET_A-4)
3A		⇑540–910	0.002	0.53–0.83	86 (A(NII) B[IV-VI] A(VIIC)); 85 (ABA)
1B		⇑1.2	0.83	0.003	84 (ET_B-2)
2B1		⇓20	20	0.08	84 (ET_B-3)
2B2		⇓26	26	0.009	83 (ET_B-C)
3B		⇓61	61	0.24	84 (ET_B-4)
4B		⇓13	12.8	0.03	85 (BAB)
5B		⇓260	260	0.09	83 (ET_B-BC)

[a]Summary of BQ 123 binding-affinity changes observed with chimeras between ET_A and ET_B receptor subtypes. The approximate composition of each receptor chimera is indicated by its ET_A (dark-line) and ET_B (light-line) components. The change in ET-3 binding affinity for ET-receptor chimeras is expressed as fold increases (up arrow) or decreases (down arrow) relative to the parental ET-receptor subtype. The change in ET-3 affinity of an ET-receptor chimera relative to its parental ET-receptor subtype is expressed as a K_i of the receptor chimera/K_i of parent wild-type receptor. The similarity in binding-affinity relative to the opposite receptor subtype is expressed as K_i of the receptor chimera/K_i of nonparent wild-type receptor.

K_i values within a factor of two of wild-type hET_B receptor values *(85,86)* (3A; Table 3). In contrast, the reciprocal ET chimera, TM 4-E2-TM 5, TM 6-E3 of hET_A receptor within an hET_B receptor framework, displays only a 13-fold decrease in ET-3 affinity relative to wild-type hET_B receptor *(85)* (chimera 4B; Table 3). These dramatic nonreciprocal effects on ET-3 binding affinity of symmetrical ET-receptor chimeras suggests that ET-3 affinity for the hET_A receptor is not directly modulated by the presence of specific residues within TMs 4–6, but that indirect effects, such as changes in receptor conformation, may be responsible.

Such an explanation is also consistent with the observation that the influence of hET_A receptor TM 2–3 on ET-3 binding affinity is dependent on the receptor-sequence context. Simple replacement of TM 2–3 of hET_B receptor by corresponding hETA receptor residues does not affect ET-3 binding affinity *(84)* (chimera 1B; Table 3). However addition of this hET_A receptor region into an ET chimera containing E2 and TM 5 of hET_A receptor within an hET_B receptor framework (chimera 2B2; Table 3) results in chimera 5B *(83)*, which has a 10-fold lower ET-3 affinity than chimera 2B2. Therefore, these data also suggest that residues of the hET_A receptor within TM 2–3 do not directly engage ET-3.

Taken together, the ET receptor chimera studies have defined different receptor regions that influence the binding affinities of BQ 123 (TMs 1–3) and ET-3 (TMs 4–6) Detailed analysis of reciprocal chimera constructs indicate TMs 1–3 affect BQ 123 binding in a reciprocal manner consistent with a direct interaction of this region of hET_A receptor with BQ 123. The effects on ET-3 affinity, however, are not reciprocal and depend on sequence context, suggesting that at least some effects on ET-3 affinity may be indirect and owing to alterations in receptor folding or helix packing.

6.2. The Extracellular Receptor Regions

Given the large molecular volume of the endothelin and sarafotoxin peptides, extracellular-receptor regions (AT, E1, E2, and E3) seem likely to contribute to peptide agonist-binding affinity and selectivity. Early studies investigating the importance of the AT of the hET_A receptor *(88)* to ET-1 binding found that deletion of residues (25–49) of the amino terminus did not affect ET-1 binding, whereas deletion of residues (25–76) leaving approximately five residues preceding TM 1, resulted in an hET_A receptor variant that had no detectable ET-1 binding. This deletion variant was detected in detergent treated cells by immunofluorescence *(88)*, confirming that the lack of observable ET-1 binding was not owing to lack of receptor expression. Reciprocal chimeras that exchange the AT region between ET-receptor subtypes have ET-3 and BQ 123 selectivities that are identical to their respective wild-type receptors *(86)*, suggesting that AT does not contribute to peptide-ligand selectivity.

The receptor-binding contribution of extracellular loop residues, which differ between ET_A and ET_B receptors, has also been examined (Lee et al., manuscript in preparation). Of the various sequence differences between ET-receptor subtypes in these regions (Fig. 3), it has been shown that simultaneous deletion of T263 and A264 located in E2 of the hET_B receptor decreases the binding affinity of sarafotoxin 6c without affecting the binding affinities of other sarafotoxins or any of the endothelin isopeptides (Lee et al., manuscript in preparation).

Although these studies do not provide compelling evidence implicating the extracellular regions of ET receptors as important for the high-affinity binding or selectivity of peptide ligands, this is not an area of the receptor that has received thorough investigation. Future studies will continue to examine the influence of nonconserved residues; however, a role for conserved residues should also be considered.

6.3. Transmembrane Domains

Within the GPCR family, site-directed mutagenesis studies have implicated residues located in TM regions as important for the binding of low-mol-wt nonpeptide, peptide, and small-protein ligands to their respective GPCRs *(89–94)*. Identification of sequence differences among closely related receptors has been the main strategy for the selection of mutation sites. More recently, three-dimensional receptor models based on the structure of bacteriorhodopsin (BR) have been used not only to rationalize previous results, but to proactively select mutant targets *(85,95)*.

6.3.1. GPCR Models and Structure–Function Hypotheses

ET-receptor models constructed using the structure of BR determined by cryoelectron microscopy *(96)* and an assignment of putative TM domains defined by multiple-sequence alignments have been used in the selection of ET-receptor mutation sites *(85,95)*. Figure 6 depicts a van der Waals surface of the TM domains of one such model of the hET_A receptor viewed from the extracellular surface *(85)*.

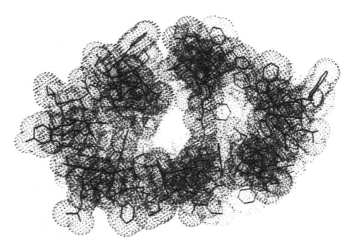

Fig. 6. Model of human-ET$_A$ receptor. The model is viewed from the extracellular surface and shown with a van der Waals surface; TM 1 is at 9 o'clock with TMs 2–7 following counter clockwise. The putative-receptor cavity shown on the left is bounded by TMs 1, 2, 3, 6, and 7 and is part of a proposed ligand-binding site.

From this perspective, two putative receptor cavities are apparent; the larger and deeper cavity is defined by TMs 1, 2, 3, 6, and 7 and a smaller, more shallow cavity defined by TMs 3, 4, 5, and 6 (Fig. 6).

In conjunction with the receptor models, two strategies have been used to develop hypotheses concerning the importance of receptor residues to agonist-peptide selectivity and high-affinity binding of nonpeptide antagonists. In the first strategy, it was hypothesized that certain receptor regions important for ligand binding may be conserved throughout the GPCR superfamily *(97–99)*. By analogy to the binding-site aspartate residues conserved within TM 3 of the bioactive-amine receptors *(89)*, two residues conserved within TM 3 of ET$_A$ and ET$_B$ were identified as potentially important for ligand binding, Q165/Q181 and K166/K182 of hET$_A$/hET$_B$, respectively *(99)*. Interestingly, these residues contribute to defining the large receptor cavity shown in Fig. 6. The second strategy considered receptor residues that differ between hET$_A$ and hET$_B$ receptors and reside within the large putative-receptor cavities (Fig. 6). Y129/H150 (in TM 2 of hET$_A$/hET$_B$, respectively) *(85,95)* and T359/S376 (in TM 7 of hET$_A$/hET$_B$, respectively) are two such sites speculated to be potential contributors to ligand binding and peptide agonist selectivity *(85)*.

6.3.2. The Conserved Role of TM 3 Residues

Mauzy and Zhu *(97,98)*, identified a lysine residue, conserved in all ET_A and ET_B receptors (Fig. 3), which is located one position downstream from the binding-site aspartate residues conserved within TM 3 of all bioactive amine receptors. Replacement of this lysine residue (K181) by aspartate in the rat ET_B receptor differentially decreased the apparent binding affinities of ET-1, ET-2, ET-3, and S6C without affecting the maximal IP-hydrolysis rates at saturating concentrations of agonist peptides. In the human receptor, the analogous residue (K182) was investigated for its potential importance to agonist peptide selectivity and to high affinity binding of nonpeptide antagonists *(99)*. Substitution of K182 by basic, acidic, or uncharged residues resulted in hET_B receptor variants with decreased affinities for agonist peptides ET-2 (11–47-fold), ET-3 (70–300-fold), S6C (90–900-fold), and IRL-1736 (>5000-fold), no detectable affinity for SB (±) 209670 (>770-fold) or Ro 46 2005 (>50-fold), and wild-type ET-1 affinities (Table 4; *99*). Further results were consistent with the direct interaction of the two-indane carboxyl group of SB 209670 (Fig. 1) with K182 within TM 3 of hET_B receptor *(99)*. These collective data indicate that K182 of hETB is important for peptide agonist selectivity and high-affinity binding of nonpeptide antagonists.

The roles of the conserved TM 3 residues Q165/Q181 and K166/K182 in hET_A/hET_B receptors, respectively, in the binding of peptide agonists, the peptide antagonist BQ 123, and structurally distinct nonpeptide antagonists (SB (±) 209670, Ro-47 0203 and BMS 182874) have now been determined (Longton, et al., manuscript in preparation) and are summarized in Fig. 7. In each ET-receptor subtype, replacement of either glutamine or lysine reduces the binding affinity of the nonpeptide antagonists examined by approx 2–3 orders of magnitude and decreases the binding affinity of at least one agonist peptide by 1–3 orders of magnitude. With the exception of K166R in hET_A receptor, these decreased ligand affinities occur in the absence of a significantly altered ET-1 affinity (Fig. 7) suggesting that the observations are not owing to global changes in receptor conformation.

6.3.3. The Receptor Subtype-Specific Role of TM 2 and TM 7 Residues

The combination of ET-receptor models with sequence differences between the hET_A and hET_B receptors suggested that residues in TM 2 (Y129 hET_A/H150 hET_B) and TM 7 (T359 hET_A/S376 hET_B)

Table 4
Ligand Affinites for hET$_B$ and K182 hET$_B$ Variants[a]

Receptor	Peptide agonists, K$_i$ (nM)						Nonpeptide, antagonists K$_i$ (nM)	
	ET-1	ET-2	ET-3	S6C	IRL 1736	(±)–SB 209670	Ro 46-2005
hETB	0.012	0.018	0.013	0.030	0.063	15	200
K182R	0.014	0.19	0.91	2.64	306	≥7000[b]	>10,000
K182A	0.042	0.86	2.56	25.1	566	>10,000	>10,000
K182D	0.022	0.29	1.45	26.4	384	>10,000	>10,000
K182E	0.025	0.45	1.46	6.0	9600	>10,000	>10,000
K182M	0.037	0.70	3.59	23.9	1900	>10,000	>10,000

[a]Competitive binding between [^{125}I]ET-1 and unlabeled ligands was performed as described (99). The K$_i$ values were calculated from IC$_{50}$ values determined from nonlinear regression of the competition; the K$_i$ values listed are the average of between two and four determinations using membranes prepared from two independent HEK 293 transfections.

[b]Lower limits of the K$_i$ values for antagonist binding to K182X hET$_B$ are derived from the maximum concentration of ligand utilized or the estimated IC$_{50}$ value.

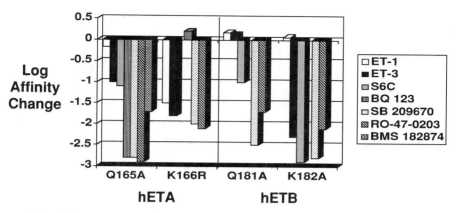

Fig. 7. Importance of TM 3 residues to peptide and nonpeptide ligand binding. The apparent affinities of the indicated ligands were determined by [^{125}I] ET-1 competition binding to Q165A hET$_A$, K166R hET$_A$, Q181A hET$_B$, K182A hET$_B$, and wild-type hET$_A$ and hET$_B$. The log of the affinity changes relative to the wild-type values are plotted as a function of the unlabeled competitor ligands. (**Note:** A decrease in affinity relative to wild-type is represented by a negative number.)

may contribute either to ligand binding or to the differences in agonist peptide selectivity observed between ET-receptor subtypes *(85)*.

Y129 within TM 2 of the hET$_A$ receptor was replaced by residues of varying size, hydrogen-bonding capability, and aromatic character, and the binding affinities for peptide agonists and BQ 123 were determined for the resulting hET$_A$ receptor variants (Table 5). Replacement of Y129 leads to hET$_A$ variants with ~140-fold increased affinities for ET-3 and S6C, 2–3 orders of magnitude lower affinities for the hET$_A$ selective peptide antagonist BQ 123 for all hET$_A$ variants except Y129F; but near wild-type affinities for ET-1 and ET-2. These results indicate that substitution of Y129 increases the "ET$_B$-like character" of the resulting hET$_A$ variants and suggests that Y129 is positioned within TM 2 of hET$_A$ to interact with both peptide agonists and antagonists. The data also support the location of Y129 within a putative-receptor cavity as predicted by the hET$_A$ receptor models *(85,95)*.

The hET$_A$ receptor model was further explored in the region of Y129 and an aspartate residue conserved between ET-receptor subtypes and located one helical turn toward the extracellular surface from Y129 was selected for mutagenesis. (Fig. 10). Figure 8 summarizes the change in ligand-binding affinities of TM 2 receptor vari-

Table 5

Ligand Affinites for hET$_A$ and Y129 hET$_A$ Variants[a]

Receptor	ET-1	ET-2	ET-3	S6C	BQ 123	IRL 1620
wt hET$_A$	0.018	0.058	6.35	222	13	>1000[b]
Y129F hET$_A$	0.012	0.012	0.031	2.95	76	105
Y129K hET$_A$	0.016	0.016	0.041	2.59	2400	ND
Y129A hET$_A$	0.021	0.034	0.100	1.60	>10,000[b]	43
Y129N hET$_A$	0.018	0.021	0.040	1.48	>10,000[b]	ND
Y129S hET$_A$	0.017	0.016	0.016	0.68	>10,000[b]	20
Y129Q hET$_A$	0.019	0.023	0.037	0.82	1240	ND
Y129H hET$_A$	0.017	0.025	0.062	0.56	1820	ND

[a]Apparent K_i of peptide (nM)-competitive binding between [^{125}I]ET-1 and unlabeled ligands was performed as described (85). The K_i values were calculated from IC$_{50}$ values determined from nonlinear regression of the competition; the K_i values listed are the average of between two and five determinations using membranes prepared from two independent HEK 293 transfections.

[b]Lower limits of the K_i values are derived from the maximum concentration of ligand utilized. ND: not determined.

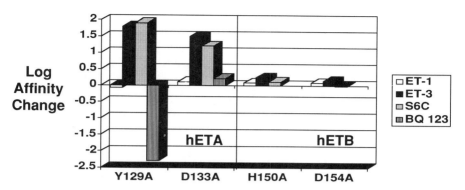

Fig. 8. Importance of TM 2 residues to peptide-ligand binding. The apparent affinities of the indicated ligands were determined by [^{125}I] ET-1 competition binding to Y129A hET$_A$, D133A hET$_A$, H150A hET$_B$, D154A hET$_B$, and wild-type hET$_A$ and hET$_B$. The log of the affinity changes relative to the wild-type values are plotted as a function of the unlabeled competitor ligands. (**Note:** A decrease in affinity relative to wild-type is represented by a negative number.)

ants in which Y129 or D133 of hET$_A$ receptor and H150 or D154 of hET$_B$ receptor have been replaced (ref. *85*; Longton et al., manuscript in preparation). Similar to the affect of the Y129 mutation, replacement of D133 in the hET$_A$ receptor increases the affinities of ET-3 and S6C without changing the binding affinity of ET-1 or, in the latter instance, the affinity of BQ 123. In contrast, replacement of the analogous residues within TM 2 of hET$_B$ (H150 and D154) has little effect on the binding affinities of the peptide agonists tested (Fig. 8). Thus, for the hET$_A$ receptor, the helical face of TM 2 containing Y129 and D133 is apparently solvent accessible and, unlike the corresponding region in hET$_B$, is utilized for engaging various peptide ligands either directly or indirectly.

In TM7, T359 and S376 within the hET$_A$ receptor and hET$_B$ receptor, respectively, were identified as potential contributors to differences in either ligand-binding or agonist peptide-binding selectivity *(85)*. To determine the importance of these residues, the Thr/Ser residues were replaced by Ala and because the adjacent residues differ between the hET$_A$ receptor (M360) and the hET$_B$ receptor (L377), the double mutants of each receptor subtype were also constructed (Longton et al., manuscript in preparation). The changes in binding affinity relative to wild-type receptor are summarized in Fig. 9. TM 7 variants of the hET$_A$ receptor have increased affinities for ET-3 and

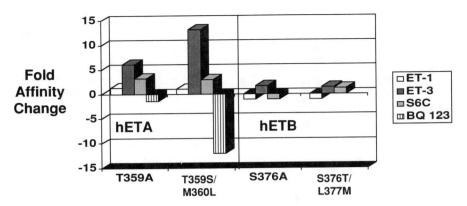

Fig. 9. Importance of TM 7 residues to peptide-ligand binding. The apparent affinities of the indicated ligands were determined by [^{125}I] ET-1 competition binding to T359A hET$_A$, T359S/M360L hET$_A$, S376A hET$_B$, S376T/l377M hET$_B$, and wild-type hET$_A$ and hET$_B$. The affinity changes relative to the wild-type values are plotted as a function of the unlabeled competitor ligands. (**Note:** A decrease in affinity relative to wild-type is represented by a negative number.)

S6C. In contrast, replacement of the analogous residues in TM 7 of hET$_B$ does not significantly affect the binding affinities of the agonist peptides tested (Fig. 9).

6.4. Conclusions: A Binding Site Model

6.4.1. Transmembrane Location of Binding Site Residues

Mutational studies combining the use of ET-receptor models and protein engineering technology have identified ET-receptor residues that contribute to peptide agonist-binding selectivity and high-affinity binding of nonpeptide antagonists. The side-chains of the hET$_A$ receptor residues which affect the binding affinities of certain agonist peptides or nonpeptide antagonists are highlighted in Fig. 10A,B. Fig. 10A is a view from the plane of the membrane; the positions of the highlighted sidechains indicate that TM 2 residues (Y129 and D133), TM 3 residues (Q165 and K166), and TM 7 residues (T359 and M360) are located deep within the TM domains of the hET$_A$ receptor. Fig. 10B is the same set of side-chains viewed from the extracellular surface of the receptor. The receptor models and mutational results suggest that at least a part of the binding site for peptide and nonpeptide ligands resides in a receptor cavity defined by

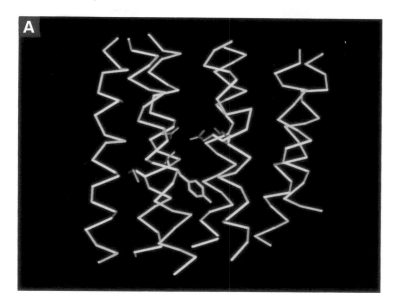

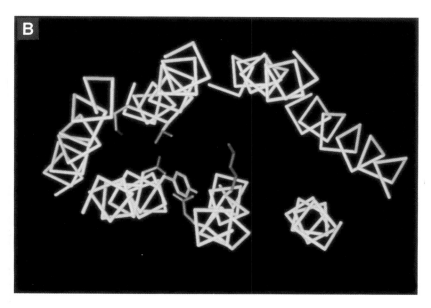

Fig. 10. Transmembrane residues of hET$_A$ important for ligand binding. Y129 in TM 2 (yellow), K166 in TM 3 (green), and D133, Q165, and T359 M360 in TMs 2, 3, and 7, respectively, (purple) are presented on a carbon representation of hET$_A$ viewed from the plane of the membrane **(A)** or from the extracellular surface **(B)**.

TMs 2, 3, and 7 (Figs. 6 and 10B). It is interesting to note that recent NMR results propose that the 11-cis retinal chromophore within rhodopsin is bounded by TMs 2, 3, 6, and 7 *(100)*.

In contrast to the hET_A receptor, only residues in TM 3 have thus far been observed to play a role in ligand binding to the hET_B receptor. The differential importance of TM 2 and TM 7 residues between ET-receptor subtypes may suggest that the ligand binding site of the hET_B receptor is distinct, but overlapping the binding site within the hET_A receptor. Although possible, this explanation appears unlikely for the binding of highly homologous ligands to receptor subtypes, which maintain 77% overall sequence homology. A more plausible alternative is that the overall structure and topology of the ET receptors are similar, but differ in more subtle details, leading to altered presentation of either conserved or nonconserved residues and consequently impart nonidentical molecular contacts between a ligand and an ET-receptor subtype.

6.4.2. Overlap of Binding Sites for Agonist Peptides and Nonpeptide Antagonists

Substitution of TM 3 residues conserved between ET receptors significantly alters the binding affinities of both agonist peptides and nonpeptide antagonists (Table 4, Fig. 7). These observations suggest that the binding sites for peptide and nonpeptide ligands overlap at least within TM 3 of ET receptors, and is supportive of the use of structure-based, peptidomimetic strategies in the development of the nonpeptide antagonist SB (±) 209670 *(10,101)*.

This apparent overlap of the binding sites for peptide and nonpeptide ligands within the ET receptor *(95,99)* (Table 4, Fig. 7) contrasts with the conclusions from studies of the CCK-B, NK1, and AT1 receptors where the binding sites for peptide and non-peptide ligands appear to be distinct *(93,102–107)* and, at least for NK1, to be expressed on mutually exclusive receptor-conformational states *(108)*. The emerging literature thus suggests that peptide-binding GPCRs do not exhibit a common relationship with respect to peptide and nonpeptide ligand-binding sites, observations that are relevant to the discovery of receptor antagonists.

6.4.3. Implications for a Conserved Binding Region in G Protein-Coupled Receptors

Residues in TM 3 that are conserved between ET-receptor sub-types, Q165/Q181 and K166/K182 in hET_A/hET_B receptors, respectively, are important for peptide and nonpeptide ligand-binding to both receptor subtypes (Fig. 7). For a number of other receptors belonging to the G protein-coupled family, residues corresponding to either Q165/181 or K166/182 in TM 3 of ET receptors have been found to be important for the binding of small molecules, peptides, or proteins to their respective receptors. An aspartate residue, analogous to Q165/181 of hET$_A$ and hET$_B$ and conserved in all bioactive-amine receptors, is important for high affinity binding of agonists and antagonists *(72,89,109–112)*. Replacement of the analogous residue, V108, in the rat angiotensin II receptor (AT1B) with isoleucine reduces the binding affinity of the nonpeptide antagonist Dup 753 by 40 fold, but does not affect the binding affinity of the peptide ligand, saralasin *(93)*. Replacement of the analogous residue in the μ opioid receptor, D147, with alanine or asparagine eliminates binding of peptide and nonpeptide ligands and DAMGO/morphine-induced function; whereas the D147E receptor variant maintains near wild-type binding affinities and DAMGO/morphine-mediated function *(91)*. Tyrosine 106, the residue of thyrotropin releasing hormone (TRH) receptor analogous to K166/182 of hET$_A$/hET*B* receptor, respectively, directly interacts with a carbonyl of the pyroglutamic-acid moiety of TRH *(92)*. Finally, simultaneous replacement of K117 and E118 within the A type (nonpermissive) IL-8 receptor eliminates binding of IL-8, a 72-residue polypeptide *(94)*. Collectively these observations indicate that this region of TM 3 is part of a general binding site conserved between divergent GPCRs *(90,99)*.

7. Future Directions

Drug discovery efforts in recent years have benefited from the availability of cloned, human ET-receptor subtypes. However, the selectivity profile required for a therapeutic agent is still unclear. Human clinical trials for existing compounds may clarify the situation; however, a key component of future molecular-biological efforts will be to clone and express subtypes of the endothelin receptors if the pharmacological evidence with animal tissues supporting their existence is predictive of human pathophysiology.

The endothelin-receptor system was the first for which site-directed mutagenesis studies provided evidence for a commonality of binding sites among peptide agonists and both peptide and nonpeptide antagonists. Subsequently, evidence for other peptide-receptor systems has been presented to support what has hitherto been considered an unlikely paradigm (*vide supra*). These observations are clearly important to the use of peptidomimetic hypotheses for the design of small molecule antagonists of both current and, as yet, unknown GPCRs. Although mutagenesis studies are indirect and subject to interpretation, it is currently the only research avenue that identifies potential ligand-receptor interactions short of a high resolution three-dimensional structure. When such structures exist, mutagenesis studies will continue to play a pivotal role in identification of energetically important interactions over the ligand-receptor surface *(113)*.

References

1. Hickey, K. A., Rubanyi, G., Paul, R. J., and Highsmith, R. F. (1985) Characterization of a coronary vasoconstrictor produced by cultured endothelial cells. *Am. J. Physiol.* **248:**C550–C556.
2. Gillespie, M. N., Owsaoyo, J. O., McMurtry, I. F., and O'Brien, R. F. (1986) Sustained coronary vasoconstriction provoked by a peptidergic substance from endothelial cell culture. *J. Pharm. Exp. Ther.* **236:**339–343.
3. Yanagisawa, M., Kurihara, H., Kimura, S., Tomobe, Y., Kobayashi, M., Mitsui, Y., Yazaki, Y., Goto, K., and Masaki, T. A. (1988) A novel potent vasoconstrictor peptide produced by vascular endothelial cells. *Nature* **332:**411–415.
4. Janes, R. W., Peapus, D. H., and Wallace, B. A. (1994) The crystal structure of human endothelin. *Nature Struct. Biol.* **1:**311–319.
5. Andersen, N. H., Chen, C., Marschner, T. M., Stanley R. Krystek, J., and Bassolino, D. A. (1992) Conformational isomerism of endothelin in acidic aqueous media: a quantitative NOESY analysis. *Biochemistry* **31:**1280–1295.
6. Arai, H., Hori, S., Aramori, I., Ohkubo, H., and Nakanishi, S. (1990) Cloning and expression of a cDNA encoding an endothelin receptor. *Nature* **348:**730–732.
7. Sakurai, T., Yanagisawa, M., Takuwa, Y., Miyazaki, H., Kimura, S., Goto, K., and Masaki, T. (1990) Cloning of a cDNA encoding a non-isopeptide-selective subtype of the endothelin receptor. *Nature* **348:**732–735.
8. Ihara, M., Noguchi, K., Saeki, T., Fururoda, T., Tsuchida, S., Kimura, S., Fukami, T. R., Ishikawa, K., Nishikibe, M., and Yano, M. (1991) Biological profiles of highly potent novel endothelin antagonists selective for the ETA receptor. *Life Sci.* **50:**247–255.
9. Clozel, M., Breu, V., Burri, K., Cassal, J. M., Fischli, W., Hirth, G., Loffler, B. M., Muller, M., Neidhart, W., and Ramuz, H. (1993) Pathophysiological role of endothelin revealed by the first orally active endothelin receptor antagonist. *Nature* **365:**759–761.

10. Elliott, J. D., A. M., L., Cousins, R. D., Gao, A., Leber, J. D., Erhard, K. F., Nambi, P., Elshourbagy, N. Y., Kumar, C., Lee, J. A., Bean, J. W., DeBrosse, C. F., Eggleston, D. S., Brooks, D. P., Feuerstein, G., Ruffolo, R. R., Weinstock, J., Gleason, J. G., Peishoff, C. E., and Ohlstein, E. H. (1994) 1,3-Diarylindane-2-carboxylic acids, potent and selective non-peptide endothelin receptor antagonists. *J. Med. Chem.* **37**:1553–1557.

11. Ohlstein, E. H., Nambi, P., Douglas, S. A., Edwards, R. M., Gellai, M., Lago, A., Leber, J. D., Cousins, R. D., Gao, A., Frazee, J. S., Peishoff, C. E., Bean, J. W., Eggleston, D., Elshourbagy, N., Kumar, C., Lee, J. A., Yue, T.-L., Louden, C., Brooks, D. P., Weinstock, J., Feuerstein, G., Poste, G., R. R. Ruffalo, J., Gleason, J. G., and Elliott, J. D. (1994) SB 209670, A rationally designed potent nonpeptide endothelin receptor antagonist. *Proc. Natl. Acad. Sci. USA* **91**:8052–8056.

12. Roux, S. P. C., M., Sprecher, U., Gray, G., and Clozel, J. P. (1993) Ro 47-0203, A new endothelin receptor antagonist reverses chronic vasospasm in experimental subarachnoid hemorrahage. *Circulation* **88**:I170.

13. Stein, P. D., Hunt, J. T., Floyd, D. M., Moreland, S., Dickinson, K. E. J., Mitchell, C., Liu, E. C.-K., Webb, M. L. M., N., Dickey, J., McMullen, D., Zhang, R., Lee, V. G., Serafino, R., Delaney, C., Schaeffer, T. R., and Kozlowski, M. (1994) The discovery of sulfonamide endothelin antagonists and the development of the orally active ETA antagonist 5-(dimethylamino)-N-(3,4-dimethyl-5-isoxazolyl)-1-naphthalene-sulfonamide. *J. Med. Chem.* **37**:329–331.

14. Baynash, A. G., Hosoda, K., Giaid, A., Richardson, J. A., Emoto, N., Hammer, R. E., and Yanagisawa, M. (1994) Interaction of endothelin-3 with endothelin-B receptor is essential for development of epidermal melanocytes and enteric neurons. *Cell* **79**:1277–1285.

15. Hosoda, K., Hammer, R. E., Richardson, J. A., Baynash, A. G., Cheung, J. C., Giaid, A., and Yanagisawa, M. (1994) Targeted and natural (piebald-lethal) mutations of endothelin-B receptor gene produce megacolon associated with spotted coat color in mice. *Cell* **79**:1267–1276.

16. Kurihara, Y., Kurihara, H., Suzuki, H., Kodama, T., Maemura, K., Nagai, R., Oda, H., Kuwaki, T., Cao, W. H., Kamada, N., et al. (1994) Elevated blood pressure and craniofacial abnormalities in mice deficient in endothelin-1. *Nature* **368**:703–710.

17. Probst, W. C., Snyder, L. A., Schuster, D. I., Brosius, J., and Sealfon, S. C. (1992) Sequence alignment of the G-protein coupled receptor superfamily. *DNA Cell Biol.* **11**, 1–20.

18. Takayanagi, R., Ohnaka, K., Takasaki, C., Ohashi, M., and Nawata, H. (1991) Multiple subtypes of endothelin receptors in porcine tissues: characterization by ligand binding, affinity labeling and regional distribution. *Regul. Peps.* **32**:23–37.

19. Bax, W. A. and Saxena, P. R. (1994) The current endothelin receptor classification: time for reconsideration? *Trends Pharmacol. Sci.* **15**:379–386.

20. Sokolovsky, M. (1992) Structure-function relationships of endothelins, sarafotoxins, and their receptor subtypes. *J. Neurochem.* **59**:809–821.

21. Takai, M., Umemura, I., Yamasaki, K., Watakabe, T., Fujitani, Y., Oda, K., Urade, Y., Inui, T., Yamamura, T., and Okada, T. (1992) A potent and specific agonist, Suc-[Glu9,Ala11,15]-endothelin-1(8–21), IRL 1620, for the ETB receptor. *Biochem. Biophys. Res. Comm.* **184:**953–959.

22. Arai, H., Nakao, K., Takaya, K., Hosoda, K., Ogawa, Y., Nakanishi, S., and Imura, H. (1993) The human endothelin-B receptor gene. Structural organization and chromosomal assignment. *J. Biol. Chem.* **268:**3463–3470.

23. Cheng, H. F., Su, Y. M., Yeh, J. R., and Chang, K. J. (1993) Alternative transcript of the nonselective-type endothelin receptor from rat brain. *Mol. Pharm.* **44:**533–538.

24. Hosoda, K., Nakao, K., Tamura, N., Arai, H., Ogawa, Y., Suga, S., Nakanishi, S., and Imura, H. (1992) Organization, structure, chromosomal assignment, and expression of the gene encoding the human endothelin-A receptor. *J. Biol. Chem.* **267:**18,797–18,804.

25. Mizuno, T., Saito, Y., Itakura, M., Ito, F., Ito, T., Moriyama, N., Hagiwara, H., and Hirose, S. (1992) Structure of the bovine ETB receptor gene. *Biochem. J.* **287:**305–309.

26. Shyamala, V., Moulthrop, T. H. M., Stratton-Thomas, J., and Tekamp-Olson, P. (1994) Two distinct human endothelin b receptors generated by alternate splicing from a single gene. *Cell. Mol. Biol. Res.* **40:**285–296.

27. Breathnach, R. and Chambon, P. (1981) Organization and expression of eukaryotic split genes coding for proteins. *Ann. Rev. Biochem.* **50:**349–383.

28. Maniatis, T., Goodbourn, S., and Fischer, J. A. (1987) Regulation of inducible and tissue-specific gene expression. *Science* **23:**1237–1245.

29. Kadonaga, J. T., Jones, K. A., and Tijan, R. (1986) Promoter-specific activation of RNA polymerase II transcription by Sp1. *Trends Biochem. Sci.* **11:**20–23.

30. Fowlkes, D. M., Mullis, N. T., Comeau, C. M., and Crabtree, G. R. (1984) Potential basis for regulation of the coordinately expressed fibrinogen genes: homology in the 5' flanking regions. *Proc. Natl. Acad. Sci. USA* **81:**2313–2316.

31. Murre, C., McCaw, P. S., Vaessin, H., Caudy, M., Jan, L. Y., Jan, Y. N., Cabrera, C. V., Buskin, J. N., Hauschka, S. D., Lassar, A. B., et al. (1989) Interactions between heterologous helix-loop-helix proteins generate complexes that bind specifically to a common DNA sequence. *Cell* **58:**537–544.

32. Bergsma, D. J., Elshourbagy, N., and Kumar, C. (1995) Molecular biology of endothelin receptors, in *Endothelin Receptors from the Gene to the Human* (Ruffolo, R. R., ed.), CRC, Boca Raton, FL, pp. 37–58.

33. Goto, K. and Warner, T. D. (1995) Endothelin versatility. *Nature* **375:**539–540.

34. Puffenberger, E. G., Hosoda, K., Washington, S. S., Nakao, K., deWit, D., Yanagisawa, M., and Chakravart, A. (1994) A missense mutation of the endothelin-B receptor gene in multigenic Hirschsprung's disease. *Cell* **79:**1257–1266.

35. Hosoda, K., Nakao, K., Hiroshi, A., Suga, S., Ogawa, Y., Mukoyama, M., Shirakami, G., Saito, Y., Nakanishi, S., and Imura, H. (1991) Cloning and expression of human endothelin-1 receptor cDNA. *FEBS Letts.* **287**:23–26.

36. Ogawa, Y., Nakao, K., Arai, H., Nakagawa, O., Hosoda, K., Suga, S., Nakanishi, S., and Imura, H. (1991) Molecular cloning of a non-isopeptide-selective human endothelin receptor. *Biochem. Biophys. Res. Comm.* **178**:248–255.

37. Davenport, A. P., O'Reilly, G., and Kuc, R. E. (1995) Endothelin ETA and ETB mRNA and receptors expressed by smooth muscle in the human vasculature: majority of the ETA sub-type. *Brit. J. Pharmacol.* **114**:1110–1116.

38. Brooks, D. P., DePalma, P. D., Pullen, M., and Nambi, P. (1994) Characterization of canine renal endothelin receptor subtypes and their function. *J. Pharmacol. Exp. Ther.* **268**:1091–1097.

39. Gellai, M., DeWolf, R., Pullen, M., and Nambi, P. (1994) Distribution and functional role of renal ET receptor subtypes in normotensive and hypertensive rats. *Kid. Int.* **46**:1287–1294.

40. Telemaque, S., Gratton, J. P., Claing, A., and D'Orleans-Juste, P. (1993) Endothelin-1 induces vasoconstriction and prostacyclin release via the activation of endothelin ETA receptors in the perfused rabbit kidney. *Eur. J. Pharmacol.* **237**:275–281.

41. Terada, Y., Tomita, K., Nonoguchi, H., and Marumo, F. (1992) Different localization of two types of endothelin receptor mRNA in microdissected rat nephron segments using reverse transcription and polymerase chain reaction assay. *J. Clin. Invest.* **90**:107–112.

42. Kohan, D. E., Hughes, A. K., and Perkins, S. L. (1992) Characterization of endothelin receptors in the inner medullary collecting duct of the rat. *J. Biol. Chem.* **267**:12,336–12,340.

43. Hasegawa, K., Fujiwara, H., Doyama, K., Inada, T., Ohtani, S., Fujiwara, T., Hosoda, K., Nakao, K., and Sasayama, S. (1994) Endothelin-1-selective receptor in the arterial intima of patients with hypertension. *Hypertension* **23**:288–293.

44. Wang, X., Douglas, S. A., and Ohlstein, E. H. (1996) The use of quantitative RT-PCR to demonstrate the increased expression of endothelin-related mRNA's following angioplasty-induced neointima formation in the rat. *Circ. Res.* **78**:322–328.

45. Elshourbagy, N. A., Korman, D. R., Wu, H. L., Sylvester, D. R., Lee, J. A., Nuthalanganti, P., Bergsma, D. J., Kumar, C. S., and Nambi, P. (1993) Molecular characterization and regulation of the human endothelin receptors. *J. Biol. Chem.* **268**:3873.

46. Dashwood, M. R., Allen, S. P., Luu, T. N., and Muddle, J. R. (1994) The effect of the ETA receptor antagonist, FR 139317, on [^{125}I]-ET-1 binding to the atherosclerotic human coronary artery. *Brit. J. Pharmacol.* **112**:386–389.

47. Li, H., Chen, S. J., Chen, Y. F., Meng, Q. C., Durand, J., Oparil, S., and Elton, T. S. (1994) Enhanced endothelin-1 and endothelin receptor gene expression in chronic hypoxia. *J. Appl. Physiol.* **77**:1451–1459.

48. Li, H., Elton, T. S., Chen, Y. F., and Oparil, S. (1994) Increased endothelin receptor gene expression in hypoxic rat lung. *Am. J. Phys.* **266:**553–560.

49. Takeda, M., Iwasaki, S., Hellings, S. E., Yoshida, H., Homma, T. and Kon, V. (1994) Divergent expression of ETA and ETB receptors in response to cyclosporine in mesangial cells. *Am. J. Pathol.* **144:**473.

50. Nakamura, T., Ebihara, I., Fukui, M., Osada, S., Tomino, Y., Masaki, T., Goto, K., Furuichi, Y., and Koide, H. (1995) Modulation of glomerular endothelin and endothelin receptor gene expression in aminonucleoside-induced nephrosis. *J. Am. Soc. Nephrol.* **5:**1585–1590.

51. Nakamura, T., Ebihara, I., Fukui, M., Osada, S., Tomino, Y., Masaki, T., Goto, K., Furuichi, Y., and Koide, H. (1993) Renal expression of mRNAs for endothelin-1, endothelin-3 and endothelin receptors in NZB/ W F1 mice. *Renal Phys. Biochem.* **16:**233–243.

52. Nambi, P., Pullen, M., Wu, H. L., Nuthulaganti, P., Elshourbagy, N., and Kumar, C. (1992) Dexamethasone down-regulates the expression of endothelin receptors in vascular smooth muscle cells. *J. Biol. Chem.* **267:**19,555–19,559.

53. Elshourbagy, N. A., Lee, J. A., Korman, D. R., Nuthalaganti, P., Sylvester, D. R., Dilella, A. G., Sutiphong, J. A., and Kumar, C. S. (1992) Molecular cloning and characterization of the major endothelin receptor subtype in porcine cerebellum. *Mol. Pharm.* **41:**465–473.

54. Lin, H. Y., Kaji, E. H., Winkel, G. K., Ives, H. E., and Lodish, H. F. (1991) Cloning and functional expression of a vascular smooth muscle endothelin 1 receptor. *Proc. Natl. Acad. Sci. USA* **88:**3185–3189.

55. Saito, Y., Mizuno, T., Itakura, M., Suzuki, Y., Ito, T., Hagiwara, H., and Hirose, S. (1991) Primary structure of bovine endothelin ETB receptor and identification of signal peptidase and metal proteinase cleavage sites. *J. Biol. Chem.* **266:**23,433–23,437.

56. Adachi, M., Yang, Y. Y., Furuichi, Y., and Miyamoto, C. (1991) Cloning and characterization of cDNA encoding human A-type endothelin receptor. *Biochem. Biophys. Res. Comm.* **180:**1265–1272.

57. Nakamuta, M., Takayanagi, R., Sakai, Y., Sakamoto, S., Hagiwara, H., Mizuno, T., Saito, Y., Hirose, S., Yamamoto, M., and Nawata, H. (1991) Cloning and sequence analysis of a cDNA encoding human non-selective type of endothelin receptor. *Biochem. Biophys. Res. Comm.* **177:**34–39.

58. Ogawa, Y., Nakao, K., Arai, H., Nakagawa, O., Hosoda, K., Suga, S., Nakanishi, S., and Imura, H. (1991) Molecular cloning of a non-isopeptide-selective human endothelin receptor. *Biochem. Biophys. Res. Comm.* **178:**248–255.

59. Sakamoto, A., Yanagisawa, M., Sakurai, T., Takuwa, Y., Yanagisawa, H., and Masaki, T. (1991) Cloning and functional expression of human cDNA for the ETB endothelin receptor. *Biochem. Biophys. Res. Comm.* **178:**656–663.

60. Kumar, C., Mwangi, V., Nuthulaganti, P., Wu, H. L., Pullen, M., Brun, K., Aiyar, H., Morris, R. A., Naughton, R., and Nambi, P. (1994) Cloning and characterization of a novel endothelin receptor from Xenopus heart. *J. Biol. Chem.* **269:**13,414–13,420.

61. Karne, S., Jayawickreme, C. K., and Lerner, M. R. (1993) Cloning and characterization of an endothelin-3 specific receptor (ETC receptor) from Xenopus laevis dermal melanophores. *J. Biol. Chem.* **268:**19,126–19,133.

62. Dohlman, H. G., Bouvier, M., Benovic, J. L., Caron, M. G., and Lefkowitz, R. J. (1987) The multiple membrane spanning topography of the β2-adrenergic receptor. Localization of the sites of binding, glycosylation, and regulatory phosphorylation by limited proteolysis. *J. Biol. Chem.* **262:**14,282–14,288.

63. Wang, H., Lipfert, L., Malbon, C. C., and Bahouth, S. (1989) Site-directed anti-peptide antibodies define the topography of the beta-adrenergic receptor. *J. Biol. Chem.* **264:**14,424–4,431.

64. O'Dowd, B. F., Hnatowich, M., Regan, J. W., Leader, W. M., Caron, M. G., Lefkowitz, R. J., and Bouvier, M. (1989) Palmitoylation of the human b2-adrenergic receptor. *J. Biol. Chem.* **264:**7564–7569.

65. Ovchinnikov, Y. A., Abdulaev, N. G., and Bogachuk, A. S. (1988) Two adjacent cysteine residues in the C-terminal cytoplasmic fragment of bovine rhodopsin are palmitylated. *FEBS Letts.* **254:**89–93.

66. Haendler, B., Hechler, U., Becker, A., and Schleuning, W. D. (1993) Extracellular cysteine residues 174 and 255 are essential for active expression of human endothelin receptor ETB in Escherichia coli. *J. Cardiovas. Pharmacol.* **22:**54–56.

67. Nambi, P., Kumar, C., and Ohlstein, E. H. (1995) Signal transduction processes involved in endothelin-mediated responses, in *Endothelin Receptors from the Gene to the Human* (Ruffolo, R. R., ed.), CRC, Boca Raton, FL, pp. 59–78.

68. Aramori, I. and Nakanishi, S. (1992) Coupling of two endothelin receptor subtypes to differing signal transduction in transfected Chinese hamster ovary cells. *J. Biol. Chem.* **267:**12,468–12,474.

69. Takagi, Y., Ninomiya, H., Sakamoto, A., Miwa, S., and Masaki, T. (1995) Structural basis of G protein specificity of human endothelin receptors. A study with endothelinA/B chimeras. *J. Biol. Chem.* **270:**10,072–10,078.

70. Hashido, K., Adachi, M., Gamou, T., Wantanabe, T., Furuichi, Y., and Miyamoto, C. (1993) Identification of specific intracellular domains of the human eta receptor required for ligand binding and signal transduction. *Cell. Mol. Biol. Res.* **39,** 3–12.

71. Fraser, C. M., Chung, F. Z., Wang, C. D., and Venter, J. C. (1988) Site-directed mutagenesis of human beta-adrenergic receptors: substitution of aspartic acid-130 by asparagine produces a receptor with high-affinity agonist binding that is uncoupled from adenylate cyclase. *Proc. Natl. Acad. Sci. USA* **85,** 5478–5482.

72. Fraser, C. M., Wang, C. D., Robinson, D. A., Gocayne, J. D., and Venter, J. C. (1989) Site-directed mutagenesis of m1 muscarinic acetylcholine receptors: conserved aspartic acids play important roles in receptor function. *Mol. Pharm.* **36:**840–847.

73. Nussenzveig, D. R., Thaw, C. N., and Gershengorn, M. C. (1994) Inhibition of inositol phosphate second messenger formation by intracellular

loop one of a human calcitonin receptor. Expression and mutational analysis of synthetic receptor genes. *J. Biol. Chem.* **269**:28,123–28,129.

74. Nussenzveig, D. R., Mathew, S., and Gershengorn, M. C. (1995) Alternative splicing of a 48-nucleotide exon generates two isoforms of the human calcitonin receptor. *Endocrinology* **136**:2047–2051.

75. Senogles, S. E. (1994) The D2 dopamine receptor isoforms signal through distinct Gi alpha proteins to inhibit adenylyl cyclase. A study with site-directed mutant Gi alpha proteins. *J. Biol. Chem.* **269**:23,120–23,127.

76. Spengler, D., Waeber, C., Pantaloni, C., Holsboer, F., Bockaert, J., Seeburg, P. H., and Journot, L. (1993) Differential signal transduction by five splice variants of the PACAP receptor. *Nature* **365**:170–175.

77. Vanetti, M., Vogt, G., and Hollt, V. (1993) The two isoforms of the mouse somatostatin receptor (mSSTR2A and mSSTR2B) differ in coupling efficiency to adenylate cyclase and in agonist-induced receptor desensitization. *FEBS Letts.* **331**:260–266.

78. Namba, T., Sugimoto, Y., Negishi, M., Irie, A., Ushikubi, F., Kakizuka, A., Ito, S., Ichikawa, A., and Narumiya, S. (1993) Alternative splicing of C-terminal tail of prostaglandin E receptor subtype EP3 determines G-protein specificity. *Nature* **365**:166–170.

79. Irie, A., Sugimoto, Y., Namba, T., Asano, T., Ichikawa, A., and Negishi, M. (1994) The C-terminus of the prostaglandin-E-receptor EP3 subtype is essential for activation of GTP-binding protein. *Eur. J. Biochem.* **224**:161–166.

80. Pickering, D. S., Thomsen, C., Suzdak, P. D., Fletcher, E. J., Robitaille, R., Salter, M. W., MacDonald, J. F., Huang, X. P., and Hampson, D. R. (1993) A comparison of two alternatively spliced forms of a metabotropic glutamate receptor coupled to phosphoinositide turnover. *J. Neurochem.* **61**:85–92.

81. Ohlstein, E. H., Nambi, P., and Ruffolo, R. R. (1995) Endothelin receptor subclassification, in *Endothelin Receptors from the Gene to the Human* (Ruffolo, R. R., ed.), CRC, Boca Raton, FL, pp. 15–36.

82. Adachi, M., Furuichi, Y., and Miyamoto, C. (1994) Identification of a ligand-binding site of the human endothelin-A receptor and specific regions required for ligand selectivity. *Eur. J. Biochem.* **220**:37–43.

83. Adachi, M., Furuichi, Y., and Miyamoto, C. (1994) Identification of specific regions of the human endothelin-B receptor required for high affinity binding with endothelin-3. *Biochim. Biophys. Acta* **1223**: 202–208.

84. Becker, A., Haendler, B., Hechler, U., and Schleuning, W. D. (1994) Mutational analysis of human endothelin receptors ETA and ETB identification of regions involved in the selectivity for endothelin 3 or cyclo-(D-Trp-D-Asp-Pro-D-Val-Leu). *Eur. J. Biochem.* **221**:951–958.

85. Lee, J. A., Elliott, J. D., Sutiphong, J. A., Friesen, W. J., Ohlstein, E. H., Stadel, J. M., Gleason, J. G., and Peishoff, C. E. (1994) Tyrosine 129 is important to the peptide ligand affinity and selectivity of human endothelin a receptor. *Proc. Natl. Acad. Sci. USA* **91**:7164–7168.

86. Sakamoto, A., Yanagisawa, M., Sawamura, T., Enoki, T., Ohtani, T., Sakurai, T., Nakao, K., Toyo-oka, T., and Masaki, T. (1993) Distinct subdomains of human endothelin receptors determine their selectivity to endothelinA-selective antagonist and endothelinB-selective agonists. *J. Biol. Chem.* **268:**8547–8553.

87. Adachi, M., Yang, Y. Y., Trzeciak, A., Furuichi, Y., and Miyamoto, C. (1992) Identification of a domain of ETA receptor required for ligand binding. *FEBS Letts.* **311:**179–183.

88. Hashido, K., Gamou, T., Adachi, M., Tabuchi, H., Watanabe, T., Furuichi, Y., and Miyamoto, C. (1992) Truncation of N-terminal extracellular or C-terminal intracellular domains of human ETA receptor abrogated the binding activity to ET-1. *Biochem. Biophys. Res. Comm.* **187:**1241–1248.

89. Strader, C. D., Sigal, I. S., Register, R. B., Candelore, M. R., Rands, E., and Dixon, R. A. (1987) Identification of residues required for ligand binding to the beta-adrenergic receptor. *Proc. Natl. Acad. Sci. USA* **84:**4384–4388.

90. Schwartz, T. W. (1994) Locating ligand-binding sites in 7TM receptors by protein engineering. *Curr. Opin. Biotech.* **5:**434–444.

91. Surratt, C. K., Johnson, P. S., Moriwaki, A., Seidleck, B. K., Blaschak, C. J., Wang, J. B., and Uhl, G. R. (1994) Mu opiate receptor. Charged transmembrane domain amino acids are critical for agonist recognition and intrinsic activity. *J. Biol. Chem.* **269:**20,548–20,553.

92. Perlman, J. H., Thaw, C. N., Laakkonen, L., Bowers, C. Y., Osman, R., and Gershengorn, M. C. (1994) Hydrogen bonding interaction of thyrotropin-releasing hormone (TRH) with transmembrane tyrosine 106 of the TRH receptor. *J. Biol. Chem.* **269:**1610–1613.

93. Ji, H., Leung, M., Zhang, Y., Catt, K. J., and Sandberg, K. (1994) Differential structural requirements for specific binding of nonpeptide and peptide antagonists to the AT1 angiotensin receptor. *J. Biol. Chem.* **268:**16,533–16,536.

94. Hebert, C. A., Chuntharapai, A., Smith, M., Colby, T., Kim, J., and Horuk, R. (1993) Partial functional mapping of the human interleukin-8 type A receptor. Identification of a major ligand binding domain. *J. Biol. Chem.* **268:**18,549–18,553.

95. Krystek, S. R., Jr., Patel, P. S., Rose, P. M., Fisher, S. M., Kienzle, B. K., Lach, D. A., Liu, E. C., Lynch, J. S., Novotny, J., and Webb, M. L. (1994) Mutation of peptide binding site in transmembrane region of a G protein-coupled receptor accounts for endothelin receptor subtype selectivity. *J. Biol. Chem.* **269,** 12,383–12,386.

96. Henderson, R., Baldwin, J. M., Ceska, T. A., Zemlin, F., Beckmann, E., and Downing, K. H. (1990) Model for the structure of bacteriorhodopsin based on high-resolution electron cryo-microscopy. *J. Mol. Biol.* **213:**899–929.

97. Zhu, G., Wu, L. H., Mauzy, C., Egloff, A. M., Mirzadegan, T., and Chung, F. Z. (1992) Replacement of lysine-181 by aspartic acid in the third transmembrane region of endothelin type B receptor reduces its affinity to

endothelin peptides and sarafotoxin 6c without affecting G protein coupling. *J. Cell Biochem.* **50:**159–164.

98. Mauzy, C., Wu, L. H., Egloff, A. M., Mirzadegan, T., and Chung, F. Z. (1992) Substitution of lysine-181 to aspartic acid in the third transmembrane region of the endothelin (ET) type B receptor selectively reduces its high-affinity binding with ET-3 peptide. *J. Cardiovas. Pharmacol.* **12:**S5–S7.

99. Lee, J. A., Brinkmann, J. A., Longton, E. D., Peishoff, C. E., Lago, M. A., Leber, J. D., Cousins, R. D., Gao, A., Stadel, J. M., Kumar, C. S., Ohlstein, E. H., Gleason, J. G., and Elliott, J. D. (1994) Lysine 182 of endothelin b receptor modulates agonist selectivity and antagonist affinity: evidence for the overlap of peptide and non-peptide ligand binding sites. *Biochemistry* **33:**14,543–14,549.

100. Han, M. and Smith, S. O. (1995) NMR Constraints on the location of the retinal chromophore in rhodopsin and bathorhodopsin. *Biochemistry* **34:**1425–1432.

101. Elliott, J. D., Lago, M. A., and Peishoff, C. E. (1995) Endothelin receptor anatgonist, in *Endothelin Receptors from the Gene to the Human* (Ruffolo, R. R., ed.), CRC, Boca Raton, FL, pp. 79–107.

102. Gether, U., Johansen, T. E., Snider, R. M., Lowe, J. A. D., Nakanishi, S., and Schwartz, T. W. (1993) Different binding epitopes on the NK1 receptor for substance P and non-peptide antagonist. *Nature* **362:**345–348.

103. Gether, U., Yokota, Y., Emonds, A. X., Breliere, J. C., Lowe, J. A. d., Snider, R. M., Nakanishi, S., and Schwartz, T. W. (1993) Two nonpeptide tachykinin antagonists act through epitopes on corresponding segments of the NK1 and NK2 receptors. *Proc. Natl. Acad. Sci. USA* **90:**6194–6198.

104. Fong, T. M., Cascieri, M. A., Yu, H., Bansal, A., Swain, C., and Strader, C. D. (1993) Amino-aromatic interaction between histidine 197 of the neurokinin-1 receptor and CP 96345. *Nature* **362:**350–353.

105. Beinborn, M., Lee, Y. M., McBride, E. W., Quinn, S. M., and Kopin, A. S. (1993) A single amino acid of the cholecystokinin-B/gastrin receptor determines specificity for non-peptide antagonists. *Nature* **362:**348–350.

106. Huang, R. R. C., Yu, H., Strader, C. D., and Fong, T. M. (1994) Interaction of substance P with the second and seventh transmembrane domains of the neurokinin-1 receptor. *Biochemistry* **33:**3007–3013.

107. Schambye, H. T., Hjorth, S. A., Bergsma, D. J., Sathe, G., and Schwartz, T. W. (1994) Differentiation between binding sites for angiotensin II and nonpeptide antagonists on the angiotensin II type 1 receptors. *Proc. Natl. Acad. Sci. USA* **91:**7046–7050.

108. Rosenkilde, M. M., Cahir, M., Gether, U., Hjorth, S. A., and Schwartz, T. W. (1994) Mutations along transmembrane segment II of the NK-1 receptor affect substance P competition with non-peptide antagonists but not substance P binding. *J. Biol. Chem.* **269:**28,160–28,164.

109. Strader, C. D., Sigal, I. S., Candelore, M. R., Rands, E., Hill, W. S., and Dixon, R. A. (1988) Conserved aspartic acid residues 79 and 113 of the b-adrenergic receptor have different roles in receptor function. *J. Biol. Chem.* **263:**10,267–10,271.

110. Wang, C. D., Buck, M. A., and Fraser, C. M. (1991) Site-directed mutagenesis of alpha 2A-adrenergic receptors: identification of amino acids involved in ligand binding and receptor activation by agonists. *Mol. Pharm.* **40:**168–179.

111. Wang, C. D., Gallaher, T. K., and Shih, J. C. (1993) Site-directed mutagenesis of the serotonin 5-hydroxytrypamine2 receptor: identification of amino acids necessary for ligand binding and receptor activation. *Mol. Pharm.* **43:**931–940.

112. Ho, B. Y., Karschin, A., Branchek, T., Davidson, N., and Lester, H. A. (1992) The role of conserved aspartate and serine residues in ligand binding and in function of the 5-HT1A receptor: a site-directed mutation study. *FEBS Letts.* **312:**259–262.

113. Clackson, T. and Wells, J. A. (1995) A hot spot of binding energy in a hormone-receptor interface. *Science* **267:**383–386.

114. Devereux, J., Haeberli, P., and Smithies, O. (1984) A comprehensive set of sequence analysis programs for the VAX. *Nucleic Acids Res.* **12:**387–395.

Chapter 3

Molecular Biology of Endothelin-Converting Enzyme (ECE)

Ryoichi Takayanagi, Keizo Ohnaka, Wei Liu, Takeshi Ito, and Hajime Nawata

1. Introduction

Endothelin (ET) was originally isolated from culture media of aortic endothelial cells as a potent vasoconstrictive peptide *(1)*. An active form of ET, consisting of 21 amino-acid residues, is generated from an inactive form of big ET-1 by a specific enzyme, called endothelin-converting enzyme (ECE). Accelerated production of ET-1 in damaged vascular endothelial cells was strongly suggested to be involved in the development of various fatal cardiovascular disorders, such as acute myocardial infarction, acute renal failure, and posthemorrhagic cerebral vasospasm. The design of specific inhibitors of ECE, along with those of ET receptors, may lead to the development of new treatments for these diseases. Accordingly, many investigators have focused on the identification and characterization of ECE. This chapter describes a history from the discovery of ECE to molecular characterization of this enzyme.

From: *Endothelin: Molecular Biology, Physiology, and Pathology*
Edited by R. F. Highsmith © Humana Press Inc., Totowa, NJ

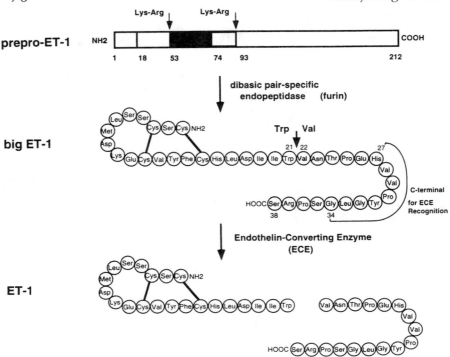

Fig. 1. Biosynthetic pathway of human ET-1. Trp[21] at P1 position and the sequence from His[27] to Gly[34] are important for recognition by ECE. The residue at P1' position needs to be hydrophobic.

2. Biosynthetic Pathway of Endothelin

2.1. Processing of Big ET Isopeptides

Following analysis of the amino-acid structure deduced from the cDNA encoding prepro-endothelin-1 *(1)*, a biosynthetic pathway for endothelin-1 was proposed as shown in Fig. 1. An intermediate form, termed big endothelin-1 (big ET-1) consisting of 38 amino-acid residues in the human, is initially produced from proendothelin-1 by a dibasic pair-specific endopeptidase. Big ET-1 is then converted to the mature peptide through an unusual proteolytic cleavage between Trp[21] and Val[22] by a proposed ECE. The vasoconstrictive potency of big ET-1 is almost negligible *(2)*, indicating that conversion to ET-1 is essential for this intermediate form to have an effect in vivo. The other two ET isoforms, named ET-2 and

ET-3, are also thought to be processed from the corresponding big ET isopeptides, big ET-2 and big ET-3 *(3)*.

2.2. Processing of Pro-ET-1

The processing of pro-ET-1 to yield big ET-1 has been reported to involve furin, one of the mammalian subtilisin-like proprotein convertases *(4)*. When pro-ET-1 was incubated with furin, only big ET-1 was produced despite the presence of multiple furin-cleavage signals in pro-ET-1. Moreover, a specific inhibitor of furin, decanoyl-Arg-Val-Lys-Arg chloromethylketone, abolished production of ET-1 in cultured endothelial cells.

3. Identification of Physiologically Relevant ECE

3.1. Aspartic Protease

In 1990, several groups found that a pepstatin A-sensitive aspartic protease displayed apparent ECE activity *(5,6)*. Furthermore, the aspartic protease type of ECE activity was extensively purified from bovine adrenal chromaffin granules and proven to be cathepsin D *(7)*. However, because cathepsin D is only active at an acidic pH and has been shown to cleave the Asn^{18}-Ile^{19} bond of big ET-1 in addition to the Trp^{21}-Val^{22} bond, questions arose regarding the actual role of an aspartic protease in ET-1 biosynthesis.

3.2. Neutral Metalloprotease

Ohnaka et al. first reported the presence of an apparent ECE activity with pH optimum at pH 7.0, in addition to that at pH 3.0, in the homogenate of cultured bovine aortic endothelial cells *(8)*. The activity at pH 3.0 was completely inhibited by pepstatin A, whereas the activity at pH 7.0 was not affected by various type-specific protease inhibitors except for the inhibitors of metalloprotease, such as metal-chelating agents and phosphoramidon. Intriguingly, thiorphan, an alternative metalloprotease inhibitor, did not inhibit the neutral ECE activity *(9,10)*. Phosphoramidon (but not thiorphan) inhibited dose-dependently the release of ET-1 by blocking the conversion of endogenous big ET-1 to ET-1 in intact cultured endothelial cells (Fig. 2) *(10,11)*. In addition, pepstatin A entered cultured endothelial cells at a sufficient concentration to inhibit an aspartic protease, but it did not affect ET-1 release from endothelial cells *(12)*. Similarly,

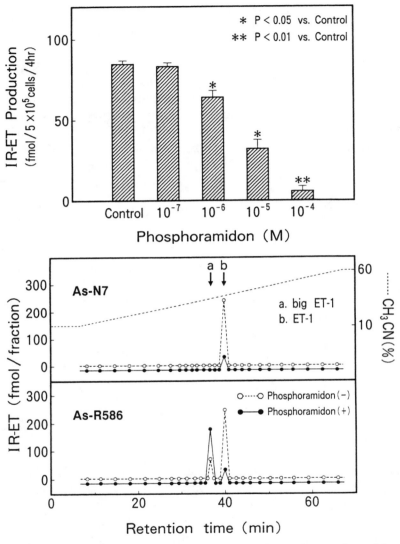

Fig. 2. Effect of phosphoramidon on ET-1 release from cultured bovine aortic endothelial cells **(top)** and analyses of culture media by reverse phase HPLC **(bottom)**. The culture media (1.5 mL) incubated for 4 h with the endothelial cells in the presence and absence of 10^{-4} *M* phosphoramidon were applied to an ODS-120T column (Tosoh), and the eluates were subjected to radioimmunoassay *(8)*. Antisera of As-N7 crossreact with ET-1 but not big ET-1, and antisera of As-R586 crossreact with both big ET-1 and ET-1.

E-64 and leupeptin did not inhibit ET-1 release. Regarding in vivo studies, iv injection of big ET-1 has been shown to exert a potent pressor effect in rats accompanied by elevation of the level of circulating ET-1 *(13)*. The pressor effect was abolished by phosphoramidon but not by thiorphan, kelatorphan, E-64, or leupeptin *(14,15)*. The pressor effect of ET-1 itself is not inhibited by phosphoramidon. These investigations strongly suggest that a phosphoramidon-sensitive, neutral metalloprotease is the most probable candidate for the physiological ECE.

4. Purification and Characterization of ECE

To purify ECE, Ohnaka et al. prepared the membrane fractions from porcine aortic intima, because phosphoramidon-sensitive ECE activity is located almost entirely in this fraction of endothelial cells *(10)*. The ECE was solubilized with Lubrol PX from the membrane fraction and was purified by sequential chromatography on DEAE-agarose, *Ricinus communis* agglutinin 120-agarose, peanut agglutinin-agarose, Mono Q, and TSKG-3000SWXL columns *(16)*. The membrane-bound form of ECE has a high affinity for *R. communis* agglutinin *(17)*, which provided a key to its purification. An approx 12,000-fold purification of the membrane fraction enzyme was achieved. The purified enzyme had a very narrow neutral pH optimum (pH 6.8–7.2) and was inhibited by EDTA, 1,10-phenanthroline, and phosphoramidon (IC_{50} = 0.8 μM) but not by thiorphan or other type-specific protease inhibitors. Addition of Zn^{2+} completely reversed the inactivation of ECE by EDTA, suggesting that this enzyme may be a zinc-containing metalloprotease. The purified enzyme showed the highest affinity for big ET-1 among big ET isopeptides, and the K_m for big ET-1 was 3.3 ± 0.3 μM. The purified ECE showed an isoelectric point (pI) of 4.1. Using this finding of an acidic pI, a simple isoelectric focusing method for obtaining ECE from cultured human endothelial cells was developed *(18)*. The molecular mass was estimated to be 120 kDa by sodium dedecylsulfate-polyacrylamide gel electrophoresis (SDS-PAGE) under reducing conditions *(16)*. Crosslinking experiments further revealed that a physiological form of ECE is a dimer *(19)*, the subunits of which are linked by one disulfide bond *(20)*. A monomer itself can catalyze the ECE activity, but it is approximately one-fifth of that achieved by a dimer *(20)*.

Table 1
Hydrolysis Rates of Big ET Analogs by Purified Porcine Aortic ECE

Substrate	Amino Acid Sequence	Specific Activity (%)
	10 20 30	
big ET-1 (1-38)	CSCSSLMDKECVYFCHLDIIWVNTPEHVVPYGLGSPRS	100
big ET-1 (1-31)	CSCSSLMDKECVYFCHLDIIWVNTPEHVVPY	0
big ET-1 (17-26)	LDIIWVNTPE	0
big ET-1 (16-37)	HLDIIWVNTPEHVVPYGLGSPR	273
big ET-1 (18-34)	DIIWVNTPEHVVPYGLG	246 (100)
[Ala20] big ET-1 (18-34)	DI**A**WVNTPEHVVPYGLG	326 (132)
[Ala21] big ET-1 (18-34)	DII**A**VNTPEHVVPYGLG	21 (9)
[Phe21] big ET-1 (18-34)	DII**F**VNTPEHVVPYGLG	42 (17)
[Ala22] big ET-1 (18-34)	DIIW**A**NTPEHVVPYGLG	22 (9)
[Phe22] big ET-1 (18-34)	DIIW**F**NTPEHVVPYGLG	1185 (482)
[big ET-2 (18-34)]	DIIWVNTPE**QTA**PYGLG	39 (16)
[Ala31] big ET-1 (18-34)	DIIWVNTPEHVVP**A**GLG	11 (4)

The purified ECE (20 ng) and each of the big ET analogs (10 μM) were incubated at pH 7.0 for 1 h at 37°C, and the products were analyzed on an ODS column (16). Boxed residues are distinct from corresponding residues in big ET-1.

5. Big Endothelin Structure Essential for Specific Processing by ECE and That for Inhibition of ECE

5.1. Substrate Specificity

The structure-substrate specificity in big ET-1 was amenable to investigation using the purified ECE (Table 1), because the use of the purified enzyme can exclude nonspecific processing of big ET-1 by other proteases (16). The amino-terminal cyclic structure of big ET-1 appears to interfere with access of the converting enzyme to big ET-1 (21), because the deletion of the disulfide-loop structure (big ET-1[16–37]) enhanced the hydrolysis rate more than two times. Deletion of the sequence of Gly^{32} to Ser^{38} (big ET-1[1–31]) from big ET-1[1–38] completely abolished the substrate activity, but not deletion of the sequence of Ser^{35} to Arg^{37} (big ET-1[18–34]) from big ET-1[16–37]. The replacement of His^{27}-Val^{28}-Val^{29} with Gln-Thr-Ala ([Gln^{27}, Thr^{28}, Ala^{29}] big ET-1[18–34], namely, big ET-2[18–34]) and Tyr^{31} with Ala ([Ala^{31}] big ET-1[18–34]) relative to big ET-1[18–34] markedly reduced the hydrolysis rates. These results suggest that the carboxyl-terminal sequence of His[27] to Gly[34] is important for recognition by the converting enzyme, and also that a low rate of cleavage of big ET-2 compared with that of big ET-1 is mainly owing to the presence of the sequence of Gln[27]-Thr[28]-Ala[29] in the carboxyl terminus. Replacement of Ile[20] by Ala in big ET-1[18–34] slightly increased the hydrolysis rate, whereas replacement of Trp[21] by Ala[21] or another aromatic amino acid of Phe[21] caused a large decrease in the hydrolysis rate, suggesting that the presence of Trp at P1 position is important but Ile at P2 is not essential. Replacement of Val[22] by Ala decreased the hydrolysis rate, whereas the substitution to Phe[22] greatly increased the cleaving rate, which was about 12 times as much as that of big ET-1[1–38]. Therefore, hydrophobic amino acids may be necessary at the P1' position. These results are summarized in Fig. 1. The fact that ECE recognizes a relatively long carboxyl-terminal amino acid sequence in addition to the processing site is unique, in contrast to neutral endopeptidase (NEP) 24.11, which only recognizes hydrophobic amino acid residues at the processing site.

5.2. Inhibition of ECE Activity by [Phe[21]] Big ET-1[18–34]

Among various big ET analogs listed in Table 1, [Phe[21]] big ET-1[18–34] showed a significant inhibition of big ET-1 cleavage, and the hydrolysis rate of big ET-1[1–38] was suppressed to about 15% of the original rate in the presence of [Phe[21]] big ET-1[18–34] at 100 μM (Fig. 3A). Analyses by Lineweaver-Burk plots as a function of the big ET-1 concentration revealed [Phe[21]] big ET-1[18–34] as a typical competitive inhibitor (K_i = 15.8 μM) (Fig. 3B), also suggesting that ECE recognizes the amino acid residue at the P1 position of big ET-1. Although [d-Val[22]] big ET-1[16–38] has been reported to depress the cellular conversion of big ET-1 to ET-1 *(22)*, the authors could not observe the inhibitory effect of this big ET-1 analog using either the purified ECE (Fig. 3A) or ECE cDNA-transfected cells.

6. Molecular Characterization of the ECE Gene

6.1. Cloning and Functional Characterization of ECE cDNA

ECE was also purified from rat lung *(23)* and bovine adrenal tissues *(24)* during its isolation from porcine aortic intima *(16)*, and ECE cDNAs were then cloned based on the partial amino-acid

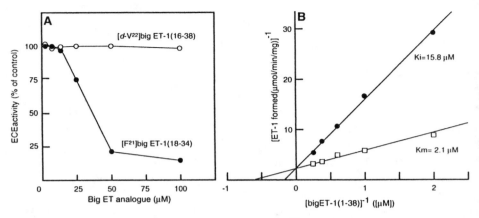

Fig. 3. Inhibition of ECE activity by [Phe²¹] big ET-1(18–34) **(A)** and Lineweaver-Burk plots of big ET-1 hydrolysis rates as a function of the big ET-1 concentration in the presence (●) and absence (○) of [Phe²¹] big ET-1(18–34) **(B)**. (A) Human big ET-1(1–38) (0.5 µM) was incubated with the purified porcine ECE at pH 7.0 for 1 h at 37°C in the absence and presence of [Phe²¹] big ET-1(18–34) (●) or [d-Val²²] big ET-1(16–38) (○) at the concentrations indicated. The ECE activities are expressed as percentages of that of control. (B) human big ET-1(1–38) at various concentrations was incubated with the purified ECE at pH 7.0 at 37°C for 10–120 min in the presence (●) and absence (□) of 50 µM [Phe²¹] big ET-1(18–34). The amounts ET-1 formed were assayed by a specific radioimmunoassay *(8)*.

sequences *(24,25)*. Because the amino acid sequence deduced from the bovine ECE cDNA contained partial sequences that we obtained from the purified porcine aortic ECE, we prepared a cDNA probe from human adrenal total RNA by reverse transcription-polymerase chain reaction (RT-PCR), setting primers based on a cDNA structure of the bovine adrenal ECE (Fig. 4). Two types of clones (α and

---

Fig. 4. *(opposite page)* Nucleotide and deduced amino-acid sequence of human ECE-1β cDNA cloned in pHECE1B. The cDNA insert of cloned pHECE1B consists of 2793 bp nucleotides. The deduced amino acid sequence (single-letter code) is shown below the cDNA sequence. The putative transmembrane domain is doubly underlined. The putative zinc-binding and catalytic domain is boxed. The potential *N*-glycosylation sites are underlined. The sense and antisense PCR primers, which were set based on the bovine ECE cDNA to prepare a screening probe, are marked with overbar (sense) and underbars (antisense).

```
                                                      AAACAAGCCTCGTCGGGGCCGAGC
                                            CACCCCTGAGACAGGAGGCAGCCCTG          -121
                                                                                  -1

M  P  L  Q  G  L  L  G  L  Q  R  N  P  F  L  Q  G  K  R  G  P  G  L  T  S        120
S  P  L  L  P  P  S  L  Q  V  N  F  H  S  P                                       40

R  S  G  Q  R  C  W  A  A  A  R  T  Q  V  E  K  R  L  V  V  L  L  A  A  G  L       240
V  A  C  L  L  A  A  L  G  I  Q  Y  Q                                              80

T  R  S  P  S  V  C  L  S  E  A  C  V  S  V  T  S  S  I  L  S  S  M  D  P  T       360
V  D  P  C  H  D  F  F  S  Y  A  C  G  G                                          120

W  I  K  A  N  P  V  P  D  G  H  S  R  W  G  T  F  S  N  L  W  E  H  N  Q  A       480
I  I  K  H  L  L  E  N  S  T  A  S  V  S                                          160

E  A  E  R  K  A  Q  V  Y  Y  R  A  C  M  N  E  T  R  I  E  E  L  R  A  K  P       600
L  M  E  L  I  E  R  L  G  G  W  N  I  T                                          200

G  P  W  A  K  D  N  F  Q  D  T  L  Q  V  V  T  A  H  Y  R  T  S  P  F  F  S       720
V  Y  V  S  A  D  S  K  K  N  S  N  S  N  V                                       240

I  Q  V  D  Q  S  G  L  G  L  P  S  R  D  Y  Y  L  N  K  T  E  N  E  K  V  L       840
T  G  Y  L  N  Y  M  V  Q  L  G  K  L  L                                          280

G  G  G  D  E  E  A  I  R  P  Q  M  Q  Q  I  L  D  F  E  T  A  L  A  N  I  T       960
I  P  Q  E  K  R  R  D  E  E  L  I  Y  H                                          320

K  V  T  A  A  E  L  Q  T  L  A  P  A  I  N  W  L  P  F  L  N  T  I  F  Y  P      1080
V  E  I  N  E  S  E  P  I  V  V  Y  D  K                                          360

E  Y  L  E  Q  I  S  T  L  I  N  T  T  D  R  C  L  L  N  N  Y  M  I  W  N  L      1200
V  R  K  T  S  S  F  L  D  Q  R  F  Q  D                                          400

A  D  E  K  F  M  E  V  M  Y  G  T  K  K  T  C  L  P  R  W  K  F  C  V  S  D      1320
T  E  N  N  L  G  F  A  L  G  P  M  F  V                                          440

K  A  T  F  A  E  D  S  K  S  I  A  T  E  I  L  E  I  K  K  A  F  E  E  S  L      1440
S  T  L  K  W  M  D  E  E  T  R  K  S                                             480

N  A  M  R  F  F  N  F  S  W  R  V  T  A  D  Q  L  R  K  A  P  N  R  D  Q  W      1560
S  M  T  P  P  M  V  N  A  Y  Y  S  P  T                                          520

F  D  D  Q  G  R  E  Y  D  K  D  G  N  L  R  P  W  W  K  N  S  S  V  E  A  F      1680
K  R  Q  T  E  C  M  V  E  Q  Y  S  N  Y                                          560

K  N  E  I  V  F  P  A  G  I  L  Q  A  P  F  Y  T  R  S  S  P  K  A  L  N  F      1800
G  G  I  G  V  V  V  G  H  E  L  T  H  A                                          600

S  V  N  G  E  P  V  N  G  R  H  T  L  G  E  N  I  A  D  N  G  G  L  K  A  A      1920
Y  R  A  Y  Q  N  W  V  K  K  N  G  A  E                                          640

H  S  L  P  T  L  G  L  T  N  N  Q  L  F  F  L  G  F  A  Q  V  W  C  S  V  R      2040
T  P  E  S  S  H  E  G  L  I  T  D  P  H                                          680

S  P  S  R  F  R  V  I  G  S  L  S  N  S  K  E  F  S  E  H  F  R  C  P  P  G      2160
S  P  M  N  P  P  H  K  C  E  V  W                                                720

                                                                                 2280
                                                                                  758

                                                                                 2400
                                                                                 2520
                                                                                 2640
                                                                                 2650
                                                                       GGAATACACT
```

83

β isoforms, mentioned in Section 6.2.) were obtained after screening of a cDNA library prepared from human umbilical vein endothelial cells. One of the two types of clones encodes 758 amino-acid residues (β isoform), which was 95 and 92% identical to those of bovine and rat ECE, respectively (Fig. 4). The membrane fractions were prepared from CHO-K1 cells transfected with expression plasmids containing the human ECE cDNA, and solubilized. These extracts displayed the big ET-1-converting activity (0.21 ± 0.01 nmol of ET-1 formed/mg protein/h, mean ± SD, n = 3), whereas those prepared from cells transfected with mock plasmids did not (<1 pmol/mg/h). The sensitivities to various protease inhibitors and the pH optimum of the ECE activity were consistent with those observed in the purified enzyme. The predicted molecular weight of the human ECE protein was 85,832. The difference between this value and the apparent molecular weight (120 kDa) of the purified ECE on SDS-PAGE appears to be owing to sugar-side chains, because the predicted ECE sequence has 10 possible consensus sequences for N-linked glycosylation sites. The deduced ECE protein structure has no apparent N-terminal signal sequence. Hydropathy analysis showed that ECE contains a single putative transmembrane domain of 21 amino acids (amino acids 57–77) near the N-terminal region. A consensus sequence of a zinc-binding motif, His-Glu-X-X-His (in which X represents a hydrophobic amino-acid residue), which is common to catalytic sites of metalloproteases, is found at amino acids 595–599 of the human ECE. A significant similarity was detected among the sequences of ECE, NEP, and the human Kell blood-group protein, a putative neutral endopeptidase *(24,25)*. These results suggest a single family of enzymes and that ECE may have cellular topology similar to that of NEP and the Kell blood group protein, which span the membrane once and contain the large C-terminal catalytic domain possibly facing outside the plasma membrane or inside the Golgi apparatus and secretory vesicles (Fig. 5). Furthermore, it has been shown that the introduction of mutations into a zinc-binding motif in ECE results in complete loss of activity *(20)*. Several amino acid residues other than the catalytic site, known to be essential for substrate-binding of NEP, are also conserved in ECE. However, mutagenesis in these residues did not affect ECE activity *(20)*. These observations along with the substrate specificity (Table 1) indicate that ECE recognizes big ET-1 in a manner far different from that of NEP.

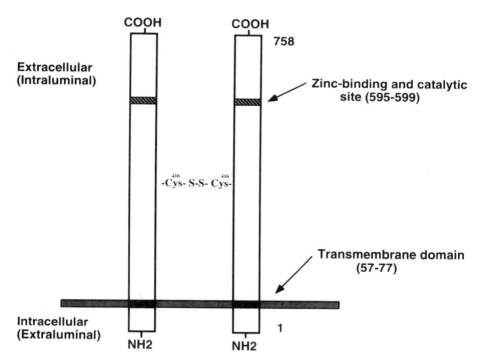

Fig. 5. Predicted structure of a native form of human ECE-1β. The dimeric structure is formed by one disulfide bond probably via Cys[416] [Cys[412] in rat *(20)*], and the C-terminal catalytic domain is facing outside the plasma membrane or intraluminal side.

6.2. Genomic Organization of the ECE Gene

The ECE cDNAs have been cloned from libraries prepared from various species and tissues *(24–29)*. They are now called ECE-1 and classified into two isoforms *(30)*, ECE-1α and ECE-1β (Fig. 6), which differ only in their N-terminal regions through alternative splicing of one ECE-1 gene *(31)*. Although their enzymatic properties are identical, their tissue distributions are different. The human ECE-1 gene is composed of 19 exons that span more than 68 kB and is located on the 1p36 band of the human genome *(31)*. The promoter region of ECE-1α has features characteristic of a housekeeping gene, whereas the promoter region of ECE-1β contains a CAAT box and potential binding sites for various transcription factors, such as the glucocorticoid receptor. These results suggest the constitutive expression of ECE-1α and the regulatory expression of ECE-1β.

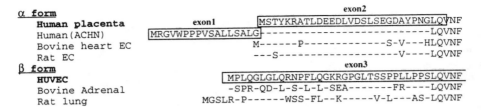

Fig. 6. Comparison between the N-terminal structures of ECE-1α and ECE-1β. Deduced N-terminal sequences reported (24–30) are compared. Amino-acids identical to those of human ECE are indicated by a dash. The human ECE-1 sequences are boxed based on their origins of exons of ECE-1 gene *(31)*.

7. ECE-1 Gene-Knockout Mice

Following the cloning of ECE-1 cDNAs, another metallo-protease called ECE-2 was cloned *(32)*. Structurally ECE-2 belongs to a NEP-ECE-Kell family, and the enzymatic properties are identical to those of ECE-1 except for an acidic pH optimum at pH 5.5. Although prior observations strongly suggested that ECE-1 is a physiological ECE functioning in vivo, there still remained the possibility that ECE-2 or another unidentified enzyme might play a functional role. This question was finally answered by the targeted disruption of the mouse ECE-1 gene *(33)*. ECE-1-knockout mice expressed the same phenotype as that manifested by ET-1 gene-knockout mice, which is a fatal craniofacial malformation owing to a failure of the normal development of the first branchial arch-derived connective tissue *(34)*. ECE-2 gene-knockout mice, however, did not manifest such a phenotype. Furthermore, the ECE-1-knockout mice presented the phenotype observed in ET-3 gene-knockout mice, a defect of myenteric ganglion neurons and melanin pigment in the choroidal layer of the retina *(35)*. These observations indicate that big ET-3 is also converted to ET-3 in vivo by ECE-1 and suggest that ECE-1 may be responsible for the conversion of all big ET isopeptides. Although ECE-1 is indispensable for the synthesis of ET isopeptides during growth and differentiation, it has been reported that hemorrhage- and hypoxia-induced ET-1 release in vivo is not inhibited by phosphoramidon *(36)*. Thus, further studies may be necessary to elucidate the role of ECE-1 in pathological conditions.

8. Cellular Localization of ECE-1

ECE-1 mRNAs are present in a variety of tissues, with high expression in vascular endothelial cells, ovary, testis, and adrenal gland *(19,24–26,31)*. The location where processing of big ET-1 occurs has been controversial. Harrison et al. *(37)* suggested the intracellular vesicle for the site for conversion, because it was shown by immunofluorescence that big ET-1 and ET-1 were localized within intracellular vesicles. Using similar methods, Takahashi et al. *(19)* showed that ECE was clustered along the plasma membrane in ECE-1-transfected COS cells and that the COS cells rapidly and efficiently cleaved big ET-1 added to the culture media, suggesting the plasma membrane for the conversion site. We also previously showed that intact cultured endothelial cells can convert exogenously added big ET-1 to ET-1, and that this conversion process is specifically inhibited by phosphoramidon *(38)*. Xu et al. *(24)* reported that when WS79089B (FR901533), a recently isolated inhibitor of ECE-1 *(39)*, was added to the culture media of ECE-1-transfected CHO cells, it prevented the conversion of added big ET-1 but not the secretion of ET-1 from the cells, suggesting that endogenous big ET-1 is converted intracellularly. It is thought that phosphoramidon enters the cells but not WS79089B.

The jellyfish *Aequorea* green fluorescent protein (GFP) has been recently applied as a visible signal in living cells *(40)*. We have constructed an expression vector encoding GFP fused to the N-terminus of human ECE-1α, and transfected to COS-7 cells (Fig. 7). The transfection of a vector encoding GFP alone resulted in a diffuse distribution of GFP-derived fluorescence in the cell, including the nucleus (Fig. 7A). GFP fused to intact ECE-1α was distributed in the whole membrane structures, including the plasma membrane (Fig. 7B), whereas GFP fused to the ECE-1α lacking a putative transmembrane domain was distributed in the cytosol and near the nucleus where the Golgi complex is often located. These observations indicate that ECE-1 is localized at both the plasma and intracellular membranes, and that a predicted transmembrane domain functions for the localization of ECE-1 to the membranes. Thus, ECE- 1 may process big ET peptides at both the plasma membrane and inside of the cell. Moreover, translocation of the GFP-fused ECE-1, which can properly catalyze the big ET-conversion, occurs from the plasma membrane to the inside of a cell. This finding is supported by our unpublished data as well as studies of Barnes et al. *(41)*,who used immunostaining of fixed cells.

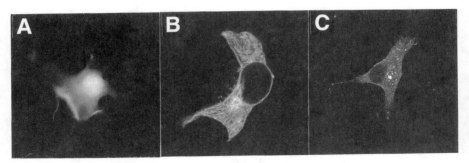

Fig. 7. Intracellular localization of the green fluorescence protein (GFP) expressed in COS-7 cells by transfection with expression vectors containing cDNAs encoding GFP alone **(A)**, GFP fused to intact ECE-1α **(B)** and GFP fused to ECE-1α lacking a putative transmembrane domain **(C)**. Cloned human ECE-1α cDNA was ligated to 3'-terminal region of GFP cDNA at the restriction sites of *Sal*I and *Hin*dIII, respectively, of ECE-1α cDNA in the pCMX/GFP vector *(40)* to prepare expression vectors encoding GFP fused to ECE-1α (Ser^{19}-Trp^{770}) and GFP fused to ECE-1α (Ala^{103}-Trp^{770}). The constructs were transfected to COS-7 cells by lipofection, and cultured cells were directly observed by a ZEISS LSM-410 confocal laser scanning microscope. (A) three-dimensionally constructed picture; and (B,C) tomograms.

Finally, it would appear that most of the basic molecular biology and physiology of ECE have been clarified over the past seven years. However, further clarification of the precise mechanism of big ET processing and pathophysiology of ECE is needed in future work.

Acknowledgment

We gratefully thank R. F. Highsmith for providing us a chance to discuss the molecular biology and physiology of ECE.

References

1. Yanagisawa, M., Kurihara, H., Kimura, S., Tomobe, Y., Kobayashi, M., Mitsui, Y., Yazaki, Y., Goto, K., and Masaki, T. (1988) A novel potent vasoconstrictor peptide produced by vascular endothelial cells. *Nature* **332:**411–415.
2. Kashiwabara, T., Inagaki, Y., Ohata, H., Iwamatsu, A., Nomizu, M., Morita, A., and Nishikori, K. (1989) Putative precursors of endothelin have less vasoconstrictor activity *in vitro* but a potent pressor effect *in vivo*. *FEBS Lett.* **247:**73–76.

3. Inoue, A., Yanagisawa, M., Kimura, S., Kasuya, Y., Miyauchi, T., Goto, K., and Masaki, T. (1989) The human endothelin family: three structurally and pharmacologically distinct isopeptides predicted by three separate genes. *Proc. Natl. Acad. Sci. USA* **86:**2863–2867

4. Denault, J.-B., Claing, A., D'Orléans-Juste, P., Sawamura, T., Kido, T., Masaki, T., and Leduc, R. (1995) Processing of proendothelin-1 by human furin convertase. *FEBS Lett.* **362:**276–280.

5. Matsumura, Y., Ikegawa, R., Takaoka, M., and Morimoto, S. (1990) Conversion of porcine big endothelin to endothelin by an extract from the porcine aortic endothelial cells. *Biochem. Biophys. Res. Commun.* **167:** 203–210.

6. Wu-Wong, J. R., Budzik, G. P., Devine, E. M., and Opgenorth, T. J. (1990) Characterization of endothelin converting enzyme in rat lung. *Biochem. Biophys. Res. Commun.* **171:**1291–1296.

7. Sawamura, T., Kimura, S., Shinmi, O., Sugita, Y., Yanagisawa, M., Goto, K., and Masaki, T. (1990) Purification and characterization of putative endothelin converting enzyme in bovine adrenal medulla: evidence for a cathepsin D-like enzyme. *Biochem. Biophys. Res. Commun.* **168:** 1230–1236.

8. Ohnaka, K., Takayanagi, R., Yamauchi, T., Okazaki, H., Ohashi, M., Umeda, F., and Nawata, H. (1990) Identification and characterization of endothelin converting activity in cultured bovine endothelial cells. *Biochem. Biophys. Res. Commun.* **168:**1128–1136.

9. Okada, K., Miyazaki, Y., Takada, J., Matsuyama, K., Yamaki, T., and Yano, M. (1990) Conversion of big endothelin-1 by membrane-bound metalloendopeptidase in cultured bovine endothelial cells. *Biochem. Biophys. Res. Commun.* **171:**1192–1198.

10. Ohnaka, K., Takayanagi, R., Ohashi, M., and Nawata, H. (1991) Conversion of big endothelin isopeptides to mature endothelin isopeptides by cultured bovine endothelial cells. *J. Cardiovasc. Pharmacol.* **17,** **Suppl.:**S17–S19.

11. Ikegawa, R., Matsumura, Y., Tsukahara, Y., Takaoka, M., and Morimoto, S. (1990) Phosphoramidon, a metalloendopeptidase inhibitor, suppresses the secretion of endothelin–1 from cultured endothelial cells by inhibiting a big endothelin–1 converting enzyme. *Biochem. Biophys. Res. Commun.* **171:**669–675.

12. Shields, P. P., Gonzales, T. A., Charles, D., Gilligan, J. P., and Stern, W. (1991) Accumulation of pepstatin in cultured endothelial cells and its effect on endothelin processing. *Biochem. Biophys. Res. Commun.* **177:**1006–1012.

13. D'Orléans-Juste, P., Lidbury, P. S., Warner, T. D., and Vane, J. R. (1990) Intravascular big endothelin increases circulating levels of endothelin-1 and prostanoids in the rabbit. *Biochem. Pharmacol.* **39:**R21–R22.

14. Matsumura, Y., Hisaki, K., Takaoka, M., and Morimoto, S. (1990) Phosphoramidon, a metalloproteinase inhibitor, suppresses the hypertensive effect of big endothelin-1. *Eur. J. Pharmacol.* **185:**103–106.

15. McMahon, E. G., Palomo, M. A., Moore, W. M., McDonald, J. F., and Stern, M. K. (1991) Phosphoramidon blocks the pressor activity of porcine big endothelin-1-(1–39) in vivo and conversion of big endothelin-1-(1-39) to endothelin-1-(1–21) in vitro. *Proc. Natl. Acad. Sci. USA* **88:**703–707.

16. Ohnaka, K., Takayanagi, R., Nishikawa, M., Haji, M., and Nawata, H. (1993) Purification and characterization of a phosphoramidon-sensitive endothelin-converting enzyme in porcine aortic endothelium. *J. Biol. Chem.* **268:**26,759–26,766.

17. Ohnaka, K., Nishikawa, M.,Takayanagi, R., Haji, M., and Nawata, H. (1992) Partial purification of phosphoramidon-sensitive endothelin converting enzyme in porcine aortic endothelial cells: high affinity for *Ricinus communis* agglutinin. *Biochem. Biophys. Res. Commun.* **185:** 611–616.

18. Corder, R., Khan, N., and Harrison, V. J. (1995) A simple method for isolating human endothelin converting enzyme free from contamination by neutral endopeptidase 24.11. *Biochem. Biophys. Res. Commun.* **207:**355–362.

19. Takahashi, M., Fukuda, K., Shimada, K., Barnes, K., Turner, A. J., Ikeda, M., Koike, H., Yamamoto, Y., and Tanzawa, K. (1995) Localization of rat endothelin-converting enzyme to vascular endothelial cells and some secretory cells. *Biochem. J.* **311:**657–665.

20. Shimada, K., Takahashi, M., Turner, A. J., and Tanzawa, K. (1996) Rat endothelin-converting enzyme-1 forms a dimer through Cys412 with a similar catalytic mechanism and a distinct substrate binding mechanism compared with neutral endopeptidase-24.11. *Biochem. J.* **315:**863–867.

21. Okada, K., Arai, Y., Hata, M., Matsuyama, K., and Yano, M. (1993) Big endothelin-1 structure important for specific processing by endothelin-converting enzyme of bovine endothelial cells. *Eur. J. Biochem.* **218:**493–498.

22. Morita, A., Nomizu, M., Okitsu, M., Horie, K., Yokogoshi, H., and Roller, P. P. (1994) D-Val^{22} containing human big endothelin-1 analog, [D-Val^{22}] big ET-1[16–38], inhibits the endothelin converting enzyme. *FEBS Lett.* **353:**84–88.

23. Takahashi, M., Matsushita, Y., Iijima, Y., and Tanzawa, K. (1993) Purification and characterization of endothelin-converting enzyme from rat lung. *J. Biol. Chem.* **268:**21,394–21,398.

24. Xu, D., Emoto, N., Giaid, A., Slaughter, C., Kaw, S., deWit, D., and Yanagisawa, M. (1994) ECE-1: a membrane-bound metalloprotease that catalyzes the proteolytic activation of big endothelin-1. *Cell* **78:**473–485.

25. Shimada, K., Takahashi, M., and Tanzawa, K. (1994) Cloning and functional expression of endothelin-converting enzyme from rat endothelial cells. *J. Biol. Chem.* **269:**18,275–18,278.

26. Schmidt, M., Kröger, B., Jacob, E., Seulberger, H., Subkowski, T., Otter, R., Meyer, T., Schmalzing, G., and Hillen, H. (1994) Molecular characterization of human and bovine endothelin converting enzyme (ECE-1). *FEBS Lett.* **356:**238–243.

27. Ikura, T., Sawamura, T., Shiraki, T., Hosokawa, H., Kido, T., Hoshikawa, H., Shimada, K., Tanzawa, K., Kobayashi, S., Miwa, S., and Masaki, T. (1994) cDNA cloning and expression of bovine endothelin converting enzyme. *Biochem. Biophys. Res. Commun.* **203:**1417–1422.

28. Shimada, K., Matsushita, Y., Wakabayashi, K.,Takahashi, M., Matsubara, A., Iijima, Y., and Tanzawa, K. (1995) Cloning and functional expression of human endothelin-converting enzyme cDNA. *Biochem. Biophys. Res. Commun.* **207:**807–812.

29. Yorimitsu, K., Moroi, K., Inagaki, N., Saito, T., Masuda,Y., Masaki, T., Seino, S., and Kimura, S. (1995) Cloning and sequencing of a human endothelin converting enzyme in renal adenocarcinoma (ACHN) cells producing endothelin-2. *Biochem. Biophys. Res. Commun.* **208:**721–727.

30. Shimada, K., Takahashi, M., Ikeda, M., and Tanzawa, K. (1995) Identification and characterization of two isoforms of an endothelin-converting enzyme-1. *FEBS Lett.* **371:**140–144.

31. Valdenaire, O., Rohrbacher, E., and Mattei, M.-G. (1995) Organization of the gene encoding the human endothelin-converting enzyme (ECE-1). *J. Biol. Chem.* **270:**29,794–29,798.

32. Emoto, N. and Yanagisawa, M. (1995) Endothelin-converting enzyme-2 is a membrane-bound, phosphoramidon-sensitive metalloproteinase with acidic pH optimum. *J. Biol. Chem.* **270:**15,262–15,268.

33. Yanagisawa, H. and Yanagisawa, M. (1996) Endothelin and the differentiation of the neural crest: analysis by gene-targeting (Japanese). *Folia Endocrinolog. Japon.* **72:**739.

34. Kurihara, Y., Kurihara, H., Suzuki, H., Kodama, T., Maemura, K., Nagai, R., Oda, H., Kuwaki, T., Cao, W., Kamada, N., Jishage, K., Ouchi, Y., Azuma, S., Toyoda, Y., Ishikawa, T., Kumada, M., and Yazaki, Y. (1994) Elevated blood pressure and craniofacial abnormalities in mice deficient in endothelin-1. *Nature* **368:**703–710.

35. Baynash, A. G., Hosoda, K., Giaid, A., Richardson, J. A., Emoto, N., Hammer, R. E., and Yanagisawa, M. (1994) Interaction of endothelin-3 with endothelin-B receptor is essential for development of epidermal melanocyte and enteric neurons. *Cell* **79:**1277–1285.

36. Vemulapalli, S., Chiu, P. J. S., Griscti, K., Brown, A., Kurowski, S., and Sybertz, E. (1994) Phosphoramidon does not inhibit endogenous endothelin-1 release stimulated by hemorrhage, cytokines and hypoxia in rats. *Eur. J. Pharmacol.* **257:**95–102.

37. Harrison, V. J., Barnes, K., Turner, A. J., Wood, E., Corder, R., and Vane, J. R. (1995) Identification of endothelin 1 and big endothelin 1 in secretory vesicles isolated from bovine aortic endothelial cells. *Proc. Natl. Acad. Sci. USA* **92:**6344–6348.

38. Ohnaka, K., Takayanagi, R., Yamauchi, T., Umeda, F., and Nawata, H. (1991) Cultured bovine endothelial cells convert big endothelin isopeptides to mature endothelin isopeptides. *Biochem. Int.* **23:**499–506.

39. Tsurumi, Y., Ohhata, N., Iwamoto, T., Shigematsu, N., Sakamoto, K., Nishikawa, M., Kiyoto, S., and Okuhara, M. (1994) WS79089A, B and C, new endothelin converting enzyme inhibitors isolated from Streptosporangium roseum. NO. 79089. Taxonomy, fermentation, isolation, physico-chemical properties and biological activities. *J. Antibiotics* **47:**619–630.

40. Ogawa, H., Inouye, S., Tsuji, F. I., Yasuda, K., and Umesono, K. (1995) Localization, trafficking, and temperature-dependence of the *Aequorea* green fluorescent protein in cultured vertebrate cells. *Proc. Natl. Acad. Sci. USA* **92:**11,899–11,903.

41. Barnes, K., Shimada, K., Takahashi, M., Tanzawa, K., and Turner, A. J. (1996) Metallopeptidase inhibitors induce an up-regulation of endothelin-converting enzyme levels and its redistribution from the plasma membrane to an intracellular compartment. *J. Cell. Sci.* **109:**919–928.

Chapter 4

Endothelin Receptor-Signaling Mechanisms in Vascular Smooth Muscle

E. Radford Decker and Tommy A. Brock

1. Introduction

The local regulation of tissue blood flow depends on a delicate balance of physical and chemical stimuli acting on the vascular endothelium, the innermost lining of all blood vessels. By virtue of its location at the blood–tissue interface in vivo, vascular endothelium is ideally suited to play a pivotal role in vascular tone regulation. It is now well-documented that endothelial cells produce several vasoactive substances that activate or inhibit underlying smooth muscle cells in the blood vessel wall. Vascular smooth muscle cell (VSMC) stimulation leads to relaxation/contraction via a series of biochemical and morphological events that are responsible directly for mediating changes in vessel diameter. To date, endothelin is one of the most potent stimulators of both vascular and nonvascular smooth muscle contraction that has been identified.

Although Hickey et al. *(1)* were the first to describe in 1985 an unidentified factor (endothelium-derived constricting factor) that caused a slowly developing, long-lasting vasoconstriction of coronary arteries, it was not until three years later that Yanagisawa and coworkers *(2)* determined the identity of the factor. In what is now a hallmark paper, these investigators reported the purification and cloning of a disulfide-bonded, 21 amino acid vasoconstrictor peptide from cultured endothelial cells and renamed the molecule endothelin (ET).

From: *Endothelin: Molecular Biology, Physiology, and Pathology*
Edited by R. F. Highsmith © Humana Press Inc., Totowa, NJ

Subsequently, it was determined that human ET constitutes a family of highly potent autocrine and paracrine vasoactive polypeptides consisting of three distinct gene products (ET-1, ET-2, and ET-3) *(3)*. Endothelin-1 was initially discovered as an endothelial cell product, but ET-2 and ET-3 have subsequently been found in a wide variety of cells and tissues. In addition, multiple receptor subtypes have been described, which in part explains the multiplicity of biological actions that have been ascribed to ET in the literature.

An extensive literature has emerged in recent years that describes the biological activities and intracellular mechanisms evoked by ET in a wide variety of diverse cell types. In this overview, we summarize what is currently known about ET receptor signal transduction mechanisms in VSMCs. Because intracellular free calcium concentration ($[Ca^{2+}]_i$) is a key determinant of vascular smooth muscle contractility and is a principal mechanism by which ET appears to mediate its cellular actions, our emphasis will be to review the molecular mechanisms underlying calcium signaling. Other signal transduction pathways involved in ET action on VSMCs which potentially modulate $[Ca^{2+}]_i$ or are activated in response to $[Ca^{2+}]_i$ changes, will also be discussed.

2. Signal-Transduction Mechanisms

In VSMCs, the two primary biological consequences of ET stimulation are contraction and mitogenesis. A general scheme of the intracellular-signaling cascade resulting from ET binding to its cell-surface receptor on vascular smooth muscle is illustrated in Fig. 1. The interaction between ET receptors and a specific guanine nucleotide regulatory protein (G protein) leads to the activation of multiple-effector proteins. In particular, phospholipase C activation results in the rapid hydrolysis of the membrane inositol phospholipid, phosphatidylinositol 4,5-bisphosphate, yielding inositol 1,4,5-triphosphate (IP_3) and *sn*1,2-diacylglycerol (DAG). A common event elicited by ET-receptor activation in many cell types is a biphasic increase in $[Ca^{2+}]_i$. The rapid rise in IP_3 initiates calcium (Ca^{2+}) release from intracellular storage sites. This burst of IP_3-dependent Ca^{2+} release activates other Ca^{2+}-dependent processes which lead to cell membrane depolarization and sustained extracellular Ca^{2+} influx. Diacylglycerol is believed to be the physiological stimulus for protein kinase C (PKC) activation. Several cellular actions of ET-1 can be mimicked by phorbol esters, potent and persistent activators of PKC.

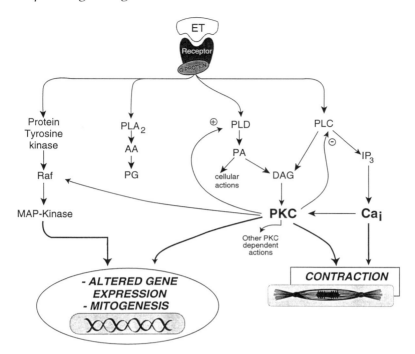

Fig. 1. General scheme of ET-1 signal transduction pathways in vascular smooth muscle. ET, Endothelin-1; G protein, guanine nucleotide binding protein; PLC, phospholipase C; IP_3, inositol 1,4,5 trisphosphate; Ca_i, intracellular Ca^{2+} concentration; DAG, diacylglycerol; PKC, protein kinase C; PLD, phospholipase D; PA, phosphatidic acid; PLA_2, phospholipase A_2; AA, arachidonic acid; PG, prostaglandin; PTKs, protein tyrosine kinases; MAP-kinase, mitogen activated protein kinase.

2.1. Endothelin-Receptor Subtypes

Molecular cloning of ET receptors have shown that they belong to the rhodopsin superfamily of G protein-coupled receptors containing seven transmembrane spanning domains *(4,5)*. To date, cDNAs of three distinct high-affinity ET receptor subtypes, designated ET_A, ET_B, and ET_C receptors have been identified in different species *(3)*. The human cDNAs for ET_A receptors and ET_B are approx 55% homologous. ET receptors are defined pharmacologically by their relative affinities for ET-1, ET-2, and ET-3. Mammalian ET_A receptors show an equal affinity for ET-1 and ET-2 and much lower affinity for ET-3, whereas mammalian ET_B receptors demonstrate an equal affinity for all three peptides. An ET_C receptor has been cloned from *Xeno-*

pus laevis melanocytes which shows increased specificity for ET-3 *(6)* and exhibits 50% amino acid sequence homology with ET_A and ET_B receptors. A homolog of this receptor subtype has not been identified in mammals.

Endothelin administered to anesthetized animals elicits a biphasic change in systemic arterial pressure, i.e., a rapid, transient hypotensive effect followed by a sustained hypertensive action *(7)*. The hypotensive effect appeared to be mediated via an ET_B receptor (ET-3=ET-2=ET-1), whereas the hypertensive effect exhibited properties that implicated an ET_A receptor. These data and subsequent molecular analysis were interpreted as evidence that two distinct ET receptors existed within the vasculature: ET_A receptors were located on smooth muscle cells and their activation resulted in vasoconstriction, whereas ET_B receptor activation on vascular endothelium was linked to the release of nitric oxide and/or prostaglandins and resulted in vasodilatation *(3)*.

However, more recent studies using pharmacologically selective ET_A or ET_B receptor antagonists have shown this simplistic view of receptor distribution within blood vessels to be incorrect (for review *see 8,9*). Using the ET_A receptor selective antagonists BQ-123 and FR139317 and the ET_B receptor specific agonist sarafrotoxin S6c, a better understanding of the role of ET receptors in different vascular beds has been obtained. For example, ET-1-induced contractile responses in rat thoracic aorta and coronary artery, rabbit carotid artery, human coronary, omental and pulmonary arteries and thoracic aorta, and rat mesenteric artery appear to be mediated entirely by ET_A receptors. In these vascular tissues, ET-1 exerts a greater contractile effect than ET-3, BQ-123 blocks the ET-1 induced contractions, and sarafrotoxin S6c exhibits no contractile effects. By contrast, ET-1-induced contractions of canine and pig coronary arteries, and rabbit jugular vein appear to be mediated via ET_B receptors. In these tissues, ET-1 and ET-3 are equipotent and sarafrotoxin S6c causes vasoconstriction, whereas BQ-123 does not antagonize the effects of ET-1, ET-3 or sarafrotoxin S6c. Finally, there are vascular beds in which ET responses are mediated via a mixture of ET_A and ET_B receptors. These include rat renal vasculature, rabbit pulmonary artery and saphenous vein , and human internal mammary artery. Thus, it appears that the contribution of ET_A vs ET_B receptors involved in vasoconstriction may differ depending upon the vascular bed being examined within an animal.

Another degree of complexity arises from the potential heterogeneity of ET_B receptor subtypes. Although there is no molecular biological evidence supporting the existence of ET_{B1} and ET_{B2} receptor subtypes, there are several examples of pharmacological *(10,11)* and radioligand binding *(12)* studies using ET_B antagonists that support their existence. Using a nonselective ET-receptor antagonist PD142893, Warner et al. *(10)* have presented the most compelling evidence that nitric oxide release from endothelial cells is mediated by an ET_{B1} receptor and that ET_{B2} receptors mediate VSMC contraction.

2.2. Guanine Nucleotide Regulatory Proteins

In all eukaryotic organisms, heterotrimeric G proteins play an important role in the transduction of extracellular signals to the cell interior. It has been estimated that at least a third of all signal transduction processes involve heterotrimeric G proteins. These protein complexes consist of α (molecular mass = $39 - 46$ kDa), β (37 kDa), and γ (8 kDa) subunits *(13,14)*. The G_α subunit binds guanine nucleotides (GDP and GTP) and contains intrinsic GTPase activity. The GDP-bound form of the G_α subunit binds tightly to the $G_{\beta\gamma}$ subunits. When GTP replaces the GDP bound to the G_α subunit, the G_α subunit dissociates from the $G_{\beta\gamma}$ subunits. The $G_{\beta\gamma}$ subunits exist as a tightly associated unit and dissociate only after denaturation. A negative feedback loop exists owing to the intrinsic GTPase activity of the α-subunit, which hydrolyzes the GTP to GDP. If GTPγS, a nonhydrolyzable GTP analog, binds to the G_α subunit, G_α becomes continuously active owing to the inability of the GTPase activity of the α-subunit to hydrolyze this form of GTP. Although the G_α subunit serves as a major regulator of many cellular proteins, it is also well-documented that $G_{\beta\gamma}$ can also positively regulate effector proteins, such as K^+ channels, adenylate cyclase, PLCβ, phospholipase A_2, phosphoinositide 3-kinase and β-adrenergic receptor kinases *(13)*. To date, more than 20 different G_α subunits, five G_β subunits, and six G_γ subunits have been cloned *(13,14)*.

As stated earlier, the ET receptors belong to the rhodopsin superfamily of G protein-coupled receptors *(5,9)*. In membranes prepared from A10 cells, an aortic smooth muscle cell line, ET-1-stimulated phosphoinositide hydrolysis was dependent on the presence of GTPγS and the binding of ET-1 to these membranes was inhibited by GTPγS in a dose-dependent manner *(15)*. Additionally, two different bacterial exotoxins have proven to be useful tools to characterize the

G proteins involved in ET signal transduction. The first is *Bordetella pertussis* toxin (PTX), which catalyzes the ADP-ribosylation of a cysteine located four amino acids from the carboxyl terminus of α subunits belonging to the G_i family, G proteins originally described to be involved in mediating adenylate cyclase inhibition *(14)*. This covalent modification disrupts G_α function, thus blocking the signaling pathway. Pertussis toxin-sensitive G proteins have been implicated in ET-1 signaling in some, but not all, VSMC types. For example, PTX significantly inhibits ET-1-induced phosphoinositide hydrolysis in cultured VSMCs *(16)* and mesangial cells *(17,18)*, as well as ET-1-induced contraction and $^{45}Ca^{2+}$ uptake in pig coronary artery *(19)*. By contrast, PTX-insensitive phosphoinositide turnover has been reported in cultured VSMCs *(15)* or A10 cells *(20)* and in pig coronary artery *(19)*. Pertussis toxin also failed to suppress the contraction of rat mesenteric arteries *(21)*.

The second toxin is *Vibrio cholera* toxin, which catalyzes the ADP ribosylation of specific arginine residues 201 and 174 in the α subunits G_s and G_t, G proteins originally described to be involved in mediating adenylate cyclase and transducin stimulation, respectively *(14,22)*. This event inhibits the intrinsic GTPase activity of the α-subunit, thus locking it into the activated mode. ET-1 has been reported in rat VSMCs containing ET_A receptors to cause a dose-dependent increase in cAMP production, which is PTX insensitive and CTX-sensitive *(23)*. In contrast, ET_B receptor stimulation in endothelial cells leads to PTX-sensitive increase in cyclic AMP levels *(23)*. These studies confirm results using ET_A and ET_B receptor-transfected Chinese hamster ovary (CHO) cells *(24)*. Therefore, the activation of adenylate cyclase in these preparations most likely involves G_s. Collectively, these studies suggest that in different types of VSMCs, ET receptors appear to be connected through multiple G proteins. Further experiments will be needed to elucidate the exact nature of the G proteins involved in ET-receptor activation in human vascular tissue.

2.3. Phospholipid Signaling Mechanisms

2.3.1. Phospholipase C

Eight mammalian inositol phospholipid-specific phospholipase C isozymes have been identified and can be divided into three structural classes (PLCβ1-4, γ1,2, δ1,2) at the cDNA level *(25)*. When stimulated, PLC primarily hydrolyzes phosphatidylinositol 4,5-bisphosphate (PIP$_2$) resulting in the activation of two ubiquitous second messengers, inositol 1,4,5-triphosphate (IP_3) and *sn*1,2-diacyl-glycerol (DAG). IP_3 activates specific receptors on intracellular Ca^{2+} stores resulting in Ca^{2+} release, whereas DAG plays an integral role in protein kinase C (PKC) activation *(26)*. Although all three classes of PI-PLCs show dependence on Ca^{2+} in vitro, the Ca^{2+} requirement may not be physiologically important because agonists can increase IP_3 production in the presence of low levels of intracellular calcium in vivo. The PLC isoforms also differ in their regulation by hetero-trimeric G proteins and protein tyrosine kinases. Receptor-activated G proteins have been shown to activate PLC-β1, PLC-β2, and PLC-β3 using the G_q family of PTX-insensitive G proteins *(25)*. Interestingly, PLCβ can be activated by both α_q and $\beta\gamma$ subunits. The rank order of PLC activation by α_q is PLC-β1 $\geq$ PLC-β3 > PLC-β4 > PLC-β2 while the rank order of activation by $\beta\gamma$ is PLC-β3 $\geq$ PLC-β2 > PLC-β1 *(25)*. $\beta\gamma$ does not activate PLC-β4. It has been suggested recently that PTX-sensitive PLC-β activation may result from $G_{\beta\gamma}$. PLC-γ is involved in the signaling cascade initiated by growth factor receptor tyrosine kinases (*see* ref. *25*). In general, PLC-β-induced $[Ca^{2+}]_i$ increases induced by G-protein activation occur more rapidly and transiently as compared to PLC-γ-induced $[Ca^{2+}]_i$ increases induced by growth factor receptor-induced tyrosine phosphorylation.

Early experiments demonstrated that ET-1 caused a rapid rise in IP_3 levels in isolated canine *(27)* and porcine *(28,29)* coronary arteries which was paralleled by an increase in $^{45}Ca^{2+}$ uptake followed by vascular contraction. Similar studies of VSMCs in culture *(20,30,31,33)* and isolated vessels *(34,35)* have shown a similar rapid activation of PI turnover following ET-1 stimulation. This increase in PI hydrolysis has been shown to lead to increased IP_3 levels within 10 s of stimulation *(34)*. The rise in IP_3 induces Ca^{2+} release from intracellular storage sites *(see below)*. The experiments with PTX discussed previously indicate that there are two different components that can activate PLC in response to ET. Thus, the PTX-insensitive pathway most likely involves the activation of PLC-β by a member of the G_q family. While PLC-β can be activated by the $\beta\gamma$ dimer, a much higher concentration is required for activation by α_q. Receptor-mediated G_i activation, the high abundance PTX-sensitive G protein family, would release $\beta\gamma$ subunits which in turn could activate PLC-β. This latter pathway may explain the PTX-sensitive pathways for ET-1-stimulated PIP_2 hydrolysis. It is most likely that the PLC-β3 form is responsible for both the PTX-sensitive and -insensitive ET-stimulated PIP_2 hydrolysis in rabbit vascular smooth muscle because PLC-β1 was not detected by Northern or Western blotting *(36)*.

2.3.2. Phospholipase D

Endothelin stimulation also leads to a rapid, biphasic rise in DAG levels, which is sustained for up to 20 min *(20,37,38)*. Diacylglycerol levels can increase directly via PI hydrolysis or via phosphatidyl-choline hydrolysis by PLC and/or phosphatidylcholine hydrolysis by phospholipase D (PLD) and phosphatidic acid phosphohydrolase. It has been postulated for other vasoconstrictors that the biphasic nature of the DAG signal results initially from PI hydrolysis, followed by a slower and more long-lasting DAG production from phosphatidyl-choline. These sustained levels of DAG correspond temporally with sustained PLD activation *(39,40)* and play an important role in PKC activation. Although the mechanisms regulating PLD activity are unclear at the present time, there are reports that PLD can be acti-vated via PKC-dependent *(40)* and independent pathways *(41)*, as well as a protein tyrosine kinase pathway *(42)*. Phospholipase D is also postulated to play an important role in the mitogenic response observed following stimulation by ET *(43)*, however, this point is con-troversial (*see* ref. *44*).

2.3.3. Phospholipase A_2

The role of phospholipase A_2 (PLA$_2$) in the ET signaling cas-cade remains a largely unexplored area. PLA$_2$ can liberate free fatty acids such as arachidonic acid (AA) from membrane phospholipids. Arachidonic acid can be metabolized by lipoxygenase, cyclooxygenase, and epoxygenase to form leukotrienes, hydroxyei-cosatetraenoic acids, prostaglandins (PGs), thromboxanes and epoxides *(45–48)*. Endothelin-1 stimulation appears to activate the arachidonate cascade through a PKC-sensitive pathway *(40)*. Activa-tion could be through the PLA$_2$ pathway which has been shown to be activated by ET-1 in mesangial cells *(49)*. The generation of arachi-donic-acid metabolites may have multiple outcomes in VSMCs, such as modulation of ion channel activities *(50)* or activation of gene expression *(49)*.

2.4. Cytosolic Calcium Signaling Mechanisms

Endothelin-1-induced contractions are more slowly developing, are maintained for longer periods of time, and are more resistant to agonist removal when compared with contractions in response to clas-sical G protein coupled agonists, such as angiotensin II or the α_1-receptor coupled agonist phenylephrine. Recent observations provide evidence that interactions among G proteins, Ca^{2+}, and protein kinase C are important stimuli to maintain the tonic contraction phase in vascular smooth muscle *(51,52)*. It is well-documented that binding of ET to its receptor leads to a biphasic increase in $[Ca^{2+}]_i$, in which an initial rapid, transient phase is followed by a sustained elevated plateau phase. The rapid phase is owing to Ca^{2+} release from the sarcoplasmic reticulum, which is the major source and sink of Ca^{2+} in vascular smooth muscle, while the sustained phase has been shown to be dependent on Ca^{2+} influx from the extracellular space *(51)*.

2.4.1. Intracellular Ca^{2+} Mobilization

Numerous studies utilizing both intact arteries and cultured VSMCs have shown that, in the absence of extracellular Ca^{2+} or in the presence of L-type Ca^{2+} channel blockers *(3,53,54)*, the transient rise in $[Ca^{2+}]_i$ and the contractile responses to ET-1 are shorter and return to baseline more rapidly than when Ca^{2+} is present in the external solution. In these cases, the sustained contractile phase is greatly attenuated or abolished. These results demonstrate that the initial ET-1-stimulated $[Ca^{2+}]_i$ rise and contraction is attributable to Ca^{2+} release from intracellular storage sites. In rat aortic smooth muscle cells, ET-1 and ET-3 both cause a transient increase in $[Ca^{2+}]_i$, but only ET-1 causes an increase in IP_3 production *(55)*.

Significant increases in IP_3 levels occur within 10 s following ET-1 stimulation and it is well-documented that IP_3 production is responsible for intracellular Ca^{2+} mobilization in VSMCs *(3,53,54)*. Intracellular Ca^{2+} release can occur through two distinct ion channels in VSMCs, the inositol 1,4,5-triphosphate receptor channel and the ryanodine receptor channel, that are found in the sarcoplasmic reticulum *(56,57)*. The IP_3 receptor is a relatively nonselective cation channel consisting of four identical 310 kDa subunits, exhibits a biphasic sensitivity to Ca^{2+}, is desensitized by IP_3 and blocked by heparin, and is sensitive to protein kinase A phosphorylation *(56)*. Additionally, the ryanodine receptor, a homotetramer of four 560 kDa subunits, may provide an additional mechanism for Ca^{2+} release in smooth-muscle cells. Kai et al. *(58)* have documented that the initial ET-1-induced rise in $[Ca^{2+}]_i$ could also be attenuated or blocked completely by ryanodine *(59)*, or by caffeine pretreatment, a selective agonist for the ryanodine-sensitive Ca^{2+} release channel. The ryanodine receptor can be gated either by electromechanical coupling *(50,51)*, by Ca^{2+}-induced Ca^{2+} release *(50,51)* or by cyclic ADP-ribose, a molecule which has been shown to be involved in regulating the ryanodine Ca^{2+}

release channel in a variety of cells and tissues (*see* ref. *60* for a review). Thus, these results imply that ET-induced intracellular Ca^{2+} mobilization in vascular smooth muscle is the result of activation of both IP_3 and ryanodine receptor-sensitive Ca^{2+} pools.

2.4.2. Extracellular Ca^{2+} Influx

Early experiments showed that endothelium-derived contracting factor-induced contractions in isolated blood vessels are dependent on extracellular Ca^{2+} and are attenuated by verapamil *(1)*. Numerous studies have since verified that the sustained contractile actions of ET-1 are dependent on extracellular Ca^{2+} and that ET-1 stimulates $^{45}Ca^{2+}$ entry into VSMCs *(3,53,54)*. The mechanism by which extracellular Ca^{2+} enters the cell has been studied extensively, but the data remain contradictory. L-type Ca^{2+} channel antagonists with different chemical structures were found to attenuate ET-1 induced vasoconstriction in vivo and in isolated arteries in many different species *(28,29,61–63,68)*. However, several similar studies have found little if any effect of the same Ca^{2+} channel antagonists on ET-1 stimulated contraction in similar preparations *(64–67)*. Similar contradictory results were seen upon examination of Ca^{2+} influx and the sustained increases in $[Ca^{2+}]_i$ in vascular smooth muscle. Ca^{2+} channel blockers reportedly caused significant inhibition of the sustained $[Ca^{2+}]_i$ rise or $^{45}Ca^{2+}$ uptake in isolated primary cultures of VSMCs *(39,58,68–70)*. However, L-type Ca^{2+} channel blockers had little or no effect on ET-1 induced $^{45}Ca^{2+}$ uptake or sustained $[Ca^{2+}]_i$ increases in other studies *(20,59,65,71,72)*. Huang et al. *(73)* reported that dihydropyridine Ca^{2+} antagonists inhibited both the transient and sustained Ca^{2+} increase in cultured A7r5 smooth muscle cells. This effect was also observed in human umbilical artery SMCs when verapamil and nicardipine were used *(69)*. These observations imply that there is a component of the ET response, which is dependent on extracellular Ca^{2+} influx. It has been postulated that the secondary influx of extracellular Ca^{2+} can stimulate additional Ca^{2+} release from the ryanodine-sensitive sarcoplasmic reticulum pool through a mechanism involving Ca^{2+}-induced Ca^{2+} release *(50)* or a diffusible second messenger, such as cADP-ribose *(60)*.

Vascular smooth-muscle cells contain numerous types of ion channels, which influence membrane excitability and calcium permeability. Importantly, VSMCs contain two distinct Ca^{2+} influx pathways, one that utilizes voltage-dependent Ca^{2+} channels (VDCC) and the other that utilizes receptor-operated channels (ROC) *(50)*. The

VDCC most often reported in VSMCs are the L-type or dihydro-pyridine sensitive (DHP) sensitive Ca^{2+} channels. L-type Ca^{2+} channels are blocked by a variety of organic compounds, including the dihydropyridines (nifedipine, and others) and are not blocked by nickel. ET-1-activated Ca^{2+} influx via ROCs have been described as a nifedipine-insensitive and nickel-sensitive pathway.

2.4.2.1. Voltage-Dependent Ca^{2+} Channels

Two types of VDCCs have been characterized in VSMCs from mammalian arteries and veins. The first is a dihydropyridine (DHP)-sensitive L-type Ca^{2+} channel which has a unitary conductance of 20–25 pS in ~100 mM Ba^{2+} and inactivates slowly (on the order of hundreds of millisec). This channel has been characterized by patch-clamp experiments in freshly isolated VSMCs and cell lines *(74–79)*. Vascular smooth muscle L-type Ca^{2+} channels are much more sensitive to DHPs than those in cardiac muscle *(75,77)*. A low threshold, rapidly inactivating T-type Ca^{2+} channel, which has a unitary conductance of ~ 8 pS in ~100 mM Ba^{2+}, is also present *(76,77)*. This channel passes Ba^{2+} and Ca^{2+} equally well *(77,80; see* also where Ba^{2+} was less permeable than Ca^{2+} in A10 VSMCs) and is relatively insensitive to DHPs *(76–79)*. The channel is activated by small amount of depolarization (5–10 mV) and inactivates quickly (in the tens of msec range). T-type Ca^{2+} channels are blocked by Ni^{2+} *(50)*.

Yanagisawa et al. *(2)*, noting the structural similarities between ET-1 and α-scorpion toxin and the attenuation of ET-1 induced vaso-constriction by DHP Ca^{2+} channel antagonists, speculated originally that ET could be an endogenous agonist for L-type Ca^{2+} channels. This hypothesis has been repeatedly tested by several groups and results have clearly indicated that ET-1 does not compete with or displace the binding of several types of Ca^{2+} channel blockers, nor do Ca^{2+} channel antagonists interfere with ET-1 binding to isolated vessels or VSMCs *(3)*. These observations demonstrate that ET-1 does not bind directly to the channel in order to activate it. Only recently has there been a report that ET-1, but not ET-3, reduced [^{3}H]-nicardipine binding, a specific DHP-type Ca^{2+} channel antagonist, in sections of human renal artery by 85% *(81)*. Additional evidence that ET works indirectly and not through direct binding to the channel comes from patch clamp studies using the cell-attached configuration where the extracellular surface of the channel is isolated from the bath solution by the patch pipet. Addition of ET-1 to the bathing solution caused changes in L-type Ca^{2+} channel activity under these conditions *(3,61,63)*.

2.4.2.2. Receptor-Operated Ca^{2+} Channels

The term receptor operated Ca^{2+} (ROC) pathway has been used to describe any pathway for the increased Ca^{2+} influx that is not sensitive to L-type Ca^{2+} channel blockers. Low doses of ET-1 (10^{-9} M) induce vascular smooth muscle contraction which is predominantly dependent on extracellular Ca^{2+} but is not dependent on L-type Ca^{2+} channel activation *(20)*. Nickel, which typically does not block L-type Ca^{2+} channels in intact arteries *(50,64,82)*, blocks ET-1 induced contraction or $[Ca^{2+}]_i$ increases *(64,82,83)*. The nonspecific cation channel-blocker La^{3+} also affected the ET-1 induced responses *(66)*. Inoue et al. *(63)* found that ET-1 stimulated a Ca^{2+} channel that was insensitive to nifedipine. Endothelin caused a rapid transient rise of $[Ca^{2+}]_i$ in A10 cells followed by a sustained elevation. When extracellular Ca^{2+} was replaced with Mn^{2+}, intracellular fluorescence was quenched. This quenching was only partially blocked by nifedipine *(83)*. Collectively, these observations have led to the conclusion that there is an alternative pathway for Ca^{2+} influx that is not through L-type Ca^{2+} channels.

Insight into the possible channel underlying the Ca^{2+} influx through non-L-type Ca^{2+} channels can be gained by looking at experiments using other vasoconstrictors. Ruegg et al. *(84)* examined ROC using angiotensin II, vasopressin, and ATP and found no evidence of any fundamental difference in the ROC mechanism involved. Their experiments indicated that phospholipase signaling was involved, but not a PTX sensitive G protein or direct modulation by PKC. However, Van Renterghem and Lazdunski *(85)* have recently identified a small whole cell current that is stimulated by vasopressin, is selective for Ca^{2+} over monovalent cations, is not voltage-dependent, and is inhibited by Ni^{2+}. This current is probably associated with the ROC Ca^{2+} pathway for vasopressin stimulation. A similar Ca^{2+} flux pathway has been described in isolated pig aortic microsomes in which a Ca^{2+} current is activated by histamine and GTPγS *(86)*. This current is insensitive to verapamil, diltiazem, or nicardipine but is blocked by Ni^{2+} and SK&F96365. These additional ionic currents that have been described for other vasoconstrictors are also likely to be involved in mediating ET signals. The identity of the channel involved in ROC Ca^{2+} influx is still unclear. Because the characteristics of the ROC pathway are similar to the T-type calcium channel *(3,50)*, investigation using specific blockers of this channel could be useful in positively identifying this channel.

2.4.2.3. Other Ion Channels

Ion channels other than Ca^{2+} channels may also play an integral role in the ET-signaling cascade in vascular smooth muscle. Bath application of ET-1 causes an initial transient hyperpolarization followed by a sustained depolarization of VSMCs *(3,30,54,62)*. This sustained depolarization is postulated to cause the voltage-dependent L-type Ca^{2+} channels to open in the plasma membrane, allowing extracellular Ca^{2+} influx. The basis for the initial transient hyperpolarization of the cell membrane could be activation of a Ca^{2+}-dependent potassium (K_{Ca}) channel. Endothelin stimulation of isolated cells from renal resistance arteries activates an outward current through the K_{Ca} channel *(87)*. Activation of a similar K_{Ca} channel was observed with angiotensin II in mesangial cells *(88)*. This outward current is only transient, even though Ca^{2+} levels are sustained for a prolonged period. Bath addition of ET-1 (50 n*M*) caused an inhibition of K_{Ca} channel activated by Ca^{2+} entry mediated by the Ca^{2+} ionophore, A23187. The inhibition by ET-1 was mimicked by application of PMA, however, the inhibition by PMA was reduced by the addition of staurosporine (1 n*M*). In contrast, ET-1 inhibition was not reduced by up to 30 n*M* staurosporine. Also, the inhibition of the potassium current by ET-1 was not abolished by neomycin, an inhibitor of PLC *(89)*. These results indicate that ET causes an increase in K_{Ca} channel activity through release of Ca^{2+} from intracellular stores, then inactivates these channels through a PKC independent pathway.

Following a transient depolarization, the cell membrane potential may depolarize for a prolonged period. This threshold depolarization is postulated to activate the L-type Ca^{2+} channels. Depolarization could be either through the influx of cations or through the efflux of anions. The plasma membrane requires depolarization from its resting level (−40 to −50 mV) to −20 to −30 mV in order to activate the L-type voltage dependent Ca^{2+} channel (*see* Section 2.4.2.1.). Although the mechanism for depolarization is poorly understood, there are two channels that have been described in the literature either of which could depolarize the membrane. One is a Ca^{2+}-activated Cl^- channel; the other is a nonselective cation channel.

Evidence for a Ca^{2+}-activated Cl^- channel has come from numerous studies *(62,87,90)*. The Cl^- channel antagonist indanyloxyacetic acid (IAA-94) inhibited the sustained phase of the $[Ca^{2+}]_i$ increase and membrane depolarization and blocked kidney-afferent arteriole vasoconstriction in perfused rat kidney *(62)*. Takenaka et al. *(62)* hypothesized that the Cl^- channel is activated through $[Ca^{2+}]_i$ mobilization (via IP_3) that activated a Ca^{2+}-dependent Cl^- channel. In A7r5 cells, ET activates two types of Cl^- channel, one of which is Ca^{2+} activated *(91)*. The channels have a conductance of 1.8 pS and 1.0–1.3 pS channel. The 1.8 pS channel was not active when Ca^{2+} was removed from the bath in the excised inside-out patch configuration where the intracellular surface of the plasma membrane is exposed to the bath solution. In freshly isolated rat interlobar and arcuate arteries, ET-1 also activated a Ca^{2+}-dependent Cl^- current in the whole cell patch configuration *(87)*. Takenaka et al. *(62)*, using fluorescent measurements, showed that the sustained increase in $[Ca^{2+}]_i$ was blocked by IAA-94. Activation of these Cl^- channels would allow Cl^- efflux, which in turn would lead to membrane depolarization. This membrane depolarization would in turn cause the opening of VDCCs.

Depolarization of the cell membrane could also be achieved through an influx of different cations. One possible route for cation entry would be through non-selective cation channels. VanRentergham et al. *(30)* presented evidence for the activation of a cation channel by ET-1. Chen and Wagoner *(92)* also reported the existence of a nonselective cation channel that was activated by ET-1. It is permeable to the monovalent cations Na^+, K^+, Cs^+, but not to the large organic cation $Tris^+$. This channel is nifedipine insensitive, but is blocked by Ni^{2+} and dependent on extracellular Ca^{2+} in order to open. Similar whole-cell currents, which are also permeable to Ca^{2+}, have been reported in rabbit aorta. This channel demonstrated prolonged activation and was also not blocked by nifedipine *(93)*. Owing to the electrochemical driving forces, this channel would allow a flow of Na^+ ions into the cell when open under physiological conditions, resulting in membrane depolarization. Nonselective cation channels, which are permeable to Ca^{2+} may play a role in the entry of Ca^{2+} through non-L-type Ca^{2+} channels, while also serving to depolarize the membrane. The interaction of different channel types in mediating ET's effects on calcium dynamics in VSMCs is summarized in Fig. 2. Although investigation of the role of these channels is difficult without specific antagonists, their role in VSMCs needs to be examined.

2.5. Protein Kinase C Signaling Mechanisms

Although it is well-documented that ET-1 causes activation of protein kinase C (PKC), the specific role of PKC in the ET-induced signaling response is complex. Much of this complexity arises from

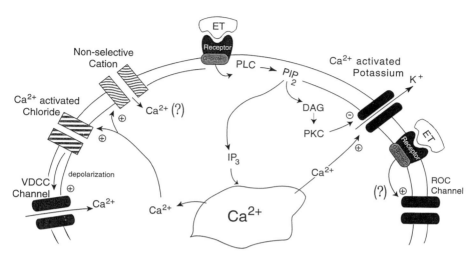

Fig. 2. Summary of ion channels involved in ET-1 Ca^{2+} signaling pathway in vascular smooth muscle. ET, Endothelin; G protein, guanine nucleotide binding protein; VDCC, voltage-dependent Ca^{2+} channel; ROC, receptor-operated Ca^{2+} channel; PIP_2, phosphatidylinositol 4,5 bisphosphate.

the diversity of the PKC isoforms. At least 11 different isozymes of PKC have been isolated from mammalian tissues *(94,95)*. These enzymes can be classified into three different groups. The first group contains the "classical" PKCs (cPKC; isoforms α, β_I, β_{II}, γ) that are activated by Ca^{2+}, phosphatidylserine, and diacylglycerol or phorbol esters. The second group consists of the "new" PKCs (nPKC; isoforms δ, ε, η, θ) that differ from cPKCs only by not requiring Ca^{2+} for activation. The third group comprises the "atypical" PKCs (aPKC; isoforms ξ, ι) which are dependent on phosphatidylserine for activation, but are not affected by Ca^{2+}, diacylglycerol or phorbol esters. The various members of the PKC family most likely differ in their sensitivity to diverse combinations of Ca^{2+}, phosphatidylserine, diacylglycerol and other phospholipid breakdown products. Of the 11 PKC isoforms isolated to date, only the PKC isoforms α, β, ε, and ξ have been found in vascular smooth muscle. PKC-α was purified from A7r5 cells *(96)* and detected by immunoblot assay in swine carotid artery *(97)*. PKC-ε and PKC-ξ have been detected in aortic smooth muscle *(98–100)*. Endothelin-1 stimulates PKC translocation from the cytosol to the membrane in cultured bovine VSMCs *(101)*. Griendling et al. *(37)* demonstrated using cultured rat aortic VSMCs that ET-1 stimulates the rapid and sustained phosphorylation of a PKC specific protein substrate. PKC activation by acute treatment with phorbol esters appears to enhance activation of L-type Ca^{2+} channels in A7r5 cells *(102,103)*.

Inhibition of endogenous PKC by staurosporine and phloretin blocks both ET-1 and phorbol ester-induced contractions *(67,68)*. Furthermore, down regulation of PKC activity by preincubation with phorbol 12,13-dibutyrate (PDBu) for 24 h prevented ET-1 induced contractions in porcine coronary arteries *(104)*. By contrast, Shimamoto and coworkers *(105)* using a more specific inhibitor of PKC action, calphostin C, found that it blocked phorbol ester-induced contraction of rat aortic rings, but had minimal effect (13% inhibition) on ET-1-induced contractions. This may be related to a inhibitory effect of PKC on L-type calcium channels in ET-1-stimulated VSMCs *(39)*.

One possible role that PKC appears to play in mediating ET action on vascular smooth muscle is to increase the sensitivity of the contractile elements to Ca^{2+}. When Ca^{2+} is removed or reduced to very low levels in the extracellular solution, ET-1 can stimulate a small, but well-maintained vascular contraction *(35,106,107,112–114)*. Application of low doses of ET-1 causes a leftward shift in the KCl dose-response curve in isolated coronary arteries *(63)* and pulmonary arteries and veins *(106)*. Experiments using L-toxin permeabilized rabbit mesenteric arteries *(108)* and chemically-skinned SMCs from the resistance arteries of the rabbit mesentery *(68)* showed that there was an increase in Ca^{2+} sensitivity via a G protein-dependent pathway involving PKC. This increase in sensitivity was attenuated, but not abolished, by the PKC inhibitor PKC_{19-36}, a peptide fragment corresponding to the autoinhibitory domain of PKC *(68)*. It has been proposed that this shift in Ca^{2+}-sensitivity may involve phosphorylation of light and heavy chain myosin, and caldesmons *(68,109,110)*. More recent studies indicate that ET-1 can also phosphorylate calponin via a PKC-dependent mechanism *(111)*. Together, these results indicate that ET-1 induces a sensitization of contractile mechanism in vascular smooth muscle through PKC-dependent and PKC-independent mechanisms.

PKC also has a prominent role in the regulation of PLC and PLD activities in many tissues *(26)*. It has been postulated that PKC may control phospholipid hydrolysis in vascular smooth muscle by acting as a switch that inhibits PLC-mediated PIP_2 hydrolysis and promotes PLD-mediated phosphatidylcholine hydrolysis. PKC activation blunts ET-1-induced PI hydrolysis in cultured cells *(115,116)*. Additionally, pretreatment with phorbol 12,13 myristate acetate causes a 33% decrease in phosphoinositide turnover, whereas pretreatment with staurosporine, a PKC inhibitor, caused a 75% increase in PI turnover in intact canine coronary artery *(117)*. These data suggest that PKC activation may negatively feedback to limit ET-1-induced PI hydrolysis. Ryu et al. *(118)* have shown that PKC phosphorylates PLC-β, but does not affect PLC-β activity. These authors suggested that PLC-β phosphorylation by PKC may affect its ability to interact with its G protein. As mentioned in Section 2.3.2., PKC is also involved in regulating PLD activity under certain conditions. In sheep pulmonary artery and the A10 VSMC line, Ro-318220 (a PKC inhibitor) blocked stimulation of PLD activity by ET-1 *(41,42)*. Endothelin stimulation of the arachidonic acid metabolism pathway was also blocked by staurosporine *(40)* indicating that PKC may be involved. These results suggest that PKC plays an important role in switching the production of DAG from a PLC pathway to a PLD pathway.

Several studies have documented that ET-1 activates the Na^+-H^+ exchanger in VSMCs *(3,53,54)*. Although this stimulation appears to be mediated in part via a PKC-dependent mechanism *(3,53,54)*, the physiological consequences of this increased Na^+-H^+ exchanger activity in VSMCs remain to be determined. PKC-induced increases in Na^+-H^+ exchanger activity in VSMCs would be expected to increase intracellular pH (pH_i) *(52–54)*, as well as to increase intracellular Na^+ content *(119)*, two important events in regulating vascular contractility and $[Ca^{2+}]_i$. However, ET-1-induced increases in pH can only be shown using bicarbonate-free buffers in cultured VSMCs *(53,120)*. An increase in intracellular Na^+ content could lead to increases in $[Ca^{2+}]_i$ via an increase in Na^+-Ca^{2+} exchanger activity *(119)*. Endothelin-1-induced $[Ca^{2+}]_i$ transients are not affected by inhibiting Na^+-H^+ exchanger activity *(120)*, suggesting that Na^+-Ca^+ exchange is not involved in mediating the effects of ET-1 on $[Ca^{2+}]_i$. Hubel and Highsmith *(120)* have also recently shown that ET-1-stimulated Na^+-H^+ exchange is secondary to an increase in $[Ca^{2+}]_i$. Although external Na^+ removal inhibits ET-1-induced contraction by 50% in rat aorta *(121)*, this phenomenon is most likely explained if Na^+ influx causes membrane depolarization leading to a secondary opening of L-type Ca^{2+} channels and Ca^{2+} influx.

2.6. Tyrosine Kinase Signaling Mechanisms

The involvement of tyrosine protein kinases in G protein coupled receptor-signaling cascades in VSMCs has been appreciated only recently. Koide et al. *(122)* showed that ET-1-induced tyrosine phosphorylation occurs on at least five proteins of about 79, 77, 73, 45, and 40 kDa in cultured aortic VSMCs. The 40 and 45 kDa proteins were shown to be mitogen-activated protein (MAP) kinases ($p44_{mapk}$ and $p42_{mapk}$) which were activated within five min of ET addition *(122)*. More recently, Wilkes et al. *(42)* showed that blocking tyrosine kinase activity with the inhibitor ST271 attenuates ET-1-stimulated PLD activation in the A10 VSMC line. The mechanism by which ET and other G protein kinase receptors stimulate tyrosine phosphorylation is unclear because the cytoplasmic regions of these typical seven transmembrane-spanning receptors lack any intrinsic protein tyrosine kinase domain. However, activation of other G protein coupled receptors, such as angiotensin II and vasopressin, has also been shown to increase tyrosine phosphorylation *(123)*. It has recently been demonstrated that ET is mitogenic for VSMCs in vitro and in vivo *(124)*. Several classes of nonreceptor protein tyrosine kinases have recently been identified that are believed to participate in cell proliferation *(125)*. These preliminary findings have led to the proposal that tyrosine kinase activation plays an important, but still undefined, role in both the contractile and mitogenic responses of VSMCs to ET. Endothelin most likely plays an important role in the long-term activation of mitogenic pathways via activation of both PKC and nonreceptor tyrosine protein kinases.

3. Conclusions

Since the discovery of an endothelium-derived contracting factor ten years ago, there has been an explosive growth of knowledge concerning ET in the cardiovascular system. Initial emphasis was focused at gaining a better understanding of the molecular mechanisms underlying ET-signal transduction. We now know that the three ET isopeptides can interact with at least two receptor subtypes in VSMCs and endothelial cells. Depending on the vascular bed, smooth-muscle cells can contain either ET_A receptors, ET_B receptors or a mixture of both subtypes and their activation results in vasoconstriction. ET_B receptor activation on vascular endothelium is linked to nitric oxide release and vasodilatation. Although Ca^{2+} is an integral component of the ET signaling cascade, it is clear that ET's cellular actions are complex and still incompletely understood. PKC, as well as nonreceptor protein tyrosine kinases, appear to be intrinsically involved in mediating diverse biological responses in VSMCs, such as contraction and mitogenesis. Thus, there is a clear need for additional studies to elucidate PKC and tyrosine kinase pathways in the ET-signaling cascade in VSMCs. Finally, the availability of highly selective ET_A and ET_B receptor antagonists will increase our understanding of the contribution of different receptor subtypes to vascular smooth muscle contraction, as well as of physiological and pathophysiological roles of the ET family in cardiovascular biology.

References

1. Hickey, K. A., Rubanyi, G. M., Paul, R. J., and Highsmith, R. F. (1985) Characterization of a coronary vasoconstrictor produced by cultured endothelial cells. *Am. J. Physiol.* **248**:C550–C556.
2. Yanagisawa, M., Kurihara, H., Kimura, S., Tomobe, Y., Kobayashi, M., Mitsui, Y., Yazaki, Y., Goto, K., and Masaki, T. (1988) A novel potent vasoconstrictor peptide produced by vascular endothelial cells. *Nature (London)* **332**:411–415.
3. Rubanyi, G. M. and Polokoff, M. A. (1994) Endothelins: molecular biology, biochemistry, pharamacology, physiology, and pathophysiology. *Pharmacol. Rev.* **46**:325–414.
4. Arai H., Nori, S., Amori, I., Ohkubu, H., and Nakanishi, S. (1990) Cloning and expression of a cDNA encoding an endothelin receptor. *Nature* **348**:730–732.
5. Sakurai, T., Yanagisawa, M., Takuwa, Y., Miyazaki, H., Kimura, S., Goto, K., and Masaki, T. (1990) Cloning of a cDNA encoding a non-isopeptide-selective subtype of the endothelin receptor. *Nature* **348**:732–735.
6. Karne, S., Ayawickreme, C. K., and Lerner, M. R. (1993) Cloning and characterization of an endothelin-3 specific receptor (ET_C) receptor from *Xenopus Laevis* dermal melanophores. *J. Biol. Chem.* **268**:19,126–19,133.
7. MacLean, M. R., Randall, M. D., and Hiley, C. R. (1989) Effects of moderate hypoxia, hypercapnia, and acidosis on haemodynamic changes induced by endothelin-1 in pithed rat. *Br. J. Pharmacol.* **98**:1055–1065.
8. Davenport, A. P. and Maguire, J. J. (1994) Is endothelin-induced vasoconstriction mediated only by Eta receptors in humans? *TIPS* **15**:9–11.
9. Bax, W. A. and Saxena, P. R. The current endothelin receptor classification: time for reconsideration? *TIPS* **15**:379–386.
10. Warner, T. D., Allcock, G. H., Corder, R., and Vane, J. R. (1993) Use of the endothelin antagonists BQ-123 and PD 142893 to reveal three endothelin receptors mediating smooth muscle contraction and the release of EDRF. *Br. J. Pharmacol.* **110**:777–782.
11. Battistini, B., O'Donnell, L. J., Warner, T. D., et al. (1994) Characterization of endothelin (ET) receptors in the isolated gallbladder of the guinea pig: evidence for an additional ET receptor subtype. *Br. J. Pharmacol.* **112**:1244–1250.

12. Teerlink, J. R., Breu, V., Sprecher, U., Clozel, M., and Clozel, J.-P. (1994) Potent vasoconstriction mediated by endothelin ET_B receptors in canine coronary arteries. *Circ. Res.* **74:**105–114.

13. Neer, E. J. (1995) Heteromeric G-proteins: organizers of transmembrane signals. *Cell* **80:**249–257.

14. Hepler, J. R. and Gilman, A. G. (1992) G-proteins. *TIBS* **17:**383–387.

15. Takuwa, Y., Kasuya, Y., Kudo, N., Yanagisawa, M., Goto, K., Masaki, T., and Yamashita, K. (1990) Endothelin receptor is coupled to phospholipase C via a pertussis toxin insensitive guanine nucleotide binding regulatory protein in vascular smooth muscle cells. *J. Clin. Invest.* **85:**653–658.

16. Reynolds, E. E., Mok, L. L., and Kurokawa, S. (1989) Phorbol ester dissociates endothelin-stimulated phosphoinositide hydrolysis and arachidonic acid release in vascular smooth muscle cells. *Biochem. Biophys. Res. Comm.* **160:**868–873.

17. Simonson, M. S. and Dunn, M. J. (1990) Cellular signaling by peptides of the endothelin gene family. *FASEB J.* **4:**2989–3000.

18. Simonson, M. S. and Dunn, M. J. (1990) Endothelin 1 stimulates contraction of rat glomerular mesangial cells and potentiates beta adrenergic mediated cyclic adenosine monophosphate accumulation. *J. Clin. Invest.* **85:**790–797.

19. Kasuya, Y., Takuwa, Y., Yanagisawa, M., Kimura, S., Masaki, T., and Goto, K. (1992) A pertussis toxin sensitive mechanism of endothelin action in porcine coronary artery smooth muscle. *Br. J. Pharmacol.* **107:**456–462.

20. Muldoon, L. L., Rodland, K. D., Forsythe, M. L., and Magun, B. E. (1989) Stimulation of phosphatidylinositol hydrolysis, diacylglcerol release and gene expression in response to endothelin, a potent new agonist for fibroblasts and smooth muscle cells. *J. Biol. Chem.* **264:**8529–8536.

21. Vigne, P., Breittmayer, J. P., Marsault, R., and Frelin, C. (1990) Endothelin mobilizes Ca^{2+} from a caffeine and ryanodine insensitive intracellular pool in rat atrial cells. *J. Biol. Chem.* **265:**6782–6787.

22. Nestler, E. J. and Duman, R. S. (1994) G-proteins and cyclic nucleotides in the nervous system, in: *Basic Neurochemistry: Molecular, Cellular, and Medical Aspects,* 5th ed. (Siegel, G. J., ed.), Raven, New York.

23. Eguchi, S., Hirata, Y., Imai, T., and Marumo, F. (1993) Endothelin receptor subtypes are coupled to adenylate cyclase via different guanyl nucleotide-binding proteins in vasculature. *Endocrinology* **132(2):**524–529.

24. Aramori, I. and Nakanishi, S. (1992) Coupling of two endothelin receptor subtypes to differeing signal transduction in transfected Chinese hamster ovary cells. *J. Biol. Chem.* **267:**12,468–12,474.

25. Lee, S. B. and Rhee, S. G. (1995) Significance of PIP_2 hydrolysis and regulation of phospholipase C isozymes. *Curr. Opin. Cell Biol.* **7:**183–189.

26. Divecha, N. and Irvine, R. F. (1995) Phospholipid signaling. *Cell* **80:**269–278.

27. Pang, D. C., John, A., Patterson, K., Botelho, L. H., and Rubanyi, G. M. (1989) Endothelin-1 stimulates phosphatidyinositol hydrolysis and

calcium uptake in isolated canine coronary arteries. *J. Cardiovasc. Pharmacol.* **13(Suppl. 5)**:S75–S79.

28. Kasuya, Y., Ishikawa, T., Yanagisawa, M., Kimura, S., Goto, K., and Masaki, T. (1989) Mechanism of contraction to endothelin in isolated porcine coronary artery. *Am. J. Physiol.* **257**:H1828–H1835.

29. Kasuya, Y., Takuwa, Y., Yanagisawa, M., Kimura, S., Goto, K., and Masaki, T. (1989) Endothelin-1 induces vasocontriction through two functionally distinct pathways in porcine coronary artery: contribution of phosphoinositide turnover. *Biochem. Biophys. Res. Commun.* **161(3):** 1049–1055.

30. Van Renterghem, C., Vigne, P., Barhanin, J., Schmid-Alliana, A., Frelin, C., and Lazdunski, M. (1988) Molecular mechanism of action of the vasoconstrictor peptide endothelin. *Biochem. Biophys. Res. Commun.* **157**:977–985.

31. Resink, T. J., Scott-Burden, T., and Buhler, F. R. (1988) Endothelin stimulates phospholipase C in cultured vascular smooth muscle cells. *Biochem. Biophys. Res. Commun.* **157**:1360–1368.

32. Araki, S., Kawahara, Y., Kariya, K., Sunako, M., Fukuzaki, H., and Takai, Y. (1989) Stimulation of phospholipase C mediated hydrolysis of phosphoinositides by endothelin in cultured rabbit aortic smooth muscle cells. *Biochem. Biophys. Res. Commun.* **159**:1072–1079.

33. Sugiura, M., Inagami, T., Hare, G. M., and Johns, J. A. (1989) Endothelin action: inhibition by a protein kinase C inhibitor and involvement of phosphoinositols. *Biochem. Biophys. Res. Commun.* **158**:170–176.

34. Rapoport, R. M., Stauderman, K. A., and Highsmith, R. F. (1990) Effects of EDCF and endothelin on phosphatidylinositol hydrolysis and contraction in rat aorta. *Am. J. Physiol.* **258**:C122–C131.

35. Ohlstein, E. H., Horohonich, S., and Hay, D. W. (1989) Cellular mechanisms of endothelin in rabbit aorta. *J. Pharmacol. Exp. Ther.* **250**:548–555.

36. Homma, Y., Sakamot, H., Tsunda, M., Aoki, M., Takenawa, T., and Ooyama, T. (1993) Evidence for involvement of phospholipase C-d_2 in signal transduction of platelet-derived growth factor in vascular smooth muscle cells. *Biochem. J.* **290**:649–653.

37. Griendling, K. K., Tsuda, T., and Alexander, R. W. (1989) Endothelin stimulates diacylglycerol accumulation and activates protein kinase C in cultured vascular smooth muscle cells. *J. Biol. Chem.* **264**:8237–8240.

38. Sunaka, M., Kawahara, Y., Kariya, K., Tsuda, T., Yokoyama, M., Fukuzaki, H., and Takai, Y. (1990) Mass analysis of 1,2 diacylglycerol in cultured rabbit vascular smooth muscle cells. Comparison of stimulation by angiotensin II and endothelin. *Hypertension* **15**:84–88.

39. Xuan, Y. T., Wang, O. L., and Wharton, A. R. (1994) Regulation of endothelin-induced Ca^{2+} mobilization in smooth muscle cells by protein kinase C. *Am. J. Physiol.* **266**:C1560–C1567.

40. Liu, Y., Geisbuhler, B., and Jones, A. W. (1992) Activation of multiple mechanisms including phospholipase D by endothelin-1 in rat aorta. *Am. J. Physiol.* **262(4 PT1):**C941–C949.

41. Plevin, R., Kellock, N. A., Wakelam, M. J., and Wadsworth, R. (1994) Regulation by hypoxia of endothelin-1 stimulated phospholipase D activity in sheep pulmonary artery cultured smooth muscle cells. *Br. J. Pharmacol.* **112(1)**:311–315.

42. Wilkes, L. C., Patel, V., Purkiss, J. R., and Boarder, M. R. (1993) Endothelin-1 stimulated phospholipase D in A10 vascular smooth muscle derived cells is dependent on tyrosine kinase. *FEBS Lett.* **322(2)**:147–150.

43. Boarder, M. R. (1994) A role for phospholipase D in control of mitogenesis. *TIPS* **15(2)**:57–62.

44. Paul, A. and Plevin, R. (1994) Evidence against a role for phospholipase D in mitogenesis. *TIPS* **15(6)**:174, 175.

45. Axelrod, J., Burch, R. M., and Jelsema, C. L. (1988) Receptor-mediated acivation of phospholipase A_2 via GTP-binding proteins: arachidonic acid and its metabolites as second messengers. *Trends Neurosci.* **11**:117–123.

46. Kim, D., Lewis, D. L., Graziadei, L., Neer, E. J., Barsagi, D., and Clapham, D. E. (1989) G-protein βγ-subunits activate the cardiac muscarinic K^+ -channel via phospholipase A_2. *Nature (Lond.)* **337**:557–560.

47. Needleman, P., Turk, J., Jakshik, B. A., Morrison, A. R., and Lefkowith, J. B. (1986) Arachidonic acid metabolism. *Ann. Rev. Biochem.* **55**:66–102.

48. Shimizu, Y. and Wolfe, L. S. (1990) Arachidonic acid cascade and signal transduction. *J. Neurochem.* **55**:1–15.

49. Schramek, H., Wang, Y., Konieczkowski, M., Simonson, M. S., and Dunn, M. J. (1994) Endothelin-1 stimulates cytosolic phospholipase A_2 activity and gene expression in rat glomerular mesangial cells. *Kidney Int.* **46**:1644–1652.

50. McDonald, T. F., Pelzer, S., Trautwein, W., and Pelzer, D. J. (1994) Regulation and modulation of calcium channels in cardiac, skeletal and smooth muscle cells. *Physiol. Rev.* **74(2)**:365–507.

51. Somlyo, A. P. and Somlyo, A. V. (1994) Signal transduction and regulation in smooth muscle. *Nature (London)* **372**:231–236.

52. Lee, M. W. and Severson, D. L. (1994) Signal transduction in vascular smooth muscle: diacylglycerol second messengers and PKC action. *Am. J. Physiol.* **267**:C659–C678.

53. Brock, T. A. and Danthuluri, N. R. (1992) Cellular actions of endothelin in vascular smooth muscle, in: *Endothelin* (Ruybanyi, G., ed.), Clinical Physiology Series, American Physiological Society, Oxford University Press, New York, pp. 103–124.

54. Pollock, D. M., Keith, T. L., and Highsmith, R. F. (1995) Endothelin receptors and calcium signaling. *FASEB J.* **9**:1196–1204.

55. Little, P. J., Neylon, C. B., Tkachuk, V. A., and Bobik, A. (1992) Endothelin-1 and endothelin-3 stimulate calcium mobilization by different mechanisms in vascular smooth muscle. *Biochem. Biophys. Res. Commun.* **183**:694–700.

56. Clapham, D. E. (1995) Calcium signaling. *Cell* **80**:259–268.

57. Marks, A. R. (1992) Calcium channels expressed in vascular smooth muscle. *Circulation* **86(Suppl. 3)**:III-61–III-67.

58. Kai, H., Kanaide, H., and Nakamura, M. (1989) Endothelin-sensitive intracellular Ca^{2+} store overlaps with a caffeine-sensitive one in rat aortic smooth muscle cells in primary culture. *Biochem. Biophys. Res. Commun.* **158:**235–243.

59. Wagner-Mann, C., Bowman, L., and Sturek, M. (1991) Primary action of endothelin on Ca^{2+} release in bovine coronary artery smooth muscle cells. *Am. J. Physiol.* **260:**C763–C770.

60. Lee, H. C., Galione, A., and Walseth, T. F. (1994) Cyclic ADP-ribose: Metabolism and calcium mobilizing function. *Vitamins and Hormones* **48:**199–257.

61. Goto, K., Kasuya, Y., Matsuki, N., Takuwa, Y., Kurihara, H., Ishikawa, T., Kimura, S., Yanagisawa, M., and Masaki, T. (1989) Endothelin activates the dihydropyridine-sensitive voltage-dependent Ca^{2+} channel in vascular smooth muscle. *Proc. Natl. Acad. Sci. USA* **86:**3915–3918.

62. Takenaka, T., Epstein, M., Forster, H., Landry, D. W., Iijima, K., and Goligorsky, M. S. (1992) Attenuation of endothelin effects by a chloride channel inhibitor, indanyloxyacetic acid. *Am. J. Physiol.* **262:**F799–F806.

63. Inoue, Y., Oike, M., Nakao, K., Kitamura, K., and Kuriyama, H. (1990) Endothelin augments unitary calcium channel currents on the smooth muscle cell membrane of guinea pig portal vein. *J. Physiol. (London)* **423:**171–191.

64. Blackburn, K. and Highsmith, R. F. (1990) Nickel inhibits endothelin induced contractions of vascular smooth muscle. *Am. J. Physiol.* **258:**C1025–C1030.

65. Charbrier, P. E., Auget, M., Roubert, P., Longchampt, M. O., Gillard, V., Guillon, J. M., DelafLotte, S., and Braquet, P. (1989) Vascular mechanisms of action of endothelin-1: effect of Ca^{2+} antagonists. *J. Cardiovasc. Pharmacol.* **13(Suppl. 5):**32–35.

66. Steffan, M. and Russell, J. A. (1990) Signal transduction in endothelin-induced contraction of rabbit pulmonary vein. *Pulm. Pharmacol.* **3:**1–7.

67. D'Orleans-Juste, P., DeNucci, G., and Vane, J. R. (1989) Endothelin-1 contracts isolated vessels independently of dihydropyridine-sensitive Ca^{2+} channel activation. *Eur. J. Pharmacol.* **165:**289–295.

68. Yoshida M., Suzuki, A., and Itoh, T. (1994) Mechanisms of vasoconstriction induced by endothelin-1 in smooth muscle of rabbit mesenteric artery. *J. Physiol.* **477:**253–265.

69. Gardner, J. P., Tokudome, G., Tomonari, H., Maher, E., Hollander, D., and Aviv, A. (1992) Endothelin induced calcium responses in human vascular smooth muscle cells. *Am. J. Physiol.* **262:**C148–C155.

70. Xuan, Y. T., Whorton, A. R., and Watkins, W. D. (1989) Inhibition by nicardipine on endothelin-mediated inositol phosphate formation and Ca^{2+} mobilization in smooth muscle cells. *Biochem. Biophys. Res. Commun.* **160:**758–764.

71. Mitsuhashi, T., Morris, R. C., Jr., and Ives, H. E. (1989) Endothelin-induced increases in vascular smooth muscle Ca^{2+} do not depend on dihydropyridine-sensitive Ca^{2+} channels. *J. Clin. Invest.* **84:**635–639.

72. Simpson, A. W. and Ashely, C. C. (1989) Endothelin evoked Ca^{2+} transients and oscillations in A10 vascular smooth muscle cells. *Biochem. Biophys. Res. Commun.* **163**:1223–1229.

73. Huang, S., Simonson, M. S., and Dunn, M. J. (1993) Mandidipine inhibits endothelin-1 induced $[Ca^{2+}]_i$ signaling but potentiates endothelin's effect on *c-fos* and *c-jun* induction in vascular smooth muscle and glomerular mesangial cells. *Am. Heart J.* **125**:589–597.

74. Wang, R., Karpinski, E., and Pang, P. K. T. (1989) Two types of calcium channels in isolated smooth muscle cells from rat tail artery. *Am. J. Physiol.* **256**:H1361–H1368.

75. Bean, B. P., Sturek, M., Puga, A., and Hermsmeyer, K. (1986) Calcium channels in muscle cells from rat mesenteric arteries: modulation by dihydropyridine drugs. *Circ. Res.* **59**:229–235.

76. Benham, C. D., Hess, P., and Tsien, R. W. (1987) Two types of calcium channels in single smooth muscle cells from rabbit ear artery studied with whole-cell and single channel recordings. *Circ. Res.* **61(Suppl. I)**:I-10–I-16.

77. Yatani, A., Seidel, C. L., Allen, J., and Brown, A. M. (1987) Whole-cell and single-channel calcium currents of isolated smooth muscle cells from saphenous vein. *Circ. Res.* **60**:523–533.

78. Friedman, M. E., Suarez-kurtz, G., Kaczorowski, G. J., Katz, G. M., and Reuben, J. P. (1986) Two calcium currents in a smooth muscle cell line. *Am. J. Physiol.* **250**:H699–H703.

79. McCarthy, R. T. and Cohen, C. J. (1989) Nimodipine block of calcium channels in rat vascular smooth muscle cell lines. Exceptionally high-affinity binding in A7r5 and A10 cells. *J. Gen. Physiol.* **94**:669–692.

80. Sturek, M. and Hermsmeyer, K. (1986) Calcium and sodium channels in spontaneously contracting vascular muscle cells. *Science* **233**:475–478.

81. Amenta, F., Rossodivita, I., and Ferrante, F. (1994) Interactions between endothelin and the dihydropyridine-type calcium channel antagonist nicardipine in human renal artery: a radioligand and autoradiographic study. *J. Auton. Pharmacol.* **14(2)**:129–136.

82. Shetty, S. S. and DelGrande, D. (1994) Inhibition by nickel of endothelin-1-induced tension and associated ^{45}Ca movement in rabbit aorta. *J. Pharmacol. Exp. Ther.* **271**:1223–1227.

83. Simpson, A. W., Stampfl, A., and Ashley, C. C. (1990) Evidence for receptor-mediated bivalent-cation entry in A10 vascular smooth muscle cells. *Biochem. J.* **267**:277–280.

84. Ruegg, U. T., Wallnofer, A., Weir, S., and Cauvin, C. (1989) Receptor-operated calcium-permeable channels in vascular smooth muscle. *J. Cardiov. Pharmacol.* **14(Suppl. 6)**:S49–S58.

85. Van Renterghem, C. and Lazdunski, M. (1994) Identification of the Ca^{2+} current activated by vasoconstrictors in vascular smooth muscle cells. *Pflugers Arch.* **429**:1–6.

86. Blayney, L. M., Gapper, P. W., and Newby, A. C. (1992) Vasoconstrictor agonists activate G-protein-dependent receptor-operated calcium channels in pig aortic microsomes. *Biochem. J.* **282**:81–84.

87. Gordienko, D. M., Clausen, C., and Goligorsky, M. S. (1994) Ionic currents and endothelin signaling in smooth muscle cells from rat renal resistance arteries. *Am. J. Physiol.* **266**:F325–F341.
88. Stockhand, J. D. and Sansom, S. C. (1994) Large Ca^{2+}-activated K^+ channels responsive to angiotensin II in cultured human mesangial cells. *Am. J. Physiol.* **267**:C1080–C1086.
89. Minami, K., Hirata, Y., Tokumura, A., Nakaya, Y., and Fukuzawa, K. (1995) Protein kinase C independent inhibition of the Ca^{2+}-activated K^+ channel by angiotensin II and endothelin-1. *Biochem. Pharmacol.* **49**:1051–1056.
90. Klockner, U. and Isenberg, G. (1991) Endothelin depolarizes myocytes from porcine coronary and human mesenteric arteries through Ca-activated chloride current. *Pflugers Arch.* **418**:168–175.
91. Van Renterghem, C. and Lazdunski, M. (1993) Endothelin and vasopressin activate low conductance chloride channels in aortic smooth muscle cells. *Pflugers Arch.* **425**:156–163.
92. Chen, C. and Wagoner, P. K. (1991) Endothelin induces a nonselective cation current in vascular smooth muscle cells. *Circ. Res.* **69**:447–454.
93. Enoki, T., Miwa, S., Sakamoto, A., Minowa, T., Komuro, T., Kobayashi, S., Ninomiya, H., and Masaki, T. (1995) Long-lasting activation of cation current by low concentration of endothelin-1 in mouse fibroblasts and smooth muscle cells of rabbit aorta. *Br. J. Pharmacol.* **115**:479–485.
94. Bell, R. M. and Burns, D. J. (1991) Lipid activation of protein kinase C. *J. Biol. Chem.* **266**:4661–4664.
95. Niskizuka, Y. (1995) Protein kinase C and lipid signaling for sustained cellular responses. *FASEB J.* **9**:484–496.
96. Stauble, B., Boscoboinik, D., and Azzi, A. (1993) Purification and kinetic properties of protein kinase C from cultured smooth muscle cells. *Biochem. Mol. Biol. Int.* **20**:203–211.
97. Singer, H. A., Oren, J. W., and Benscoter, H. (1989) Myosin light chain phosphorylation in ^{32}P-labelled rabbit aorta stimulated by phorbol-12,13-dibutyrate and phenylephrine. *J. Biol. Chem.* **264**:21,215–21,222.
98. Andrea, J. E. and Walsh, M. P. (1992) Protein kinase C of smooth muscle. *Hypertension* **20**:585–595
99. Khalil, R. A., Lajoie, C., Resnick, M. S., and Morgan, K. G. (1992) Ca^{2+}-independent isoforms of protein kinase C differentially translocated in smooth muscle. *Am. J. Physiol.* **263**:C714–C719.
100. Walsh, M. P., Andrea, J. E., Allen, B. G., Clement-Chomienne, O., Collins, E. M., and Morgan, K. G. (1994) Smooth muscle protein kinase C. *Can. J. Physiol. Pharmacol.* **72**:1392–1399.
101. Lee, T. S., Chao, T., Hu, K. Q., and King, G. L. (1989) Endothelin stimulates a sustained 1,2 diacylglycerol increase and protein kinase C activition in bovine aortic smooth muscle cells. *Biochem. Biophys. Res. Commun.* **162**:381–386.
102. Sperti, G. and Colucci, W. S. (1987) Phorbol ester-stimulated bidirectional transmembrane calcium flux in A7r5 vascular smooth muscle cells. *Mol. Pharmacol.* **32**:37–42.

103. Fisher, R. D., Speriti, G., Colucci, W. S., and Clapham, D. E. (1988) Phorbol ester increases the dihydropyridine-sensitive calcium conductance in a vascular smooth muscle cell line. *Circ. Res.* **62:**1049–1054.

104. Marala, R. B. and Mustafa, S. J. (1995) Adenosine analogues prevent phorbol ester-induced PKC depletion in porcine coronary atery via A1 receptor. *Am. J. Physiol.* **268:**H271–H277.

105. Shimamoto, H., Shimamoto, Y., Kwan, C.-Y., and Daniel, E. (1992) Participation of protein kinase C in endothelin-1 induced contraction in rat aorta: studies with a new tool, calphostin C. *Br. J. Pharmacol.* **107:**282–287.

106. Cardell, L. O., Uddman, R., and Edvinsson, L. (1990) Analysis of endothelin-1 induced contractions of guinea pig trachea, pulmonary veins and different types of pulmonary arteries. *Acta Physiol. Scand.* **139:**103–111.

107. Huang, X. N., Hisayama, T., and Takayanagi, I. (1990) Endothelin-1 induced contraction of rat aorta: contributions made by Ca^{2+} influx and activation of contractile apparatus associated with no change in cytoplasmic Ca^{2+} level. *Naunyn Schmiedibergs Arch. Pharmacol.* **341:**80–87.

108. Nishimura, J., Moreland, S., Ahn, H. Y., Kawase, T., Moreland, R. S., and VanBreeman, C. (1992) Endothelin increases myofilament Ca^{2+} sensitivity in alpha toxin permeabilized rabbit mesenteric artery. *Circ. Res.* **71:**951–959.

109. Abe, Y., Kasuya, Y., Kudo, M., Yamashita, K., Goto, K., Masaki, T., and Takuwa, Y. (1991) Endothelin-1 induced phosphorylation of the 20 kDa myosin light chain and caldesmon in porcine coronary artery smooth muscle. *Jpn. J. Pharmacol.* **57:**431–435.

110. Adam, L. P., Milio, L., Brengle, B., and Hathaway, D. R. (1990) Myosin light chain and caldesmon phosphorylation in arterial muscle stimulation with endothelin-1. *J. Mol. Cell. Cardiol.* **22:**1017–1023.

111. Mino, T., Yuasa, U., Naka, M., and Tanaka, T. (1995) Phosphorylation of calponin mediated by protein kinase C in association with contraction in porcine coronary artery. *Biochem. Biophys. Res. Commun.* **208:**397–404.

112. Kodoma, M., Kanaide, H., Abe, S., Hirano, K., Kai, H., and Nakamura, M. (1989) Endothelin induced Ca independent contraction of the porcine coronary artery. *Biochem. Biophys. Res. Commun.* **160:**1302–1308.

113. Ozaki, H., Sato, K., Sakata, K., and Karaki, H. (1989) Endothelin dissociates muscle tension from cytosolic Ca^{2+} in vascular smooth muscle of rat carotid artery. *Jpn. J. Pharmacol* **50:**521–524.

114. Sakata, K., Ozaki, H., Kwon, S. C., and Karaki, H. (1989) Effects of endothelin on the mechanical activity and cytosolic calcium level of various types of smooth muscle. *Br. J. Pharmacol.* **98:**483–492.

115. Resink, T. J., Scott-Burden, T., Weber, E., and Buhler, F. (1990) Phorbol ester promotes a sustained down-regulation of endothelin receptors and cellular responses to endothelin in human vascular smooth muscle cells. *Biochem. Biophys. Res. Commun.* **166:**1213–1219.

116. Reynolds, E. E., Mok, L. L. S., and Kurokawa, S. (1989) Phorbol ester dissociates endothelin-stimulated phosphoinositide hydrolysis and arachidonic acid release in vascular smooth muscle cells. *Biochem. Biophys. Res. Commun.* **160:**868–873.

117. Calderone, A., Rouleau, J. L., de Champlain, J., Belichard, P., and Stewart, D. J. (1993) Regulation of the endothelin-1 transmembrane signaling pathway: the potential role of agonist-induced desensitization in the coronary artery of the rapid ventricular pacing-overdrive dog model of heart failure. *J. Mol. Cell. Cardiol.* **25**:895–903.

118. Ryu, S. H., Kim, U., Wahl, M. I., Brown, A. B., Carpenter, G., Huang, K., and Rhee, S. G. (1990) Feedback regulation of phospholipase C-b by protein kinase C. *J. Biol. Chem.* **265**:17,941–17,945.

119. Mulvaney, M. J., Aalkjaer, C., and Jensen, P. E. (1991) Sodium-calcium exchange in vascular smooth muscle. *Ann. NY Acad. Sci.* **639**:498–504.

120. Hubel, C. A. and Highsmith, R. F. (1995) Endothelin-induced changes in intracellular pH and Ca^{2+} in coronary smooth muscle: role of Na^+-H^+ exchange. *Biochem. J.* **310**:1013–1020.

121. Zagulova, D. V., Pinelis, V. G., Markov, Kh. M., Storozhevykh, T. P., Medvedev, M. A., Baskahov, M. R., Chabrier, E. P., and Braque, P. (1993) The role of extracellular calcium in the vasocontriction evoked by endothelin-1. *Bull. Eksp. Biol. Med.* **116**:258–260 (abstract).

122. Koide, M., Kawahara, Y., Tsuda, T., Ishida, Y., Shii, K., and Yokoyama, M. (1992) Endothelin-1 stimulates tyrosine phosphorylation and the activities of two mitogen-activated protein kinases in cultured vascular smooth muscle cells. *J. Hypertension* **10**:1173–1182.

123. Hollenberg, M. D. (1994) Tyrosine kinase pathways and the regulation of smooth muscle contractility. *TIPS* **15**:108–111.

124. Douglas, S. A., Louden, C., Vickery-Clark, L. M., Storer, B. L., Hart, T., Feuerstein, G. Z., Elliott, J. D., and Ohlstein, E. H. (1994) A role for endogenous endothelin-1 in neointimal formation after rat carotid artery balloon angioplasty. *Circ. Res.* **75**:190–197.

125. Skobat, K. M. (1994) Tyrosine kinases: modular signaling enzymes with tunable specificities. *Chem. Biol.* **2**:509–514.

Chapter 5

Mechanisms of Endothelin-Induced Mitogenesis in Vascular Smooth Muscle

Thomas Force

1. Introduction

The study of signal transduction mechanisms of the endothelin (ET) family of vasoactive peptides is in its infancy compared to the study of growth factor activated pathways. The most proximal mechanisms activated by ETs are well known—activation of phospholipase C-β, and subsequently protein kinase C (PKC), and activation of plasma membrane Ca^{2+} channels. What is only starting to become clear is how these proximal signaling pathways, which are strikingly different from proximal mechanisms activated by growth factors, culminate in the activation of the same protein serine/threonine kinase cascade that has dominated the research on growth factor signaling over the past several years, the c-Raf-1 cascade. To understand ET-induced mitogenesis it is critical to understand how a G protein-coupled receptor activates this and potentially other kinase cascades, because it is primarily protein kinases that transduce signals from cell surface receptors to the nucleus, thus altering the transcription of genes which lead to the mitogenic response. In this chapter I will first explore the role of the ETs as growth factors and discuss candidate modulators or transducers of the mitogenic signal. Then I will focus on two major areas of ET signalling that putatively play major roles in transducing the mitogenic signal: the c-Raf-1/extracellular-signal regulated kinase (ERK), also known as mitogen-activated pro-

From: *Endothelin: Molecular Biology, Physiology, and Pathology*
Edited by R. F. Highsmith © Humana Press Inc., Totowa, NJ

tein kinase (MAP) cascade, which is critical to the mitogenic response to growth factors, and activation of nonreceptor tyrosine kinases including Src, the focal adhesion kinase (FAK), and the Janus kinase (Jak) family with their substrates, the STAT (signal transducers and activators of transcription) family of transcription factors. Finally, I will discuss possible roles for other pathways in the mitogenic response to ETs, including phosphoinositide-3 kinases and protein kinase cascades culminating in the activation of other members of the MAP kinase superfamily such as the stress-activated protein kinases (SAPKs) and p38. Because the ET_A, but not ET_B receptor appears to be primarily responsible for ET signaling in vascular smooth muscle cells (1) much of the work that will be reviewed herein derives from studies in which endothelin-1 (ET-1) was used as agonist in cells which signal primarily via the ET_A receptor. Although relatively little is known about signalling triggered by the other ETs acting via the ET_B receptor, with the recent discovery of the role of the ET_B receptor and ET-3 in megacolon (2,3) and the production of ET_B-specific antagonists, this deficiency should soon be corrected.

2. Endothelin as a Mitogen

ET-1 stimulates growth in a number of different cell lines including vascular smooth-muscle cells (4,5), glomerular-mesangial cells (the contractile cell of the renal glomerulus) (6,7), and a number of fibroblast cell lines (8,9). Although ET-1 alone in some cells is weakly mitogenic (9–11), the vast majority of experiments demonstrate that ET-1 is a comitogen, requiring the presence of low concentrations of serum (<0.5%) or insulin (<5 µg/mL) for maximal mitogenic effect (12; and extensively reviewed in 13). When low concentrations of comitogens are present, the magnitude of the mitogenic effect of ET-1 is comparable to that of EGF and PDGF. ET-1 also produces a synergistic mitogenic effect in combination with submaximal concentrations of growth factors, including EGF and PDGF, or with serum (5,10,11).

Where examined, the mitogenic effect of the endothelins in vascular smooth muscle cells and glomerular mesangial cells is mediated via the ET_A receptor (14–16). This conclusion is based on several lines of evidence: ET-3 is a much less potent mitogen than ET-1 (EC_{50} roughly two orders of magnitude greater for ET-3 vs ET-1); the ET_B-

selective agonists, sarafotoxin 6c and [Ala¹, Ala³, Ala¹¹, Ala¹⁵]ET-1 *(6–21)*, do not stimulate DNA synthesis; and the ET_A-selective antagonist BQ123 completely inhibits DNA synthesis in response to ET-1 *(15,16)*. This is not surprising since the ET_A receptor is the predominant one expressed in these cells in culture. Furthermore, the ET_A receptor appears to be the predominant one expressed in human arterial and venous vascular smooth-muscle cells *(17)*.

Reported half-maximal and maximal concentrations of ET-1 required to induce DNA synthesis in various cell lines, including smooth-muscle cell lines, have varied widely in the literature. Much of this variation is owing to the use of different comitogens, or different concentrations of comitogens, but even where similar experimental protocols were used, differences remain. These differences are probably accounted for, in part, by differences in the number of receptors expressed by the cells. Not surprisingly, Kanse et al. have reported a correlation between ET-1-induced mitogenesis and ET_A receptor number on human vascular smooth-muscle cells *(17)*. The phenotypic state of the smooth muscle cell lines used (differentiated, contractile state vs undifferentiated, proliferating state) also may lead to inconsistent results *(18)*. Simply put, we and others have observed a gradual reduction in responsiveness of glomerular-mesangial cells and A10 vascular smooth-muscle cells to ET-1, whether measured as stimulation of DNA synthesis, increases in cytosolic free $[Ca^{2+}]$, or enhanced tyrosine phosphorylation, as passage number increases. Although the reasons for this are not clear, we have found it to be a constant source of variability in experiments designed to examine the mitogenic response to ET-1.

Because of the aforementioned considerations, it is impossible to compare relative potencies of ET-1 with the other mitogenic vasoactive peptides [angiotensin II (AngII), and arginine vasopressin (AVP)] unless receptor number is known and cell type is taken into account. However, qualitatively, mitogenic responses to the three peptides are similar.

Autocrine effects of ET-1 (and AngII) on mitogenesis must also be considered *(19)*. Following exposure of primary glomerular mesangial cells to ET-1, there is increased expression of PDGF-A and PDGF-B genes and increased secretion of PDGF dimers *(7)*. PDGF secretion was detected 12 h after ET-1 and was maintained for 36 h. Similar effects have been observed in vascular smooth-muscle cells in response to AngII *(20,21)*. This "autocrine growth model" has been postulated to account for the delayed mitogenic response to

ET-1 (and AngII) compared to PDGF (48 vs 24 h) observed in rat aortic smooth muscle cells *(19)*. In support of this model, AngII-induced mitogenesis in these cells is reversed by suramin, a nonspecific growth factor antagonist *(22)*. Although this model may apply to some cell types, it is unlikely to account for all of the mitogenic effects of ET-1 because the mitogenic response is seen as early as 18 h after exposure of cells to ET-1 (T. Force, unpublished observations). Furthermore, the inhibitor of protein synthesis, cycloheximide, fails to block ET-1-induced induction of c-*fos*, indicating synthesis of PDGF, or other growth factors, is not necessary for ET-1-induced induction of this immediate-early gene (IEG) which correlates with the mitogenic response in many types of cells *(14,15)*.

2.1. Signal Transduction Pathways as Potential Modulators of the Mitogenic Response

Many signal-transduction pathways have been proposed as mediators of the mitogenic response to ET-1 (reviewed in *13,23*). When ET-1 binds to the ET_A receptor, phospholipase C-β (PLC-β) is activated, resulting in increases in inositol trisphosphate (IP_3) and diacylglycerol. Although isolated reports have appeared suggesting that the vasoactive peptides may also activate the growth factor-activated PLCγ *(24)*, this does not appear to be the case in the majority of cells (reviewed in *25*). IP_3 releases Ca^{2+} from intracellular stores when IP_3 binds to a specific receptor in the endoplasmic reticulum. Diacylglycerol, together with the increase in Ca^{2+}, activates certain isoforms of PKC. The ET-1 receptor also couples to membrane Ca^{2+} currents. Each of these proximal events, release of Ca^{2+} from internal stores, activation of PKC, and influx of Ca^{2+}, has been postulated to mediate some or all of the mitogenic response to ET-1. In addition, activation of one or more tyrosine kinases has been proposed to be a mediator of ET-1-induced mitogenesis. We will consider the evidence for each.

2.1.1. Increases in Cytosolic-Free [Ca^{2+}]

Depletion of intracellular Ca^{2+} stores can arrest cells at G0, and Ca^{2+} transients can initiate the G0 to G1 transition and gene transcription in many types of cells (*25,26* and references therein). The mechanisms for this are unclear but may involve, in part, activation of the serine/threonine phosphatase, calcineurin, or activation of Ca^{2+}/calmodulin kinase with subsequent activation of the cAMP response element binding protein (CREB) (reviewed in *26,27*). Elevation of cytosolic-free [Ca^{2+}], whether from release of intracellular stores or influx via a receptor-operated channel, a voltage-dependent channel, or capacitative entry via a Ca^{2+} release-activated current (I_{CRAC}), is one of the earliest responses of the cell to ET-1. Not surprisingly, several groups have sought to prove a connection between the [Ca^{2+}] transient and the mitogenic response. Pretreatment of cells with either of two blockers of the dihydropyridine-sensitive voltage-dependent Ca^{2+} channel, nifedipine or nicardipine, significantly reduced DNA synthesis by vascular smooth muscle cells in response to ET-1 *(11,12,28)*. Similar results were reported for HeLa cells pretreated with the Ca^{2+} chelator EGTA *(29)*. Although nonspecific effects of these agents must be considered, these data suggest Ca^{2+} influx may be an important component of the mitogenic response to ET-1. As noted, however, mechanisms of this effect are purely speculative and generation of a Ca^{2+} transient alone is not sufficient to induce mitogenesis.

2.1.2. PKC Activation

Exposure of smooth-muscle cells or fibroblasts to ET-1 induces a prolonged (>20 min) increase in diacylglycerol levels and, not surprisingly, activates PKC as determined by translocation to the membrane of kinase activity or phosphorylation of a PKC substrate *(30,31)*. Phorbol ester responsive isoforms of PKC are, in general, susceptible to "downregulation," the process of markedly reducing levels of certain isoforms of PKC by prolonged exposure (24 h or more) to high concentrations (>100 n*M*) of phorbol ester *(32)*. Most studies have suggested that downregulation of PKC attenuates the mitogenic response *(8,9,15)*, protein synthesis *(33)*, and expression of the immediate-early gene, c-*fos* *(5)* in response to ET-1. In support of a requirement for a functioning PKC pathway, various inhibitors of PKCs, including H7 and sangivamycin, have also been reported to inhibit [^{3}H]thymidine incorporation or protein synthesis *(15,33)*.

Thus one or more phorbol ester-sensitive PKC isoforms appear to be necessary for ET-1-induced mitogenesis in many types of cells. Activation of PKCs by phorbol esters do not, however, appear to be sufficient for mitogenesis in these same cells. Neither the phorbol ester, PMA, nor the cell permeant diacylglycerol analog, 1-oleoyl 2-acetyl-*sn*-glycerol (OAG), enhanced [^{3}H]thymidine uptake in glomerular mesangial cells *(15)*. Candidates for the additional factors necessary to transduce the mitogenic signal include phorbol ester-insensitive PKCs or one or more nonreceptor tyrosine kinases.

2.1.3. Tyrosine Kinase Activation

The other signal transduction pathway that appears critical to ET-1-induced mitogenesis is activation of a tyrosine kinase. It has been clear for some time that ET-1 activates one or more tyrosine kinases as evidenced by the phosphorylation on tyrosine residues of several cytosolic proteins ranging in molecular weight from 45 to 225 kDa *(32,34–36)*. Furthermore, activation of the tyrosine kinase pathway is independent of PKC downregulation and occurs despite pretreatment of cells with various PKC inhibitors, making it a candidate pathway to transduce the PKC-independent mitogenic signal *(32)*. The most convincing evidence to date that a tyrosine kinase(s) is critical to the mitogenic response to ET-1 is based on the use of two chemically unrelated tyrosine kinase inhibitors, genistein and herbimycin A. Pre-treatment of glomerular mesangial cells with either of these agents virtually eliminated the mitogenic response to ET-1 (100 n*M*) whereas daidzein, an inactive compound related to genistein, was ineffective *(15)*. Furthermore, an ET-1-induced increase in expression of the IEG, c-*fos*, is only minimally decreased by PKC downregulation but is markedly decreased by the tyrosine kinase inhibitors.

These data, taken together, indicate that one or more isoforms of phorbol ester-sensitive PKCs and one or more nonreceptor tyrosine kinases transduce the mitogenic signal to the nucleus. For the PKCs, it is likely that the effect is mediated, at least in part, by the c-Raf-1 protein kinase cascade that culminates in the activation of the ERKs, which in turn appear to transduce the signal to the nucleus and activate transcription by phosphorylating certain transcription factors. In addition to PKC-induced activation of this cascade, there may be other mechanisms whereby ET-1 activates this cascade (*see* Section 3.1.). For the tyrosine kinase pathway, at least two kinases, Src and FAK, and possibly members of a third family, the Jaks, appear to be activated by ET-1. These kinases play critical roles in the reorganization of the cytoskeleton and may mediate, in part, the phenomenon of anchorage-dependent growth. The Jaks activate the STAT family of transcription factors, which appear to be important components in the response to a wide array of cytokines *(37,38)*. In the sections to follow, I will discuss each of these pathways, what is known about their activation, and how they might play a role in the transduction of the endothelin-induced mitogenic signal to the nucleus.

3. Signal Transduction Mechanisms of Mitogenesis

3.1. The c-Raf-1/ERK Cascade

The mitogen-activated protein (MAP) kinases, p42 and p44, also known as extracellular signal regulated kinases (ERKs)-1 and -2, were initially identified as two protein kinases that became phosphorylated on tyrosine in response to insulin and other growth factors *(39)*. The ERKs, in turn, phosphorylated and activated another serine/threonine kinase, p85^{rsk}, the ribosomal S6 protein kinase *(40)*. This, plus their activation by growth factors, strongly suggested the ERKs were involved in the mitogenic response, but it was not clear how they were activated or what role they played in transducing the mitogenic signal.

It had been known for some time that expression of the viral oncogene v-*raf* led to a grossly transformed phenotype in NIH3T3 fibroblasts *(41–43)*. v-*raf* encodes a constitutively active protein serine/threonine kinase. The protooncogene product, c-Raf-1, was, like the ERKs, potently activated by growth factors. The crucial observations placing these two kinases on a protein kinase cascade and identifying c-Raf-1 as "upstream" of the ERKs greatly advanced our understanding of how the mitogenic signal might be transduced from the growth-factor receptor at the cell surface to the nucleus *(44–46)*.

A wealth of data in multiple types of cells now suggest that activation of the c-Raf-1/ERK kinase cascade (Fig. 1) is both necessary and sufficient for the mitogenic response to a variety of stimuli *(47–50)*. Dominant interfering mutants of various components of the cascade inhibit the mitogenic response to growth factors and constitutively active components activate mitogenesis or transformation, even in the absence of growth factors. It is not surprising, therefore, that ET-1 activates this cascade in fibroblasts, glomerular mesangial cells, and vascular smooth muscle cells *(51–53)*. Clearly, to understand how ET-1 signals mitogenesis, it is critical to understand this cascade and how ET-1 activates it. Although much of the pathway was elucidated in growth factor-stimulated cells, the identical pathway, at least from c-Raf-1 to the ERKs, is utilized in response to ET-1.

Using (PDGF) as an example, the cascade, as currently defined, is activated by simultaneous binding of a PDGF dimer to two receptors, forming a receptor dimer *(54)*. The dimerized receptors, with intrinsic tyrosine kinase activity, then "autophosphorylate" or, more correctly, cross-phosphorylate several tyrosine residues within the receptor *(55)*. One phosphotyrosine residue within the kinase domain

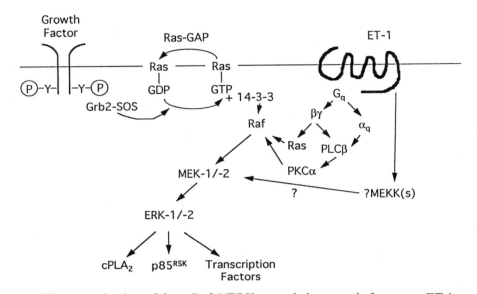

Fig. 1. Activation of the c-Raf-1/ERK cascade by growth-factors vs ET-1. On the left, the growth-factor stimulated cascade, as described in the text, is shown. Following growth factor binding, the receptors dimerize and cross phosphorylate, activating the receptor's intrinsic tyrosine kinase. Grb2 complexed with the guanine nucleotide exchange factor, mSOS, binds via its SH2 domain to a phosphotyrosine residue in the receptor. This culminates in exchange of GDP for GTP on Ras, thus activating Ras. Ras, plus another factor, probably the 14-3-3 proteins, stimulates c-Raf-1, triggering activation of the rest of the cascade. On the right, activation of the cascade by ET-1 is illustrated. Although PKCα can activate c-Raf-1, there is at least one PKC-independent, ET-1-stimulated pathway to c-Raf-1 activation, probably involving βγ-induced activation of Ras. In addition, there may be a third pathway involving activation of a MEK kinase (MEKK) which phosphorylates and activates MEK-1 (or MEK-2).

enhances catalytic activity of the receptor's tyrosine kinase. Several other phosphotyrosine residues outside the kinase domain act as docking sites for signal-transducing molecules. These signal-transducing molecules interact with the various phosphotyrosine residues on the receptor via Src homology 2 (SH2) domains, first identified in the nonreceptor tyrosine kinase, Src. These SH2 domains are composed of approx 100 amino acids and interact with phosphotyrosine residues but not unphosphorylated tyrosine residues. Which phosphotyrosine a particular SH2 domain interacts with is largely determined by the three amino acids immediately carboxy-terminal to the phosphotyrosine *(56)*.

SH2 domain-containing proteins bound to the receptor then propagate the signal by one of two mechanisms: by changing the subcellular localization of another signal-transducing protein to which the SH2 domain-containing protein is also bound, or by inducing an allosteric change in a protein, which alters its catalytic activity. The former mechanism is utilized in the growth factor-induced activation of Ras, and is mediated by the SH2-containing protein growth factor receptor bound protein 2 (Grb2) (Fig. 1). Grb2 exists in a pre-bound complex in the cytoplasm with mSOS [the guanine nucleotide exchange factor (GEF) homologous to Drosophila son of sevenless]. Grb2 and mSOS bind via interaction of the former's SH3 domain with a short proline-rich sequence in mSOS (reviewed in *57*). When, for example, the EGF receptor autophosphorylates, Grb2 binds to a specific phosphotyrosine residue via its SH2 domain, bringing mSOS to the membrane where its substrate, Ras, is located. mSOS then catalyzes the exchange of GDP for GTP on Ras, and Ras is activated. Catalytic activity of mSOS does not appear to be regulated, and thus activation of Ras appears to occur solely as a result of the change in the localization of mSOS.

GTP-loaded Ras then binds several signaling molecules, including c-Raf-1 *(58)*, rasGAP (the GTPase-activating protein that enhances the intrinsic GTPase activity of Ras, thus inactivating it), and a phosphoinositide 3 kinase (PI3K, *see* Section 3.8.). c-Raf-1 binds to Ras via a region in its N-terminus, residues 51–131, contained in the CR1 region (conserved region 1, a region conserved in mammalian, *Drosophila*, and *Caenorhabditis elegans* Raf homologs) *(58)*. If CR1 is overexpressed in cells, it functions as a dominant negative inhibitor of signal transduction induced by activated Ras or growth factors, presumably by competing with full-length c-Raf-1 for Ras-GTP *(59)*.

Additional components are required to activate c-Raf-1, however, because coincubation of purified GTP-loaded Ras with c-Raf-1 fails to activate the latter. It now seems clear that the primary function of activated Ras is simply to bring c-Raf-1 to the cell membrane, because targetting c-Raf-1 to the membrane by attaching a membrane localization signal (CAAX box plus a polybasic domain) is sufficient to activate c-Raf-1, even in the presence of dominant negative Ras *(60,61)*. However, c-Raf-1 is not fully activated in this setting unless growth factor is also added. Thus it appears that once c-Raf-1 arrives at the membrane, it interacts with an additional, mitogen-dependent factor that is responsible for full activation of c-Raf-1. Activation presumably occurs when the inhibitory amino-terminal regulatory domain of c-Raf-1, which normally masks the kinase domain, swings out of the way of the kinase domain, freeing it to interact with its target *(62)*. The importance of this regulatory domain is best seen with truncation mutants of c-Raf-1 lacking the regulatory domain, such as BXB-Raf, which is highly transforming *(44,62)*.

There are several candidate cofactors/activators of c-Raf-1 that have been identified in yeast two-hybrid screens or by coimmunoprecipitation or affinity chromatography. The most likely group are the 14-3-3 family of proteins, which have been implicated in remarkably diverse roles, including activation of enzymes involved in neurotransmitter release and of Ca^{2+}-activated phospholipase A_2, and inhibition of PKC. The β isoform, identified in a yeast two-hybrid screen, associates with the N-terminal regulatory domain of c-Raf-1 *(63)*. Each 14-3-3 molecule binds two c-Raf-1 molecules (reviewed in *64*). The 14-3-3 protein appears to allow c-Raf-1 to dimerize more effectively when it is brought to the cell membrane by GTP-bound Ras. The dimerization appears to be critical for activation of c-Raf-1 kinase activity, and may bring about crossphosphorylation of one c-Raf-1 molecule by the other *(64)*.

Although c-Raf-1 is clearly activated by ET-1, it is not clear that this activation proceeds via Ras. G protein coupled receptors, such as the m2 muscarinic receptor, the α_2-adrenergic receptor, the thrombin receptor, and the receptor for lysophosphatidic acid clearly activate guanine nucleotide exchange by Ras, resulting in an increase in the percent of GTP bound and active Ras *(65–67)*. This effect appears to be mediated primarily via a pertussis toxin sensitive G protein, possibly Gi, Go, or βγ subunits. Receptors that signal primarily via Gq do not activate Ras consistently. ET-1 stimulation of Rat-1 cells or BC3H1 smooth-muscle cells, and carbachol stimulation of Rat-1 cells transfected with the m1 muscarininc receptor do not increase Ras-GTP *(65,66)* (T. Force, unpublished observations), yet both potently activate c-Raf-1 *(51,68)*. In contrast, ET-1 does activate Ras and a dominant inhibitory mutant of Ras blocks ET-1 induction of c-*fos* in glomerular mesangial cells *(52)*, indicating that the mechanisms of ET-1-dependent activation of c-Raf-1 are cell-type specific.

Cotransfection of the m1 muscarinic receptor with a dominant inhibitory mutant of ras or with Rap1a (which antagonizes effects of Ras by competing for similar substrates) blocked ERK-2 activation in response to carbachol *(69)*. Overexpression of α subunits had no effect on ERK-2 activity but overexpression of βγ subunits alone led to marked activation of ERK-2, an effect that was prevented by expression of the Ras inhibitory proteins. These data suggest that in susceptible cells, βγ subunits may activate the c-Raf-1/ERK cascade by somehow activating Ras.

In all studies employing overexpression of dominant inhibitory mutants, caution must be exercised in interpreting inhibition of an effect (ERK-2 activation by βγ) by overexpression of a dominant negative construct (N-17Ras) as evidence that the normal protein (Ras) is involved in activation. N17-Ras has a decreased affinity for GTP and is defective in the GTP exchange process, effectively tying up GEF such as mSOS *(70)*. Thus, the dominant negative Ras protein may be simply competing with a protein on an entirely different pathway (e.g., a small G protein other than Ras or a heterotrimeric G protein) for GEFs.

Taken together, the data suggest that alternative routes to c-Raf-1 activation are employed by some G_q-linked receptors in certain types of cells. One such route of ET-1-induced c-Raf-1 activation may be via activation of PKC. c-Raf-1 can be phosphorylated and activated by PKC in vitro *(71,72)*. PKCα phosphorylates c-Raf-1 at two serine residues which may be important for kinase activation, and coexpression of PKCα and c-Raf-1 in SF9 insect cells activates c-Raf-1, albeit modestly *(72)*. This has not been a consistent observation, however *(73)*. Furthermore, mutation of the residues phosphorylated by PKCα did not prevent activation of c-Raf-1 in insect cells when co-expressed with Ras and Src *(72)*. Arginine vasopressin, which signals via the V_1 receptor and a pertussis toxin insensitive G protein coupled to phospholipase C in VSMC, activates ERKs (and presumably c-Raf-1) via a PKC-dependent pathway *(74)*. In COS cells transfected with the m1 muscarinic (G_q-linked) receptor and NIH3T3 cells stably expressing the receptor, however, carbachol-induced c-Raf-1 (and ERK-2) activation was only minimally inhibited by PKC downregulation by prolonged phorbol ester treatment or by a putatively specific PKC inhibitor, GF 109203X *(68,75)*. Furthermore, DNA synthesis and focus formation were unaffected by PKC inhibition. We have found that downregulation of susceptible PKC isoforms in glomerular mesangial cells minimally inhibits c-Raf-1 activation in response to ET-1. Although the data suggest PKC isoforms may, in some circumstances, activate c-Raf-1, the activation is modest and inconsistent. Furthermore, in many cells, it appears that G-protein-coupled receptors, including those coupled to G_q, can activate c-Raf-1 via pathways independent of the classical PKC isoforms.

Phosphatidylcholine-specific phospholipase C (PC-PLC) (reviewed in *76*), presumably acting via its primary product, diacylglycerol, has also been proposed to be a c-Raf-1 activator *(77)*. Expression of PC-PLC activates c-Raf-1 and the activation is not prevented by downregulation of PKCs. We have directly assayed species of diacylglycerol for their ability to activate c-Raf-1, and found the activation to be minimal (1.5-fold vs >100-fold for PKC) *(78)*. Thus diacyglycerol does not appear to play any direct role in the activation of c-Raf-1.

Activation of members of the Src family of nonreceptor tyrosine kinases (*see* Section 3.6.1.) has been suspected to play a direct role in activation of c-Raf-1 in some situations (T-cell-receptor activation and IL-2 stimulation) (reviewed in *(62)*. Because c-Raf-1 is not phosphorylated on tyrosine in response to ET-1 *(51)*, this mechanism plays no role in endothelin signalling, though an indirect effect of Src is possible.

Agents that increase cellular levels of cAMP have been known for some time to interfere with the actions of growth factors. This effect appears to be via inhibition of activation of the c-Raf-1/ERK cascade by inhibiting the coupling of GTP loaded Ras to c-Raf-1 *(79,80)*. The mechanism involves cAMP-induced activation of protein kinase A, which then phosphorylates c-Raf-1 on Ser43 within the regulatory domain of c-Raf-1. This phosphorylation reduces the affinity with which c-Raf-1 binds to Ras *(79)*. This raises the possibility that ET-1-induced inhibition of adenylyl cyclase could play a role in enhancing c-Raf-1 activation. Although this mechanism is unlikely to be the primary mechanism of activation of c-Raf-1, simultaneous exposure of cells to ET-1 and an activator of protein kinase A can be expected to reduce the mitogenic effect of ET-1 *(53)*.

In summary, although we know that ET-1 clearly activates c-Raf-1, the mechanism of that activation remains somewhat uncertain in most types of cells, including vascular smooth muscle cells. This is one of the critical problems which need to be solved before the mechanisms of endothelin-induced mitogenesis can be fully understood.

3.2. Downstream of c-Raf-1

Components of the signalling cascade downstream of c-Raf-1 have been identified and their mechanisms of activation determined (Fig. 2). Once activated, c-Raf-1 initiates activation of a cascade of serine/threonine kinases which culminate in signaling the nucleus. The only known physiologic substrates of c-Raf-1 are MAP/ERK

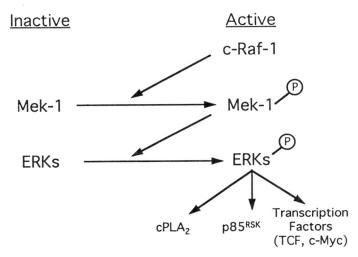

Fig. 2. The c-Raf-1/ERK serine/threonine kinase cascade. Phosphorylation of MEK-1 by active c-Raf-1 activates MEK-1, which, in turn, phosphorylates and activates ERK-1 and ERK-2. Various targets of the ERKs are also shown.

Kinase-1 (MEK-1) and MEK-2, although the former appears to be the preferred substrate *(81)*. MEK-1 is phosphorylated on two serine residues within kinase subdomain VIII by c-Raf-1 *(82)*. Expression of constitutively active forms of MEK-1, made by mutating these phosphorylation sites to acidic amino acids, which presumably function as phosphorylated residues, is sufficient to activate mitogenesis in fibroblasts *(48,49)*. These data strongly support the concept that activation of the ERKs is sufficient to activate mitogenesis and that the key downstream kinases are the ERKs, not components of a divergent pathway activated by Ras or c-Raf-1. MEK kinase-1 (MEKK-1) can also phosphorylate and weakly activate MEK-1 *(83)*. This, plus its similarity to a yeast kinase, Ste11 (for Sterile 11, so named because yeast with mutations in the gene do not mate normally in response to pheromone), which is downstream of a heterotrimeric G protein in yeast (reviewed in *84*), led some to postulate it might be the missing connection in the G protein pathway to the ERKs. Activation of MEK-1 by MEKK-1 appears to be an artefact of overexpression of MEKK-1, however, and is probably not physiologically relevant *(85)*. Rather, MEKK-1 appears to be on the pathway culminating in activation of the SAPKs (*see* Section 3.7.) *(85)*.

MEK-1, and the closely related MEK-2, are dual specificity kinases, phosphorylating tyrosine as well as serine/threonine residues. MEK-1 phosphorylates a TEY motif in subdomain VIII of ERK-1 and ERK-2 *(86)* and at present, the only known substrates of MEK-1 are ERK-1 and ERK-2.

As noted, there seems to be no question that the ERKs are major effectors of the mitogenic signal, whether generated by a growth factor or a G protein coupled receptor. They are "proline-directed" kinases, having as their consensus phosphorylation sequence motif S/TP. In contrast to the remarkable substrate specificity of c-Raf-1 and MEK-1, which probably serves to isolate this pathway from other mammalian MAP kinase pathways *(see* Section 3.7.), the ERKs have many substrates, including $cPLA_2$ and other protein kinases including the 85 kDa (but not the 70 kDa) ribosomal S6 kinase. However, this discussion will focus on those substrates that might transduce the mitogenic signal within the nucleus, the transcription factors.

3.3. Regulation of Transcription by the ERKs

3.3.1. Translocation to the Nucleus

Although the ERKs have been characterized as cytosolic proteins, following mitogenic stimulation, a portion of the cytosolic pool translocates to the nucleus *(87,88)*. Interestingly, in the PC12 chromaffin cell line, prolonged activation of the ERKs following fibroblast growth factor (FGF) leads to translocation to the nucleus of the ERKs and differentiation of the cells into sympathetic neurons, whereas exposure of cells to EGF leads to transient activation, no detectable translocation, and proliferation. In fibroblasts, however, exposure to FGF or other growth factors leads to prolonged activation and translocation of the ERKs into the nucleus, and the response is proliferative (reviewed in *50*).

Pouyssegur and coworkers have studied the time-course of ERK activation in response to growth factors and agonists with heterotrimeric G protein-coupled receptors, and determined how this correlates with the mitogenic response *(87,89)*. From their data it is clear that irrespective of the type of agonist, if the agonist leads to prolonged activation of the ERKs (> 3 h), the ERKs translocate to the nucleus. Furthermore, they found that prolonged activation and nuclear translocation correlated highly with induction of mitogenesis. The intensity and percentage of nuclei immunolabeled with anti-ERK antibody correlated well with the relative ability of various mitogens (serum, FGF, thrombin, phorbol esters, thrombin-receptor peptide) to stimulate DNA synthesis. This work was done with thrombin, which is linked to a G_i-coupled receptor, as agonist, and it is not clear that sustained activation of the ERKs is necessary for ET-1-induced mitogenesis. In Swiss 3T3 fibroblasts, ET-1 (10 nM) caused only very transient activation of the ERKs whereas basic FGF (5 ng/mL) produced sustained activation. Despite these differences, both agonists were highly mitogenic *(90)*.

Simonson and Dunn have found that exposure of glomerular mesangial cells to ET-1 induces translocation of both ERK-1 and ERK-2 into the nucleus (discussed in *87*). This is a critical observation because it confirms that following ET-1, as with the growth factors, the activated ERKs have access to those potential substrates which determine the genetic response to ET-1, transcription factors.

3.3.2. Activation of Transcription

Activation of the c-Raf-1/ERK cascade is, as noted above, both necessary and sufficient for the mitogenic response. One hallmark of the action of most mitogens is that several immediate-early genes are rapidly induced. Following exposure to ET-1, at least four of these immediate-early genes, including c-*fos*, *Egr*-1, c-*jun*, and c-*myc*, are induced. The ERKs appear to play a role in either the induction of, and/or activation of the products of, each of these genes. In this section, I will explore the likely mechanisms of these effects, and propose that the ERKs, via modulation of these and other transcription factors, play a major role in activating the complex genetic program culminating in mitogenesis.

3.3.3. Activation of AP-1 and Induction of c-*fos*

The transcription factor, AP-1, typically consists of a heterodimer of a c-Jun family member (c-Jun, JunB, or JunD) and a member of the *fos* family (c-Fos, FosB, Fra-1, or Fra-2)(reviewed in *91*). Regulation of AP-1 activity is extremely complex and can be modulated by increases in DNA binding or transactivating activities of one or both components of the dimer, or by increases in the abundance of one or more components *(91)*. AP-1 binds to a palindromic motif TGAC/GTCA present in the promoters of numerous genes and, in response to mitogens, regulates transcription of those genes. One of the genes regulated by AP-1 is the human collagenase gene *(92)*. ET-1 induces collagenase and enhances transcription from a reporter construct containing the AP-1 site of the collagenase gene fused to CAT, strongly suggesting AP-1 is activated in response to ET-1 *(14,15)*.

One mechanism of activation of AP-1 by ET-1 clearly seems to involve enhanced expression of c-*fos (14)*. c-*fos* is rapidly induced following exposure of vascular smooth muscle cells and glomerular mesangial cells to ETs *(5,12,14,15)*. Induction of c-*fos* is controlled by at least two major regulatory elements of the promoter of c-*fos*. The first, called the calcium response element (CaRE), is bound by the cAMP response element binding protein (CREB). CREB may be activated not only by increases in cAMP but also in a Ca^{2+}-dependent manner by phosphorylation of Ser 133 of CREB by calcium/calmodulin kinases *(26)*. Thus the ET-1-induced cytosolic free $[Ca^{2+}]$ transient could trigger expression of c-*fos*. The second regulatory element, called the serum response element (SRE) (Fig. 3), is a *cis*-acting element required for mitogen-induced expression of a number of immediate-early genes (reviewed in *93*). The ERKs phosphorylate a number of transcription factors but the best characterized are the ternary complex factors (TCF), Elk-1 or SAP-1, which together with Serum Response Factor (SRF) form a ternary complex at the SRE of the c-*fos* promoter and control induction *(94,95)*. TCF-Elk-1 is an Ets domain-containing transcription factor. Elk-1 contains two amino-terminal domains that mediate DNA contact and ternary complex formation, and a C-terminal domain that contains several potential ERK phosphorylation sites (S/T-P). The other component of the ternary complex, SRF, is not an ERK substrate. ERK-1 and ERK-2 readily phosphorylate Elk-1 in vitro, at the same sites that are phosphorylated in vivo in response to mitogens *(94,95)*. After mutation of these phosphorylation sites, the Elk-1 protein is no longer phosphorylated in response to mitogens and cannot enhance transcription from a reporter construct containing the SRE. Dominant negative mutants of components of the c-Raf-1/ERK cascade inhibit activation of Elk-1, strongly suggesting the ERKs are the critical modulators *(59,96)*. Phosphorylation of Elk-1 by the ERKs appears to enhance both transactivating activity and DNA-binding activity (ternary complex formation) of Elk-1, though the physiologic significance of the latter is uncertain because Elk-1 and SRF appear to exist as a prebound complex at the SRE *(95)*. These data, and the recent finding that a dominant inhibitory mutant of Ras inhibits ET-1-dependent induction of c-*fos (52)*, strongly suggest that ERK-induced activation of Elk-1 or related TCFs is in large part responsible for the induction of c-*fos* following exposure to ET-1. c-Fos then forms a stable heterodimer with c-Jun and the dimer binds to various promoter targets (e.g., collagenase) via the AP-1 motif.

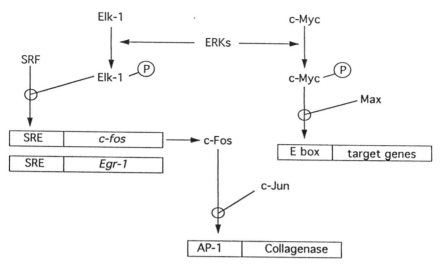

Fig. 3. Mechanisms of activation of transcription by ERK-1 and ERK-2. ERK-induced phosphorylation of Elk-1 and c-Myc increases transactivating activity of the transcription factors at target genes with promoters containing the SRE or the E box, respectively. Elk-1 and c-Myc bind to these elements as dimers with SRF and Max, respectively (dimerization is indicated by a circle). The resulting induction of c-*fos* provides one mechanism of ERK-induced AP-1 activation.

Other mechanisms could contribute to ET-1-induced activation of AP-1. Transactivating activity of c-Fos is increased by phosphorylation within the transactivation domain, catalyzed by a putative MAP kinase, the 88 kDa Fos regulating kinase (FRK) *(97)*. It is not known whether ET-1 activates this kinase, or even whether ET-1 enhances transactivating activity of c-Fos.

ET-1 could also increase AP-1 activity by modulating the abundance or activity of c-Jun. Expression of c-jun does increase following ET-1 *(14)*, although the role of increased levels of c-Jun in AP-1 activation are unclear. The DNA binding and transactivating activities of c-Jun are regulated in response to mitogens by posttranslational modifications. The carboxy-terminal region of c-Jun contains a DNA binding domain followed by a leucine zipper motif that mediates dimerization. The amino-terminal region contains a transcriptional-activation domain *(98)*. DNA binding activity is inhibited by phosphorylation of three or four sites adjacent to the DNA binding domain, and enhanced by dephosphorylation. In resting cells, these sites are generally phosphorylated. Mitogen stimulation leads to dephosphorylation of these sites and enhances DNA-binding *(99)*, although the mechanism of this dephosphorylation is unclear. It is not clear whether the ERKs are involved in regulation of c-Jun DNA-binding activity. Some evidence suggests, however, that the ERK substrate, p85 ribosomal S6 kinase, may phosphorylate and inactivate glycogen synthase kinase-3 (GSK-3) which is a candidate c-Jun DNA-binding domain kinase *(99,100)*. Inactivation of GSK-3 could, therefore, enhance DNA-binding activity of c-Jun.

c-Jun transactivating activity is markedly enhanced by phosphorylation of two serine residues, Ser63 and Ser73, within the transactivation domain *(101,102)*. Although these sites are phosphorylated in *ras* transformed cells, and are phosphorylated by the ERKs in vitro, the related MAP kinase family of stress-activated protein kinases (SAPKs) or c-Jun N-terminal kinases (JNKs) phosphorylate the residues much more readily (approximately five- to sevenfold greater at equal MAP-2 phosphorylating activity *(102)*. Furthermore, expression of dominant negative ERK mutants does not inhibit c-Jun activation in cells transformed by oncogenic *ras*. Thus it appears that the ERKs play a minor role at best in regulation of c-Jun transactivating activity. In contrast, given the recent findings suggesting that ET-1 significantly activates the SAPKs (*see* Section 3.7.), it appears that ET-1 modulation of AP-1 activity may also involve enhanced trasactivating activity of c-Jun, in addition to enhanced expression of c-*fos*, which is controlled, in turn, by the ERKs.

3.3.4. Induction of Egr-1

The SRE controls induction of another immediate-early gene, *Egr*-1, which is also induced following ET-1 *(103)* (Fig. 3). *Egr*-1 antisense oligonucleotides block protein synthesis in response to ET-1, suggesting protein synthesis may be controlled by *Egr*-1. Induction of *Egr*-1 is probably modulated by the ERKs via activation of TCF (Elk-1) *(104)*.

3.3.5. Regulation of Other Transcription Factors by the ERKs

The transcription factor, c-Myc, is also the product of an IEG and is rapidly induced in vascular smooth muscle cells and mesangial cells following exposure to mitogens including ET-1 *(5,12,14,15)*. Although no clear-cut target genes for c-Myc have been identified, the *myc* protooncogene product plays an important role in the control of proliferation, differentiation, and apoptosis. c-Myc is a basic helix-loop-helix-leucine zipper (bHLH-ZIP) transcription factor that is active when heterodimerized with Max, another bHLH-ZIP family member *(105)*. The Myc-Max dimer binds to the E-box sequence (CACGTG) and activates transcription from promoters containing this sequence. A major mode of regulation of the activity of Myc, which has a very short half-life, appears to be at the transcriptional level. Myc transcription is tightly regulated as is transcription of another bHLH-ZIP protein, Mad, which competes with Myc for Max. Thus Myc-Max activates while Mad-Max represses transcription from E box-containing target genes *(106)*.

c-Myc activity, like that of Elk-1, is also regulated by posttranslational modifications. The amino-terminus of c-Myc contains a transcriptional-activation domain *(107,108)*. Ser-62 within this domain is necessary for transactivating activity of c-Myc and is phosphorylated in vivo in response to mitogens. This residue is also phosphorylated by an ERK in vitro, and cotransfection of this ERK with the c-Myc transactivation domain fused to the GAL4 DNA-binding domain enhances transcription from a GAL4-CAT reporter construct *(108)*. These data suggest the ERKs, via phosphorylation of Ser-62, enhance transactivating activity of c-Myc and could be responsible, in part, for induction of c-Myc-dependent genes following ET-1.

In *Drosophila*, two Ets domain-containing transcription factors, yan and pointed[P2], which play a critical role in neural development and in cell fate determination in other organs, appear to be regulated by the ERK homolog, Rolled/ERKA *(109,110)*. Activity of yan, which is a transcriptional repressor, appears to be inhibited by phosphorylation whereas pointed[P2], a transcriptional activator, is activated. Because AP1/Ets motifs are major Ras-responsive elements, and serum-, TPA-, and Ras-induced expression from AP1/Ets promoters requires c-Raf-1 *(59)*, it is very likely that multiple other transcription factor targets of the ERKs will be identified in humans.

The ERKs can also phosphorylate the CREB family member, ATF-2, at sites that increase its DNA-binding activity *(111,112)*. ATF-2 mediates adenoviral E1a transformation, and probably mediates induction of c-*jun* and E-selectin. For ATF-2, like c-Jun, however, it appears that the SAPKs, not the ERKs, are the physiologic regulators of DNA-binding activity *(113)*, and the SAPKs or the related MAP kinase, p38, primarily regulate transactivating activity (*see* Section 3.7.) *(114–116)*.

The ERKs or a related kinase may also play a role in translation initiation. PHAS-I, which in the unphosphorylated form binds to the initiation factor 4E (eIF-4E) and inhibits protein synthesis, does not bind to eIF-4E when phosphorylated by the ERKs *(117)*.

In summary (Fig. 3), activation of the c-Raf-1/ERK cascade culminates in the translocation of the ERKs to the nucleus where they phosphorylate and activate two transcription factors, Elk-1 and c-Myc, which are believed to play critical roles in the mitogenic response. The existence of two Ets domain-containing transcription factors in *Drosophila* that are also ERK substrates suggests many other mammalian transcription factors will be identified which are regulated by this pathway. Identifying these substrates, how they are regulated by the ERKs, and what role they play in ET-1-induced mitogenesis, will be a fruitful and vitally important area of research.

3.4. Turning off the ERKs

ERKs are activated by phosphorylation, catalyzed by MEK-1, on a threonine and a tyrosine residue in the motif Thr-Glu-Tyr within the kinase domain. Not surprisingly, incubation of activated ERKs with serine/threonine or tyrosine phosphatases in vitro inactivates the kinase. Recently it has been convincingly demonstrated that a dual-specificity phosphatase (dephosphorylating Ser/Thr and Tyr residues), MKP-1 (MAP kinase phosphatase-1), and its human homolog, CL100, likely inactivate the ERKs by a similar mechanism in vivo *(118,119)*. Regulation of MKP-1 activity appears to be predominantly at the level of transcription and marked increases in MKP-1 mRNA are seen within the first 60 min after exposure of cells to mitogens. Most importantly, overexpression of MKP-1 inhibits Ras-induced DNA synthesis, suggesting MKP-1 is a major negative modulator of the mitogenic response to agonists, such as the growth factors, which act via Ras *(118)*. Induction of MKP-1 occurs in response to ET-1 and it is likely that it is a major counterregulatory mechanism for ET signaling as well.

The c-Raf-1/ERK cascade appears to be negatively regulated at other sites as well. I have discussed the negative modulation of Ras/c-Raf-1 by activators of PKA. In addition, MEK-1, the immediate upstream activator of the ERKs, appears to be negatively regulated by phosphorylation on two threonine residues *(120)*. Phosphorylation at these sites overrides the activating phosphorylations catalyzed by c-Raf-1. These threonine residues lie in a sequence that is predicted to be a substrate for the kinase, p34^{cdc2}, a key regulator of the cell-division cycle *(120)*. It is unlikely that p34^{cdc2} catalyzes these phosphorylations in vivo, since MEK-1 has not been shown to translocate to the nucleus.

3.5. Interaction with the Cell Cycle

Sustained, as opposed to transient, activation of the ERKs appears to be required for many cells to pass the G_1 restriction point and to enter S phase, in which cellular DNA is replicated (reviewed in *50*). Although ERK activation is clearly linked to the cell cycle, it has not been clear where the ERKs might interact with the cell cycle machinery. The D-type cyclins, which are the regulatory (activating) subunits for the cyclin-dependent kinase 4 and 6 (cdk4 and cdk6) catalytic subunits, appear to control the early stages of the transition toward S phase. A critical link between signal transduction and the cell cycle has recently been suggested by the finding that expression of dominant inhibitory mutants of MEK-1or ERK-1, or expression of the MAP kinase phosphatase, MKP-1, inhibited growth factor-dependent expression of cyclin D1. Expression of a constitutively active mutant of MEK-1 increased cyclin D1 expression *(121)*. Although the mechanisms of this effect are not clear, these data represent a clear link between activation of the ERK cascade and entry into S phase.

3.6. Tyrosine Kinase Signaling

The other major signal-transduction system activated by ET-1 that is likely to modulate the mitogenic response is the activation of tyrosine kinases. Nonreceptor tyrosine kinases known or suspected to be activated by ET-1 include Src and possibly related family members, FAK, and the Jaks, any or all of which may play important roles in the mitogenic response.

As noted, ET-1 enhances tyrosine phosphorylation of a number of cellular proteins via activation of one or more tyrosine kinases *(32,34–36)*. Furthermore, activation of the tyrosine kinase(s) appears indispensable for ET-1-induced mitogenesis in glomerular-mesangial cells expressing the ET_A receptor *(15)*. Given the apparent importance of these pathways, we will explore in detail the kinases involved (where known), and their mechanisms of regulation.

3.6.1. The Role of Src

The proteins phosphorylated in response to ET-1 and the kinase(s) potentially responsible for phosphorylating them are only now starting to be identified. The nonreceptor tyrosine kinase, Src, was the first identified tyrosine kinase that was activated in response to ET-1 *(15,122)*. Src is activated only about twofold over control by ET-1 in A10 or BC3H1 smooth muscle cells or glomerular-mesangial cells. However, this is equivalent to the degree of activation observed after the exposure of NIH3T3 cells to the potent mitogen, PDGF *(123,124)* or after exposure of macrophages to CSF-1 *(125)*.

The role played by Src in ET-1-induced mitogenesis is not clear. As noted, tyrosine kinase inhibitors reduced ET-1-stimulated ^{3}H-thymidine incorporation, but this is not necessarily owing to inhibiton of Src. Src does appear to play a vital role in the mitogenic response to growth factors because in NIH3T3 cells, a kinase-inactive Src mutant functioned as a dominant inhibitor of PDGF-activated signaling and inhibited entry of PDGF-stimulated cells into S phase *(126)*. A similar requirement for Src has been demonstrated for CSF-1- and EGF-induced mitogenesis *(126–128)*. Although Src "knock-outs" might seem to be an ideal way in which to address the role of Src in mitogenesis, Src is a member of a large family of nonreceptor tyrosine kinases, including Lyn, Fyn, and Yes, and it appears that there may be significant overlap in function of these kinases *(129)*.

Src-kinase activity is tightly negatively regulated by phosphorylation of Tyr 527, at least in part catalyzed by the carboxy-terminal Src kinase (Csk) and possibly by Src itself *(130–134)* (Fig. 4). Kinase activity is repressed by binding of the SH2 domain of Src to phosphorylated Tyr 527, in effect masking the kinase domain (reviewed in *135*). The oncogenic variant, v-Src, lacks Tyr 527 and is constitutively active as are mutants in which Tyr 527 has been mutated. Src is activated by dephosphorylation of Tyr 527 by an as yet unidentified tyrosine phosphatase. CD45 probably is responsible for activation of Src following T-cell-receptor activation and another transmembrane protein tyrosine phosphatase (RPTPα) may be involved in neuronal differentiation *(136)*, but it is most unlikely that these transmembrane tyrosine phosphatases play any role in the response to ET-1. Following dephosphorylation of Tyr 527, Tyr 416, a residue within the kinase domain, is autophosphorylated, further increasing Src kinase activity (Fig. 4). Not surprisingly, ET-1-induced Src activation in smooth muscle cells is accompanied by transient dephosphorylation of Tyr 527, and activation of Src is inhibited by the tyrosine phosphatase inhibitor, sodium orthovanadate *(122)*.

When Src is activated, its SH2 domain releases from Tyr 527 and the SH2 domain is then free to interact with phosphotyrosine residues on various receptors and signaling molecules *(123,125,137–139)*. In addition, the SH3 domain of Src may bind to various proteins, including Shc, which have proline-rich peptide motifs *(140)*. Finally, signaling proteins containing SH2 domains may complex to Src, presumably via

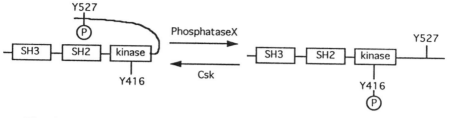

Fig. 4. Mechanisms of activation and inactivation of Src. Tyr 527 (Y527), when phosphorylated by the tyrosine kinase, Csk, interacts with the SH2 domain of Src, in effect, masking the kinase domain. Following ET-1, an unidentified phosphatase (X), dephosphorylates Tyr 527, exposing the kinase domain and allowing phosphorylation of the autophosphorylation site, Tyr 416, and interaction of both the SH2 domain and the kinase domain with Src targets.

interaction of their SH2 domains with phosphotyrosine residues on Src (reviewed in *57,141*). These multiple SH2-phosphotyrosine and SH3-proline-rich region interactions allow the assembly of multiprotein complexes containing signaling proteins, which are candidate modulators of the mitogenic signal. The importance of these complexes in mitogenic signaling is best illustrated by the observations that overexpression of any of three so-called docking proteins, Crk, Shc, or Nck, which contain SH2 and SH3 domains but no obvious enzymatic activity, induces cellular transformation *(142–145)*.

Identification of specific Src substrates or Src associated proteins that might transduce mitogenic signals has been difficult, but there are several candidates. The adaptor protein, Shc, which contains one SH2 domain, has been implicated in the regulation of Ras. In v-*src* transformed cells, Shc is found complexed with Grb2 and mSOS *(146)*. Given the membrane localization of Src, formation of this complex may serve to bring mSOS, the GEF, to the membrane where its substrate, Ras, is located. More recent studies have suggested that G_q- and G_i-linked receptors may indeed activate Ras and the c-Raf-1/ERK cascade via this mechanism, and that Src is activated by a Ca^{2+} transient-dependent activation of Pyk2 or a related tyrosine kinase *(147)*.

We have found that the SH2 domain-containing protein tyrosine phosphatase, Syp, which is highly tyrosine phosphorylated in v-*src* transformed cells *(148)*, does not appear to be regulated in response to ET-1 because Syp is not tyrosine phosphorylated (which appears to be its mechanism of activation) in response to ET-1 and does not form a complex with Src. Although there are many other proteins that interact with Src in v-*src* transformed cells *(138)*, the role of these proteins in the response to ET-1, especially the mitogenic response, are unknown. In summary, although it is likely that Src activation plays a role in ET-1-induced mitogenesis, as it does in the response to growth factors, the phosphatase responsible for activating Src in response to ET-1 is not known, nor are the substrates responsible for transducing the mitogenic signals.

3.6.2. Cytoskeletal Reorganization and the Mitogenic Response

Although the role of cytoskeletal reorganization following exposure of cells to endothelins is only beginning to be explored, it is a common feature of the response of cells to mitogens and to transformation, and therefore is likely to be a component of the mitogenic response to endothelins. In this section, I will discuss what is known about the role of Src and another nonreceptor tyrosine kinase activated by endothelins, FAK, in cytoskeletal reorganization.

Growth factor stimulation induces transient actin reorganization. Elegant work by Ridley and Hall has demonstrated that the small GTP binding protein, Rho, regulates one component of cytoskeletal reorganization, actin stress fiber and focal adhesion formation, while Rac regulates another component, plasma membrane ruffling *(149,150)*. Although not specifically explored with endothelins as yet, other agonists with heterotrimeric G protein linked receptors, including lysophosphatidic acid (LPA) and the neuropeptide, bombesin, which have many signaling pathways in common with ET-1, rapidly stimulate formation of focal adhesions and actin-stress fibers *(149–152)*. Focal adhesions are regions on the ventral-cell surface where integrin receptors interact with extracellular matrix proteins and anchor the cell to that matrix. Because in the cell, actin-filament bundles are attached, the focal adhesions modulate cell-shape change and motility. Focal adhesions are also believed to play a role in the anchorage-dependency of cell growth. Focal adhesions form at sites where actin-stress fibers terminate at the plasma membrane. Importantly, LPA- and bombesin-induced stress fiber formation, which is mediated by Rho, is independent of PKC activation, increases in $[Ca^{2+}]_i$, and increases in cAMP. Stress-fiber formation is, however, dependent on activation of one or more genistein-sensitive tyrosine kinases because genistein markedly inhibits stress-fiber formation in response to these ligands *(152)*. Furthermore, it appears that the tyrosine kinase(s) is downstream of Rho since genistein also inhibits stress fiber formation induced by microinjection of activated Rho protein *(152)*.

Src and/or FAK are likely candidates to be the tyrosine kinases required for stress-fiber and focal-adhesion formation in response to agonists with G protein-linked receptors. FAK is a tyrosine kinase which, unlike many nonreceptor tyrosine kinases, lacks SH2 and SH3 domains *(153,154)*. FAK was first recognized as a tyrosine phosphorylated protein of 125 kDa in v-*src* transformed cells. It is tyrosine phosphorylated in response to transformation with many oncogenes, but this is not a general feature of transformation because FAK is not tyrosine phosphorylated in *ras* transformed cells. Besides being activated by integrin receptor binding, FAK is phosphorylated in response to LPA, vasopressin, and bombesin *(36,155)*, and was the first protein identified that was tyrosine-phosphorylated in response to endothelin *(36,156)*.

The precise role of these kinases in actin cytoskeleton reorganization is not clear, but much evidence suggests they are involved. Src redistributes from endosomal membranes to focal adhesions in response to a variety of stimuli *(157–159)*. This redistribution appears to be directed by dephosphorylation of Tyr 527 *(160)*. As discussed in Section 3.6.1., phosphorylation of Tyr 527 inhibits Src kinase activity by causing an intramolecular association of Tyr 527 with the SH2 domain in the amino-terminal region of the protein. Mutation of Tyr 527 causes a marked redistribution of Src into focal adhesions. In cells lacking Csk, the kinase which phosphorylates Tyr 527, Src is also found predominantly in focal adhesions *(160)*. Interestingly, this redistribution of Src is independent of its kinase activity and appears to be modulated by the SH3 domain in the amino-terminal region, which is presumably freed to interact with targets in the focal adhesion when Tyr 527 is dephosphorylated. Expression of this amino-terminal (noncatalytic) region alone produces larger focal adhesion that, surprisingly, contain greater amounts of phosphotyrosine. These data indicate the amino-terminal region of Src may somehow activate one or more tyrosine kinases or inhibit a tyrosine phosphatase *(160)*.

Stimulation of BC3H1 smooth-muscle cells with ET-1 causes a redistribution of Src to a cytoskeleton-associated (Triton X-100 insoluble) fraction *(122;* and unpublished observations). Although immunofluorescence studies have not been reported, this presumably represents redistribution to focal adhesions. This redistribution of Src is inhibited by the tyrosine phosphatase inhibitor, sodium orthovanadate. These data are consistent with the findings of Kaplan et al.

(160) discussed above, and indicate ET-1 induces redistribution of Src to focal adhesions via dephosphorylation of Tyr 527.

One cannot conclude from these studies that Src or a Src family member is the critical genistein-sensitive tyrosine kinase modulating stress fiber/focal adhesion formation, but mounting evidence suggests that Src may be directly responsible for activation of FAK. FAK is targetted to the focal adhesion by a carboxy-terminal focal adhesion targeting (FAT) domain *(159)*, but activation of FAK requires additional signals. As noted, FAK is densely phosphorylated in v-*src* transformed cells. In addition, Src colocalizes with FAK (in focal adhesions). Furthermore, Src and FAK stably associate with one another and this association occurs via interaction of the SH2 domain of Src with Tyr 397, the major autophosphorylation site of FAK *(161,162)*. It has been postulated that the Src amino terminus, by associating with Tyr 397 of FAK, may protect this residue from dephosphorylation by tyrosine phosphatases, allowing for prolonged activation of FAK *(161)*. Finally, c-Src phosphorylates FAK in vitro on Tyr 576 and Tyr 577, two residues which are critical for FAK activity and are phosphorylated in v-*src* transformed cells *(163)*.

FAK is clearly activated in response to ET-1. Activation is independent of both PKC and the $[Ca^{2+}]_i$ transient *(32,164)*, but does require an intact cytoskeleton because cytochalasin D is a potent inhibitor of ET-1-induced FAK tyrosine phosphorylation. It is not clear what role FAK activation is playing in focal-adhesion formation. Hindering the assignment of a precise role to any of the proteins located within the focal adhesion is the formation of large multiprotein complexes consisting of multiple cytoskeletal proteins and multiple-signaling molecules (reviewed in *159*). For example, FAK may associate with Grb2, which in turn associates with mSOS, conceivably providing a means of activating Ras. FAK may also associate with phosphatidylinositol-3-kinase (PI-3-K) activity, probably via the p85 subunit. As noted, FAK associates with Src which, in turn, associates with the cytoskeletal protein, paxillin and, via the latter, with Csk. Finally, FAK may associate directly with paxillin and Csk. Two components of the focal adhesion, tensin and paxillin, are likely physiologic substrates of FAK because they are tyrosine phosphorylated in the focal adhesion, are substrates of FAK in vitro, and one, paxillin, associates with FAK via a region in the carboxy terminus of FAK *(159)*.

If the role of FAK in forming the focal adhesion is unclear, it is even more unclear what role FAK activation plays in transducing a mitogenic signal. Clearly, based on the findings of several laboratories using a variety of inhibitors, one or more tyrosine kinases are required for both focal-adhesion formation and DNA synthesis *(15,152,165,166)*. Many questions remain, including: which tyrosine kinases are critical, are they located in the focal adhesion, and if so, how do events occurring in the focal adhesion get transmitted to the nucleus? How does the nucleus know the cell is anchored so that DNA synthesis may proceed? FAK has not been demonstrated to translocate to the nucleus and the only likely substrates of FAK identified thus far are the two cytoskeleton-associated proteins, paxillin and the SH2 domain-containing protein, tensin, noted above *(159,166)*. Sorting out the role of the focal adhesion in the mitogenic response and what role FAK and Src may play in the formation of the focal adhesion remains a major challenge to understanding mitogenic signaling by the endothelins.

3.6.3. Role of the Jak/STAT Pathway in Endothelin-Induced Mitogenesis

The Jak/STAT pathway was first discovered as a signal transduction pathway involved in gene expression induced by interferon (IFN)-α and IFN-γ (reviewed in *37,38,167*). Members of the Jak family include Jak1, Jak2, and Tyk2, and are notable for a tyrosine kinase domain and a second kinase-like domain. This second kinase-like domain was the impetus for naming them after the Roman god of gates and doorways, Janus, who is usually depicted with two faces *(57)*. Based on somatic-cell genetic complementation experiments, the Jak family was shown to be critical in IFN responsiveness. A mutant cell line defective in IFN-α and -β signalling was rescued by transfection with genomic DNA encoding Tyk2 (reviewed in *37,38,167*). More recently, these kinases have been found to play a role in signal transduction from many cytokine receptors, including the mitogenic cytokines, erythropoietin, several interleukins, and GM-CSF and G-CSF as well as growth hormone and prolactin. Most importantly for this discussion, the vasoactive peptide, AngII, rapidly induces tyrosine phosphorylation of Jak2 and Tyk2 (but not Jak1) in rat aortic smooth muscle cells *(168)* and enhances kinase activity of Jak2.

Signal transduction through this pathway typically is initiated when a cytokine binds to its cognate receptor and induces dimerization of receptors with single chains. Jaks then associate with a juxtamembrane domain of the cytoplasmic portion of the receptors. In the case of the AngII (AT$_1$) receptor, Jak 2 appears to directly associate with the AT$_1$ receptor based on coimmunoprecipitation

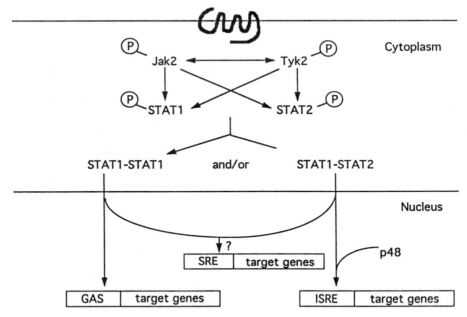

Fig. 5. Postulated mechanisms of activation of the Jak/STAT pathway by ligands with heptahelical receptors. Following occupation of the receptor with ligand, members of the Jak family of tyrosine kinases associate with the receptor. This is believed to bring the kinases into proximity so they can crossphosphorylate and activate one another. Once activated, the Jaks phosphorylate one or more STATs, which then dimerize and move to the nucleus where they activate transcription from genes with promoters containing specific elements. *See text* for details.

(Fig. 5). It is not known which portion of the receptor is the Jak-family target. After binding to the receptors, it is believed that Jaks, now in proximity, crossphosphorylate a tyrosine residue within the catalytic domain that enhances the kinase's activity. Of note, at least for IFN signaling, two different Jak family members are required, but there is no evidence of a cascade, suggesting rather that one family member crossphosphorylates the other. The kinases also phosphorylate residues within the receptor, possibly providing binding sites for other signaling molecules (e.g., Shc, p85 subunit of PI3K, and the tyrosine phosphatase, Syp) *(167)*, and for the second arm of this signaling pathway, the STATs (signal transducers and activators of transcription), which contain an SH2 (and an SH3) domain.

The STAT family includes at least six members at present. STATs, which in resting cells are largely cytoplasmic, associate with the various receptors after ligand stimulation. Interaction with and activation of STATs by the various cytokine receptors are specific, that is each receptor associates with a particular group of STATs. The specificity does not appear to be determined by which Jak family member associates but rather by the relative affinities of the STAT SH2 domain for the phosphotyrosine residue in the receptor. After the STATs associate with the receptor, they are phosphorylated, presumably by a Jak family member, at a conserved tyrosine residue in the C-terminus. Following this, the STATs dimerize. The dimerization may be driven by interaction of the SH2 domain of one STAT with the phosphotyrosine residue of the other STAT, and vice versa.

In rat aortic smooth muscle cells, AngII leads to tyrosine phosphorylation of STAT1α and β, and STAT2 with a slightly delayed time course compared to IFNs. STAT3 is phosphorylated minimally and very late following AngII *(168)*.

Following dimerization of the STATs, they move into the nucleus via an unknown mechanism. After IFN-α/β, a dimer of STAT1 and STAT2 binds to p48, a DNA-binding protein, to form a complex called ISGF3, which then binds to the interferon-stimulated response elements (ISREs, consensus sequence AGTTTCNNTTTCNC/T) within various interferon-responsive promoters and activates transcription (Fig. 5). Following IFN-γ, homodimers of STAT1α form. These dimers do not complex with p48 but probably do complex with a related DNA-binding protein that directs the complex to gamma-activated sequences (GAS, consensus sequence TTNCNNG/TAA) within promoters responsive to IFN-γ. Thus which genes are transcribed in response to a particular stimulus is determined in large part by which STATs are activated, and, in turn, which STATs are activated is determined either by STAT SH2 domain interactions with specific receptors and/or, conceivably, with a contribution of differing substrate specificities of the members of the Jak family for different STATs.

STAT1 translocation into the nucleus has been demonstrated following AngII, albeit with a markedly delayed time course compared to IFNs (30 vs 5 min), suggesting the possibility of an autocrine or paracrine mechanism *(168)*. Although direct involvement of the Jak/STAT pathway in ET-1 signaling has not been demonstrated, given the ever-expanding list of ligands that stimulate this pathway, and the direct demonstration of activation by the G_q-linked vasoactive peptide, AngII, it is highly likely that this pathway is involved in growth regulation following endothelins.

What role the Jak/STAT pathways play in growth regulation in response to vasoactive peptides is unclear, and will likely have to await the creation of dominant inhibitory mutants of various components of the pathway. IFN-α and IFN-γ are predominantly growth inhibitory in many cell types. However, certain combinations of STATs may be relatively promiscuous in their interactions with promoters. This promiscuity may explain how STATs might also mediate the proliferative response to many cytokines. For example, Darnell et al. have noted the similarity between the GAS site and the SRE, (contained in the promoters of many IEG, including c-*fos* and *Egr*-1). They found that multiple gel-shift bands are produced using an SRE oligonucleotide after growth-factor stimulation of epithelial cells, and some of the bands contain STAT1 and/or STAT3 *(37)*. Furthermore, a Sis-inducible enhancer within the c-*fos* promoter may also mediate induction of c-*fos* by stimuli which activate the Jaks *(91)*. This suggests other possible mechanisms, besides ERK activation of TCF (*see* Section 3.3.3.), for induction of c-*fos* following growth factors and, possibly, AngII and ET-1.

3.7. Role of Other MAP Kinase Signaling Cascades

Recently there has been an explosion of interest in other members of the MAP kinase superfamily of protein serine/threonine kinases. The remarkable conservation of the yeast-pheromone pathway in mammals and the multiple MAP kinase pathways in yeast suggested the existence of other MAP kinases in humans. To date, three mammalian MAP kinases, in addition to the ERKs, have been cloned, and a fourth has been tentatively identified (Fig. 6). These include the stress-activated protein kinases (SAPKs; also known as the c-Jun amino-terminal kinases or JNKs) *(114,115)*, p38, the mammalian homolog of HOG-1, a yeast kinase involved in the response to hyperosmolar stress *(116,169,170)*, and ERK-5, a kinase of unknown function *(171)*. Fos regulating kinase (Frk) has been tentatively identified as a MAP kinase based on its substrate preference, though it has not been cloned *(97)*. The SAPKs are, as their name suggests, activated by cellular stresses including inflammatory cytokines (TNFα and IL-1β), heat shock, and reperfusion of ischemic kidney or reversible ATP depletion induced by chemical anoxia in renal tubular epithelial cells *(114,172)*. Major substrates include the transcription factors c-Jun and ATF-2 and the kinases appear to increase transactivating activity of both and DNA-binding activity of

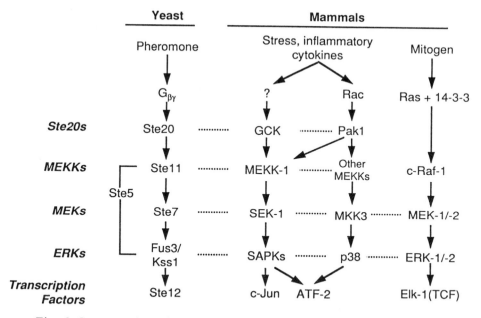

Fig. 6. Conservation of yeast MAP-kinase pathways in mammals. Three mammalian MAP-kinase cascades are aligned with components of the yeast-pheromone response pathway, which culminates in activation of two MAP kinases, Fus3 and Kss1. The small GTP-binding proteins, Ras and Rac, are in parentheses to indicate they are not kinases. c-Raf-1 is bracketed to indicate it is not homologous with either Ste11 or MEKK-1. Abbreviations not in text are: SEK-1, SAPK/ERK kinase; MKK3, MAP kinase kinase 3; GCK, germinal-center kinase *(186).*

ATF-2 *(111–113,173–175).* p38 is also activated by IL-1β and osmolar stress and substrates include Max, and possibly ATF-2 *(116,170,176).* Both the SAPKs and p38, like ERK-1 and ERK-2, are downstream of kinase cascades and their is remarkably little "crosstalk" between the three pathways. Frk is activated by mitogens and activators of Ras, and phosphorylates c-Fos at a threonine residue that increases transactivating activity *(97).* This provides another mechanism whereby transcription of AP-1 dependent genes can be regulated.

Very little has been published on the role of these other MAP kinase family members in ET signal transduction. In NIH3T3 cells expressing the m1 muscarininc acetylcholine receptor, carbachol activated the SAPKs, confirming that a G_q-linked receptor could signal via this cascade *(177).* Furthermore, constitutively active $G\alpha_q$

modestly but persistently activates the SAPKs *(178)*. Angiotensin II, via a PKC-independent pathway, potently activates the SAPKs, and the degree of activation appears to be much greater than the activation of the ERKs *(179)*. More recently, ET-1 has been reported to activate the SAPKs in airway smooth-muscle cells to a relatively similar degree as the ERKs are activated *(53)*. These data suggest that activation of the SAPKs may be a major response arm of endothelin signal transduction. Given the emerging evidence of the role of the SAPKs (and p38) in the induction of apoptosis, or programmed cell death *(180–182)*, it is unlikely that these kinases activate the mitogenic response to endothelin, and more likely that they inhibit it.

3.8. Phosphoinositide 3 Kinase

The role of the lipid products of phosphoinositide 3 kinase (PI3K), phosphatidylinositol (3,4,5)-trisphosphate and phosphatidylinositol (3,4)-bisphosphate, in cell signaling are unknown but they have been implicated in processes as diverse as membrane ruffling, the respiratory burst (superoxide generation) in neutrophils, and the regulation of cell growth (reviewed in *183*). Not surprisingly, the role, if any, of PI3K enzymes and their products in ET-signal transduction is not clear. The growth-factor receptor-associated and Ras-modulated PI3K *(184)*, which consists of an 85 kDa regulatory subunit and a 110 kDa catalytic subunit, probably plays little, if any role in ET-1 signal transduction, based on the observations that there is no tyrosine phosphorylation of p85 or any increase in PI3K activity in anti-phosphotyrosine or anti p85 immunoprecipitates from ET-1 stimulated mesangial cells (T. Force and J. V. Bonventre, unpublished observations). Recently, however, a novel PI3K activity in myeloid cells was found to be activated in a pertussis toxin-sensitive manner by fMetLeuPhe, which signals via a G protein-coupled receptor *(185)*. This PI3K activity was stimulated by G$\beta\gamma$ but not by heterotrimeric G proteins and was immunologically and chromatographically distinct from the p85/p110 growth factor-activated PI3K *(185)*. Furthermore, wortmannin, which potently inhibits the p85/p110 PI3K activity, only modestly inhibited the G$\beta\gamma$-activated PI3K. Hawkins and coworkers noted the similarities between growth factor-induced activation of PLCγ vs G protein-linked receptor activation of PLCβ, and activation of the p85/p110 PI3K vs the novel PI3K *(185)*. Although it is possible that ET-1 may activate this novel PI3K, marked production of 3 phosphorylated phosphinositides in response to agonists with G protein-linked receptors has been noted primarily in cells of myeloid origin. Furthermore, we found no accumulation of phosphatidylinositol (3,4,5)-trisphosphate in glomerular mesangial cells exposed to ET-1 but clear increases in cells exposed to PDGF (T. Force, J.V. Bonventre, unpublished observations). These data suggest that 3-phosphorylated inositides probably do not play an important role in mitogenic signaling in response to ET-1.

4. Conclusions

ET-1 has been known for many years to be a potent mitogen in vascular smooth-muscle cells, yet a picture of the pathways transducing the mitogenic signal to the nucleus has only recently begun to develop. Although sometimes based on limited data, a recurring theme has emerged: despite the marked differences in proximal signal transduction mechanisms of the G protein-coupled receptors and the growth factors, both groups of mitogens share several distal pathways. Most important among these appear to be the c-Raf-1/ERK cascade and activation of nonreceptor tyrosine kinases, both of which have been repeatedly demonstrated to be critical for growth factor-induced mitogenesis. Major questions remain, including: Are these pathways critical for ET-1-induced mitogenesis and if so, how do the endothelins activate c-Raf-1, Src, and FAK? Is the Jak/STAT pathway activated directly in vascular smooth muscle cells and if so, how? What role do other MAP kinase cascades play? Finally, given activation of similar distal pathways, what accounts for the specificity in the transcriptional response of cells to growth factors vs ET-1? Addressing these questions will advance the field of endothelin signaling beyond phenomenology.

References

1. Chun, M., Lin, H. Y., Henis, Y. I., and Lodish, H. F. (1995) Endothelin-induced endocytosis of cell surface ET-A receptors. *J. Biol. Chem.* **270:**10,855–10,860.
2. Baynash, A. G., Hosoda, K., Giaid, A., Richardson, J. A., Emoto, N., Hammer, R. E., and Yanagisawa, M. (1994) Interaction of endothelin-3 with endothelin-B receptor is essential for development of epidermal melanocytes and enteric neurons. *Cell* **79:**1277–1285.
3. Puffenberger, E. G., Hosoda, K., Washington, S. S., Nakao, K., deWit, D., Yanagisawa, M., and Chakravarti, A. (1994) A missense mutation of the endothelin-B receptor gene in multigenic Hirschsprung's disease. *Cell* **79:**1257–1266.

4. Dubin, D., Pratt, R. E., Cooke, J. P., and Dzau, V. J. (1989) Endothelin, a potent vasoconstrictor, is a vascular smooth muscle mitogen. *J. Vasc. Med. Biol.* **1:**150–154.

5. Bobik, A., Grooms, A., Millar, J. A., Mitchell, A., and Grinpukel, S. (1990) Growth factor activity of endothelin on vascular smooth muscle. *Am. J. Physiol.* **258:**C408–C415.

6. Simonson, M. S., Wann, S., Mene, P., Dubyak, G. R., Kester, M., Nakazato, Y., Sedor, J. R., and Dunn, M. J. (1989) ET stimulates phospholipase C, Na+/H+ exchange, c-fos expression, and mitogenesis in rat mesangial cells. *J. Clin. Invest.* **83:**708–712.

7. Jaffer, F. E., Knauss, T. C., Poptic, E., and Abboud, H. E. (1990) Endothelin stimulates PDGF secretion in cultured human mesangial cells. *Kidney Int.* **38:**1193–1198.

8. Muldoon, L., Pribnow, D., Rodland, K. D., and Magun, B. (1990) ET-1 stimulates DNA synthesis and anchorage-independent growth of rat-1 fibroblasts through a protein kinase C-dependent mechanism. *Cell Regul.* **1:**379–390.

9. Takuwa, N., Takuwa, Y., Yanagisawa, M., Yamashita, K., and Masaki, T. (1989) A novel vasocative peptide stimulates mitogenesis through inositol lipid turnover in Swiss 3T3 fibroblasts. *J. Biol. Chem.* **264:**7856–7861.

10. Weissberg, P. L., Witchell, C., Davenport, A. P., Hesketh, T. R., and Metcalfe, J. C. (1990) The endothelin peptides ET-1, ET-2, ET-3 and sarafotoxin S6b are co-mitogenic with PDGF for VSMC. *Atherosclerosis* **85:**257–262.

11. Hirata, Y., Takagi, Y., Fukuda, Y., and Marumo, F. (1989) ET is a potent mitogen for rat vascular smooth muscle cells. *Atherosclerosis* **78:**225–228.

12. Komuro, I., Kurihara, H., Sugiyama, T., Takaku, F., and Yazaki, Y. (1988) ET stimulates c-fos and c-myc expression and proliferation of vascular smooth muscle cells. *FEBS Lett.* **238:**249–252.

13. Battistini, B., Chailler, P., D'Orleans-Juste, P., Briere, N., and Sirois, P. (1993) Growth regulatory properties of endothelins. *Peptides* **14:**385–399.

14. Simonson, M., Jones, J., and Dunn, M. (1992) Differential regulation of fos and jun gene expression and AP-1 cis-element activity by endothelin isopeptides. *J. Biol. Chem.* **267:**8643–8649.

15. Simonson, M. S. and Herman, W. H. (1993) Protein kinase C and protein tyrosine kinase activity contribute to mitogenic signaling by endothelin-1. *J. Biol. Chem.* **13:**9347–9357.

16. Ohlstein, E. H., Arleth, A., Bryan, H., Elliott, J. D., and Sung, C. P. (1992) The selective endothelin receptor antagonist BQ123 antagonizes endothelin-1-mediated mitogensis. *Eur. J. Pharm.* **225:**347–350.

17. Kanse, S., Wijelath, E., Kanthou, C., Newman, P., and Kakkar, V. (1995) The proliferative responsiveness of human vascular smooth muscle cells to endothelin correlates with endothelin receptor density. *Lab. Invest.* **72:**376–382.

18. Serradeil-Le Gal, C., Herbert, J. M., Garcia, C., Boutin, M., and Maffrand, (1991) Importance of the phenotypic state of vascular smooth muscle cells on the binding and mitogenic activity of endothelin. *Peptides* **12:**575–579.

19. Weber, H., Webb, M. L., Serafino, R., Taylor, D. S., Moreland, S., Norman, J., and Molloy, C. J. (1994) Endothelin-1 and Angiotensin-II stimulate delayed mitogensis in cultured rat aortic smooth muscle cells: evidence for common signaling mechanisms. *Mol. Endocrinol.* **8**:148–156.

20. Naftilan, A. J., Pratt, R. E., and Dzau, V. J. (1989) Induction of platelet derived growth factor A-chain and c-myc gene expression by angiotensin II in cultured rat vascular smooth muscle cells. *J. Clin. Invest.* **83**:1419–1424.

21. Gibbons, G. H., Pratt, R. E., and Dzau, V. J. (1992) Vascular smooth muscle cell hypertrophy vs. hyperplasia. *J. Clin. Invest.* **90**:456–461.

22. Weber, H., Taylor, D. S., and Molloy, C. J. (1994) Angiotensin II induces delayed mitogenesis and cellular proliferation in rat aortic smooth muscle cells: correlation with the expression of specific endogenous growth factors and reversal by suramin. *J. Clin. Invest.* **93**:788–798.

23. Simonson, M. S. and Dunn, M. J. (1990) Cellular signaling by peptides of the endothelin gene family. *FASEB J.* **4**:2989–3000.

24. Marrero, M., Paxton, W., Duff, J., Berk, B., and Bernstein, K. (1994) Angiotensin II stimulates tyrosine phosphorylation of phospholipase c-γ1 in vascular smooth muscle cells. *J. Biol. Chem.* **269**:10,935–10,939.

25. Clapham, D. E. (1995) Calcium signalling. *Cell* **80**:259–268.

26. Ghosh, A. and Greenberg, M. E. (1995) Calcium signalling in neurons: molecular mechanisms and cellular consequences. *Science* **268**:239–247.

27. Means, A. R. (1994) Calcium, calmodulin, and cell cycle regulation. *FEBS Lett.* **347**:1–4.

28. Nakaki, T., Nakayama, M., Yamamoto, S., and Kato, R. (1989) ET-mediated stimulation of DNA synthesis in VSMC. *Biochem. Biophys. Res. Commun.* **158**:880–883.

29. Shichiri, M., Hirata, Y., Nakajima, T., Ando, K., Imai, T., Yanagisawa, M., Masaki, T., and Marumo, F. (1991) ET-1 is an autocrine/paracrine growth factor for human cancer cell lines. *J. Clin. Invest.* **87**:1867–1871.

30. Muldoon, L., Rodland, K. D., Forsythe, M. L., and Magun, B. E. (1989) Stimulation of phosphatidylinositol hydrolysis, diacylglycerol release, and gene expression in response to endothelin, a potent new agonist for fibroblasts and smooth muscle cells. *J. Biol. Chem.* **264**:8529–8536.

31. Griendling, K., Tsuda, T., and Alexander, R. W. (1989) Endothelin stimulates diacylglycerol accumulation and activates protein kinase C in cultured vascular smooth muscle cells. *J. Biol. Chem.* **264**:8237–8240.

32. Force, T., Kyriakis, J. M., Avruch, J., and Bonventre, J. V. (1991) Endothelin, vasopressin, and angiotensin II enhance tyrosine phosphorylation by protein kinase C-dependent and -independent pathways in glomerular mesangial cells. *J. Biol. Chem.* **266**:6650–6656.

33. Chua, B. H. L., Krebs, C. J., Chua, C. C., and Diglio, C. A. (1992) ET stimulates protein synthesis in SMC. *Am. J. Physiol.* **262**:E412–E416.

34. Huckle, W. R., Prokop, C. A., Dy, R. C., Herman, B., and Earp, S. (1990) Angiotensin II stimulates protein-tyrosine phosphorylation in a calcium-dependent manner. *Mol. Cell. Biol.* **10**:6290–6298.

35. Zachary, I., Sinnett-Smith, J., and Rozengurt, E. (1991) Stimulation of tyrosine kinase activity in anti-phosphotyrosine immune complexes of Swiss 3T3 cell lysates occurs rapidly after addition of bombesin, vasopressin, and endothelin to intact cells. *J. Biol. Chem.* **266**:24,126–24,133.

36. Zachary, I., Sinnett-Smith, J., and Rozengurt, E. (1992) Bombesin, vasopressin, and endothelin stimulation of tyrosine phosphorylation in Swiss 3T3 cells. *J. Biol. Chem.* **267**:19,031–19,034.

37. Darnell, J. E., Kerr, I. M., and Stark, G. R. (1994) Jak-STAT pathways and transcriptional activation in response to IFNs and other extracellular signaling proteins. *Science* **264**:1415–1421.

38. Ihle, J. N., Witthuhn, B. A., Quelle, F. W., Yamamoto, K., Theirfelder, W. E., Kreider, B., and Silvennoinen, O. (1994) Signaling by the cytokine receptor superfamily: JAKs and STATs. *TIBS* **19**:222–227.

39. Ray, B. L. and Sturgill, T. W. (1988) Insulin-stimulated microtubule-associated protein kinase is phosphorylated on tyrosine and threonine in vivo. *Proc. Natl. Acad. Sci. USA* **85**:3753–3757.

40. Sturgill, T. W., Ray, L. B., Erikson, E., and Maller, J. L. (1988) Insulin-stimulated MAP-2 kinase phosphorylates and activates ribosomal protein S6 kinase II. *Nature* **334**:715–718.

41. Rapp, U. R., Goldsborough, M. D., Mark, G. E., Bonner, T. I., Groffen, J., Reynolds, F. H., Jr., and Stephenson, J. R. (1983) Structure and biological activity of v-raf, a unique oncogene transduced by a retrovirus. *Proc. Natl. Acad. Sci. USA* **80**:4218–4222.

42. Rapp, U. R., Heidecker, G., Huleihel, M., Cleveland, J. L., Chol, W. C., Pawson, T., Ihle, J. N., and Anderson, W. B. (1988) Raf family serine/threonine protein kinases in mitogen signal transduction. *Cold Spring Harbor Symp. Quant. Biol.* **53**:173–184.

43. Rapp, U. R. (1991) Role of Raf-1 serine/threonine protein kinase in growth factor signal transduction. *Oncogene* **6**:495–500.

44. Kyriakis, J. M., App, H., Zhang, X., Banerjee, P., Brautigan, D. L., Rapp, U. R., and Avruch, J. (1992) Raf-1 activates MAP kinase-kinase. *Nature* **358**:417–421.

45. Dent, P., Haser, W., Haystead, T. A. J., Vincent, L. A., Roberts, T. M., and Sturgill, T. W. (1992) Activation of mitogen-activated protein kinase kinase by v-Raf in NIH 3T3 cells and in vitro. *Science* **257**:1404–1407.

46. Howe, L. R., Leevers, S. J., Gomez, N., Nakielny, S., Cohen, P., and Marshall, C. J. (1992) Activation of the MAP kinase pathway by the protein kinase raf. *Cell* **71**:335–342.

47. Pages, G., Lenormand, P., L'Allemain, G., Chambard, J.-C., Meloche, S., and Pouyssegur, J. (1993) Mitogen-activated protein kinases p42mapk and p44mapk are required for fibroblast proliferation. *Proc. Natl. Acad. Sci. USA* **90**:8319–8323.

48. Cowley, S., Paterson, H., Kemp, P., and Marshall, C. (1994) Activation of MAP kinase kinase is necessary and sufficient for PC12 differentiation and for transformation of NIH 3T3 cells. *Cell* **77**:841–852.

49. Mansour, S., Matten, W., Hermann, A., Candia, J., Rong, S., Fukasawa, K., Woude, G., and Ahn, N. (1994) Transformation of mammalian cells by contitutively active MAP kinase kinase. *Science* **265**:966–970.

50. Marshall, C. (1995) Specificity of receptor tyrosine kinase signalling: transient versus sustained extracellular signal-regulated kinase activation. *Cell* **80**:179–185.

51. Kyriakis, J. M., Force, T. L., Rapp, U. R., Bonventre, J. V., and Avruch, J. (1993) Mitogen regulation of c-Raf-1 protein kinase activity toward mitogen-activated protein kinase kinase. *J. Biol. Chem.* **268**:16,009–16,019.

52. Herman, W. H. and Simonson, M. S. (1995) Nuclear signaling by endothelin-1. *J. Biol. Chem.* **270**:11,654–11,661.

53. Shapiro, P. S., Evans, J. N., Davis, R. J., and Posada, J. A. (1996) The seven-transmembrane-spanning receptors for endothelin and thrombin cause proliferation of airway smooth muscle cells and activation of the extracellular regulated kinase and c-Jun NH2-terminal kinase groups of mitogen-activated protein kinases. *J. Biol. Chem.* **271**:5750–5754.

54. Heldin, C.-H. (1995) Dimerization of cell surface receptors in signal transduction. *Cell* **80**:213–223.

55. Ullrich, A. and Schlessinger, J. (1990) Signal transduction by receptors with tyrosine kinase activity. *Cell* **61**:203–212.

56. Songyang, Z., Shoelson, S. E., Chauduri, M., Gish, G., Pawson, T., Haser, W. G., King, F., Roberts, T., Ratnofsky, S., Lechleider, R. J., Neel, B. G., Birge, R. B., Fajardo, J. E., Chou, M. M., Hanafusa, H., Schaffhausen, B., and Cantley, L. C. (1993) SH2 domains recognize specific phosphopeptide sequences. *Cell* **72**:767–778.

57. Cohen, G. B., Ren, R., and Baltimore, D. (1995) Modular binding domains in signal transduction proteins. *Cell* **80**:237–248.

58. Zhang, X.-F., Settleman, J., Kyriakis, J. M., Takeuchi-Suzuki, E., Elledge, S. J., Marshall, M., Bruder, J. T., Rapp, U. R., and Avruch, J. (1993) Normal and oncogenic p21[ras] proteins bind to the amino-terminal regulatory domain of c-Raf-1. *Nature* **364**:308–313.

59. Bruder, J. T., Heidecker, G., and Rapp, U. R. (1992) Serum-, TPA-, and Ras-induced expression from Ap-1/Ets-driven promoters requires Raf-1 kinase. *Genes Devl.* **6**:545–556.

60. Leevers, S. J., Paterson, H. F., and Marshall, C. J. (1994) Requirement for Ras in Raf activation is overcome by targeting Raf to the plasma membrane. *Nature* **369**:411–414.

61. Stokoe, D., Macdonald, S. G., Cadwallader, K., Symons, M., and Hancock, J. F. (1994) Activation of Raf as a result of recruitment to the plasma membrane. *Science* **264**:1463–1467.

62. Daum, G., Eisenmann-Tappe, I., Fries, H.-W., Troppmair, J., and Rapp, U. R. (1994) The ins and outs of Raf kinases. *TIBS* **19**:474–480.

63. Li, S., Janosch, P., Tanji, M., Rosenfeld, G., Waymire, J. C., Mischak, H., Kolch, W., and Sedivy, J. M. (1995) Regulation of Raf-1 kinase activity by the 14-3-3 family of proteins. *EMBO J.* **14**:685–696.

64. Marshall, C. J. (1996) Raf gets it together. *Nature* **383:**127,128.
65. Winitz, S., Russell, M., Qian, N.-X., Gardner, A., Dwyer, L., and Johnson, G. L. (1993) Involvement of Ras and Raf in the Gi-coupled acetylcholine muscarininc m2 receptor activation of mitogen-activated protein (MAP) kinase kinase and MAP kinase. *J. Biol. Chem.* **268:**19,196–19,199.
66. Van Corven, E. J., Hordijk, P. L., Medema, R. H., Bos, J. L., and Moolenaar, W. H. (1993) Pertussis toxin-sensitive activation of p21ras by G protein-coupled receptor agonists in fibroblasts. *Proc. Natl. Acad. Sci. USA* **90:**1257–1261.
67. Ablas, J., van Corven, E. J., Hordijk, P. L., Milligan, G., and Moolenaar, W. H. (1993) Gi-mediated activation of the p21ras-mitogen-activated protein kinase pathway by α2-adrenergic receptors expressed in fibroblasts. *J. Biol. Chem.* **268:**22,235–22,238.
68. Crespo, P., Xu, N., Daniotti, J. L., Troppmair, J., Rapp, U. R., and Gutkind, J. S. (1994) Signaling through transforming G protein-coupled receptors in NIH 3T3 cells involves c-Raf activation. *J. Biol. Chem.* **269:**21,103–21,109.
69. Crespo, P., Xu, N., Simonds, W., and Gutkind, S. (1994) Ras-dependent activation of MAP kinase pathway mediated by G-protein βγ subunits. *Nature* **369:**418–420.
70. Boguski, M. S. and McCormick, F. (1993) Proteins regulating Ras and its relatives. *Nature* **366:**643–654.
71. Sozeri, O., Vollmer, K., Kiyanage, M., Frith, D., Kour, G., Mark, G. E., and Stabel, S. (1992) Activation of the c-Raf protein kinase by protein kinase C phosphorylation. *Oncogene* **7:**2259–2262.
72. Kolch, W., Heidecker, G., Kochs, G., Hummel, R., Vahldi, H., Mischak, H., Finkenzeller, G., Marme, D., and Rapp, U. R. (1993) Protein kinase Cα activates RAF-1 by direct phosphorylation. *Nature* **364:**249–252.
73. MacDonald, S. G., Crews, C. M., Wu, L., Driller, J., Clark, R., Erikson, R. L., and McCormick, F. (1993) Reconstitution of the Raf-1-MEK-ERK signal transduction pathway in vitro. *Mol. Cell. Biol.* **13:**6615–6620.
74. Kribben, A., Wieder, E. D., Li, X., Van Putten, V., Granot, Y., Schrier, R. W., and Nemenoff, R. A. (1993) AVP-induced activation of MAP kinase in vascular smooth muscle cells is mediated through protein kinase C. *Am. J. Physiol.* **265:**C939–C945.
75. Qian, N.-X., Winitz, S., and Johnson, G. L. (1993) Epitope-tagged Gq alpha subunits: expression of GTPase-deficient alpha subunits persistently stimulates phosphatidylinositol-specific phospholipase C but not mitogen-activated protein kinase activity regulated by the M1 muscarinic acetylcholine receptor. *Proc. Natl. Acad. Sci. USA* **90:**4077–4081.
76. Exton, J. H. (1994) Phosphatidylcholine breakdown and signal transduction. *Biochim. Biophys. Acta.* **1212:**26–42.
77. Cai, H., Erhardt, P., Troppmair, J., Diaz-Meco, M. T., Sithanandam, G., Rapp, U. R., Moscat, J., and Cooper, G. M. (1993) Hydrolysis of phosphatidylcholine couples Ras to activation of Raf protein kinase during mitogenic signal transduction. *Mol. Cell. Biol.* **13:**7645–7651.

78. Force, T., Bonventre, J. V., Heidecker, G., Rapp, U., Avruch, J., and Kyriakis, J. M. (1994) Enzymatic characteristics of the c-Raf-1 protein kinase. *Proc. Natl. Acad. Sci. USA* **91:**1270–1274.
79. Wu, J., Dent, P., Jelinek, T., Wolfman, A., Weber, M. J., and Sturgill, T. W. (1993) Inhibition of the EGF-activated MAP kinase signaling pathway by adenosine 3',5'–monophosphate. *Science* **262:**1065–1069.
80. Cook, S. J. and McCormick, F. (1993) Inhibition by cAMP of Ras-dependent activation of Raf. *Science* **262:**1069–1072.
81. Jelinek, T., Catling, A. D., Reuter, C. W., Moodie, S. A., Wolfman, A., and Weber, M. J. (1994) RAS and RAF-1 form a signalling complex with MEK-1 but not MEK-2. *Mol. Cell. Biol.* **14:**8212–8218.
82. Zheng, C.-F. and Guan, K.-L. (1994) Activation of MEK family kinases requires phosphorylation of two conserved Ser/Thr residues. *EMBO J.* **13:**1123–1131.
83. Lange-Carter, C. A., Pleiman, C. M., Gardner, A. M., Blumer, K. J., and Johnson, G. L. (1993) A divergence in the MAP kinase regulatory network defined by MEK kinase and Raf. *Science* **260:**315–319.
84. Herskowitz, I. (1995) MAP kinase pathways in yeast: for mating and more. *Cell* **80:**187–197.
85. Yan, M., Dai, T., Deak, J. C., Kyriakis, J. M., Zon, L. I., Woodgett, J. R., and Templeton, D. J. (1994) Activation of stress-activated protein kinase by MEKK1 phosphorylation of its activator SEK1. *Nature* **372:**798–800.
86. Payne, D. M., Rossomando, A. J., Martino, P., Erickson, A. K., Shabanowitz, J., Hunt, D. F., Weber, M. J., and Sturgill, T. W. (1991) Identification of the regulatory phosphorylation sites in pp42/mitogen-activated protein kinase (MAP kinase). *EMBO J.* **10:**885–892.
87. Lenormand, P., Sardet, C., Pages, G., L'Allemain, G., Brunet, A., and Pouyssegur, J. (1993) Growth factors induce nuclear translocation of MAP kinases (p42 and p44) but not of their activator MAP kinase kinase (p45) in fibroblasts. *J. Cell Biol.* **122:**1079–1088.
88. Gonzalez, F., Seth, A., Raden, D., Bowman, D., Fay, F., and Davis, R. (1993) Serum-induced translocation of mitogen-activated protein kinase to the cell surface ruffling membrane and the nucleus. *J. Cell Biol.* **122:**1089–1101.
89. Meloche, S., Pages, G., and Pouyssegur, J. (1992) Biphasic and synergistic activation of p44MAPK (ERK1) by growth factors: correlation between late phase activation and mitogenicity. *Mol. Endocrinol.* **6:**845–854.
90. Sakurai, T., Abe, Y., Jasytam, T., Takuwa, N., Shiba, R., Yamashita, T., Endo, T., and Goto, K. (1994) Activin A stimulates mitogenesis in Swiss 3T3 fibroblasts without activation of mitogen-activated protein kinases. *J. Biol. Chem.* **269:**14,118–14,122.
91. Karin, M. (1995) The regulation of AP-1 activity by mitogen-activated protein kinases. *J. Biol. Chem.* **270:**16,483–16,486.
92. Angel, P., Imagawa, M., Chiu, R., Stein, B., Imbra, R. J., Rahmsdorf, H. J., Jonat, C., Herrlich, P., and Karin, M. (1987) Phorbol ester inducible genes contain a common cis element recognized by a TPA-modulated trans-acting factor. *Cell* **49:**729–739.

93. Treisman, R. (1990) The SRE: A growth factor-responsive transcriptional regulator. *Sem. Cancer Biol.* **1**:47–58.
94. Marais, R., Wynne, J., and Treisman, R. (1993) The SRF accessory protein Elk-1 contains a growth factor-regulated transcriptional activation domain. *Cell* **73**:381–393.
95. Gille, H., Sharrocks, A. D., and Shaw, P. E. (1992) Phosphorylation of transcription factor p62^{TCF} by MAP kinase stimulates ternary complex formation at c-*fos* promoter. *Nature* **358**:414–416.
96. Janknecht, R., Wolfram, E. H., Pingoud, V., and Nordheim, A. (1993) Activation of ternary complex factor Elk-1 by MAP kinase. *EMBO J.* **12**:5097–5104.
97. Deng, T. and Karin, M. (1994) c-Fos transcriptional activity stimulated by H-Ras-activated protein kinase distinct from JNK and ERK. *Nature* **371**:171–175.
98. Hunter, T. and Karin, M. (1992) The regulation of transcription by phosphorylation. *Cell* **70**:375–387.
99. Boyle, W. J., Smeal, T., Defize, L. H., Angel, P., Woodgett, J. R., Karin, M., and Hunter, T. (1991) Activation of protein kinase C decreases phosphorylation of c-Jun at sites that negatively regulate its DNA-binding activity. *Cell* **64**:573–584.
100. Sutherland, C., Leighton, I. A., and Cohen, P. (1993) Inactivation of glycogen synthase kinase-3β by phosphorylation: new kinase connections in insulin and growth factor signalling. *Biochem. J.* **296**:15–19.
101. Binetruy, B., Smeal, T., and Karin, M. (1991) Ha-Ras augments c-jun activity and stimulates phosphorylation of its activation domain. *Nature* **351**:122–127.
102. Pulverer, B., Kyriakis, J. M., Avruch, J., Nikolakaki, E., and Woodgett, J. R. (1991) Phophorylation of c-jun mediated by MAP kinases. *Nature* **353**:670–674.
103. Ito, H., Hirata, Y., Hiroe, M., Tsujino, M., Adachi, S., Takamoto, T., Nitta, M., Taniguchi, K., and Marumo, F. (1991) ET-1 induces hypertrophy with enhanced expression of muscle-specific genes in cultured neonatal rat cardiomyocytes. *Circ. Res.* **69**:209–215.
104. Neyses, L., Nouskas, J., and Vetter, H. (1991) Inhibition of ET-1 induced myocardial protein synthesis by an antisense oligonucleotide against the early growth response gene-1. *Biochem. Biophys. Res. Commun.* **181**:22–27.
105. Blackwood, E. M., Kretzner, L., and Eisenman, R. N. (1992) Myc and Max function as a nucleoprotein complex. *Curr. Opin. Genet. Dev.* **2**:227–235.
106. Ayer, D. E., Lawrence, Q. A., and Eisenman, R. N. (1995) Mad-Max transcriptional repression is mediated by ternary complex formation with mammalian homologs of yeast repressor Sin3. *Cell* **80**:767–776.
107. Kato, G. J., Barret, J., VillaGarcia, M., and Dang, C. V. (1990) An amino-terminal c-Myc domain required for neoplastic transformation activates transcription. *Mol. Cell. Biol.* **10**:5914–5924.
108. Seth, A., Alverez, E., Gupta, S., and Davis, R. J. (1991) A phosphorylation site located in the NH2-terminal domain of c-Myc increases transactivation of gene expression. *J. Biol. Chem.* **266**:23,521–23,524.

109. Brunner, D., Ducker, K., Oellers, N., Hafen, E., Scholz, H., and Klambt, C. (1994) The ETS domain protein pointed-P2 is a target of MAP kinase in the sevenless signal transduction pathway. *Nature* **370**:386–389.
110. O'Neill, E. M., Rebay, I., Tjian, R., and Rubin, G. M. (1994) The activities of two Ets-related transcription factors required for Drosophila eye development are modulated by the Ras/MAPK pathway. *Cell* **78**:137–147.
111. Abdel-Hafiz, H. A., Heasley, L. E., Kyriakis, J. M., Avruch, J., Kroll, D. J., Johnson, G. L., and Hoeffler, J. P. (1992) Activating transcription factor-2 DNA-binding activity is stimulated by phosphorylation catalyzed by p42 and p54 microtubule-associated protein kinases. *Mol. Endocrinol.* **6**:2079–2089.
112. Abdel-Hafiz, H. A., Chen, C. Y., Marcell, T., Kroll, D. J., and Hoeffler, J. P. (1993) Structural determinants outside of the leucine zipper influence the interactions of CREB and ATF-2: interaction of CREB with ATF-2 blocks E1a-ATF-2 complex formation. *Oncogene* **8**:1161–1174.
113. Morooka, H., Bonventre, J. V., Pombo, C. M., Kyriakis, J. M., and Force, T. (1995) Ischemia and reperfusion enhance ATF-2 and c-Jun binding to cAMP response elements and to an AP-1 binding site from the c-jun promoter. *J. Biol. Chem.* **270**:30,084–30,092.
114. Kyriakis, J. M., Banerjee, P., Nikolakaki, E., Dai, T., Rubie, E. A., Avruch, J., and Woodgett, J. R. (1994) A MAP kinase subfamily activated by cellular stress and tumour necrosis factor. *Nature* **369**:156–160.
115. Derijard, B., Hibi, M., Wu, I. H., Barrett, T., Su, B., Deng, T., Karin, M., and Davis, R. J. (1994) JNK1: A protein kinase stimulated by UV light and Ha-Ras that binds and phosphorylates the c-Jun activation domain. *Cell* **76**:1025–1037.
116. Han, J., Lee, J. D., Bibbs, L., and Ulevitch, R. J. (1994) A MAP kinase targeted by endotoxin and hyperosmolarity in mammalian cells. *Science* **265**:808–811.
117. Lin, T.-A., Kong, X., Haystead, T., Pause, A., Belsham, G., Sonenberg, N., and Lawrence, J. (1994) PHAS-I as a link between mitogen-activated protein kinase and translation initiation. *Science* **266**:653–656.
118. Sun, H., Tonks, N. K., and Bar-Sagi, D. (1994) Inhibition of Ras-induced DNA synthesis by expression of the phosphatase MKP-1. *Science* **266**:285–288.
119. Sun, H., Charles, C., Lau, L., and Tonks, N. (1993) MKP-1 (3CH134), an immediate early gene product, is a dual specificity phosphatase that dephophorylates MAP kinase in vivo. *Cell* **75**:487–493.
120. Rossomando, A. J., Dent, P., Sturgill, T. W., and Marshak, D. R. (1994) Mitogen-activated protein kinase kinase 1 (MKK1) is negatively regulated by threonine phosphorylation. *Mol. Cell. Biol.* **14**:1594–1602.
121. Lavoie, J. N., L'Allemain, G., Brunet, A., Muller, R., and Pouyssegur, J. (1996) Cyclin D1 expression is regulated positively by the p42/44 MAPK and negatively by the p39/HOG MAPK pathway. *J. Biol. Chem.* **271**:20,608–20,616.

122. Force, T. and Bonventre, J. V. (1992) Endothelin activates Src tyrosine kinase in glomerular mesangial cells. *J. Am. Soc. Nephrol.* **3:**491.

123. Kypta, R. M., Goldberg, Y., Ulug, E. T., and Courtneidge, S. A. (1990) Association between the PDGF receptor and members of the src family of tyrosine kinases. *Cell* **62:**481–492.

124. Gould, K. and Hunter, T. (1988) Platelet-derived growth factor induces multisite phosphorylation of pp60$^{c\text{-}src}$ and increases its protein-tyrosine kinase activity. *Mol. Cell. Biol.* **8:**3345–3356.

125. Courtneidge, S. A., Dhand, R., Pilat, D., Twamley-Stein, G. M., Waterfield, M. D., and Roussel, M. F. (1993) Activation of Src family kinases by colony stimulating factor-1, and their association with its receptor. *EMBO J.* **12:**943–950.

126. Twamley-Stein, G. M., Pepperkok, R., Ansorge, W., and Courtneidge, S. A. (1993) The Src family tyrosine kinases are required for platelet-derived growth factor-mediated signal transduction in NIH3T3 cells. *Proc. Natl. Acad. Sci. USA* **90:**7696–7700.

127. Wilson, L. K., Luttrell, D. K., Parsons, J. T., and Parsons, S. J. (1989) Src tyrosine kinase, myristylation, and modulatory domains are required for enhanced mitogenic responsiveness to epidermal growth factor seen in cells overexpressing c-src. *Mol. Cell. Biol.* **9:**1536–1544.

128. Roche, S., Koegl, M., Barone, M. V., Roussel, M. F., and Courtneidge, S. A. (1995) DNA synthesis induced by some but not all growth factors requires Src family protein tyrosine kinases. *Mol. Cell. Biol.* **15:**1102–1109.

129. Soriano, P., Montgomery, C., Geske, R., and Bradley, A. (1991) Targeted disruption of the c-src proto-oncogene leads to osteopetrosis in mice. *Cell* **64:**693–702.

130. Shenoy, S., Chackalaparampil, I., Bagrodia, S., Lin, P.-H., and Shalloway, D. (1992) Role of p34^{cdc2}-mediated phosphorylations in two-step activation of pp60$^{c\text{-}src}$ during mitosis. *Proc. Natl. Acad. Sci. USA* **89:**7237–7241.

131. Chackalaparamil, I., Bagrodia, S., and Shalloway, D. (1994) Tyrosine dephosphorylation of pp60$^{c\text{-}src}$ is stimulated by a serine/threonine phosphatase inhibitor. *Oncogene* **9:**1947–1955.

132. Sabe, H., Hata, A., Okada, M., Nakagawa, H., and Hanafusa, H. (1994) Analysis of the binding of the Src homology 2 domain of Csk to tyrosine-phosphorylated proteins in the suppression and mitotic activation of c-Src. *Proc. Natl. Acad. Sci. USA* **91:**3984–3988.

133. Nada, S., Okada, M., MacAuley, A., Cooper, J. A., and Nakagawa, H. (1991) Cloning of a complementary DNA for a protein -tyrosine kinase that specifically phosphorylates a negative regulatory site of p60c-src. *Nature* **351:**69–72.

134. Chow, L. M. L., Fournel, M., Davidson, D., and Veillette, A. (1993) Negative regulation of T-cell receptor signalling by tyrosine protein kinase p50csk. *Nature* **365:**156–160.

135. Cooper, J. A. and Howell, B. (1993) The when and how of Src regulation. *Cell* **73:**1051–1054.

136. den Hertog, J., Pals, C., Peppelenbosch, M. P., Tertoolen, L. G. J., de Laat, S., and Kruijer, W. (1993) Receptor protein tyrosine phosphatase activates pp60-c-src and is involved in neuronal differentiation. *EMBO J.* **12:**3789–3798.

137. Bibbins, K. B., Boeuf, H., and Varmus, H. E. (1993) Binding of the Src SH2 domain to phosphopeptides is determined by residues in both the SH2 domain and the phosphopeptides. *Mol. Cell. Biol.* **13:**7278–7287.

138. Koch, C. A., Moran, M. F., Anderson, D., Liu, X., Mbamalu, G., and Pawson, T. (1992) Multiple SH2-mediated interactions in v-src-transformed cells. *Mol. Cell. Biol.* **12:**1366–1374.

139. Fukui, Y. and Hanafusa, H. (1991) Requirement of phosphatidylinositol-3 kinase modification for its association with p60^{src}. *Mol. Cell. Biol.* **11:**1972–1979.

140. Weng, Z., Thomas, S. M., Rickles, R. J., Taylor, J. A., Brauer, A. W., Seidel-Dugan, C., Michael, W. M., Dreyfuss, G., and Brugge, J. S. (1994) Identification of Src, Fyn, and Lyn SH3-binding proteins: implications for a function of SH3 domains. *Mol. Cell. Biol.* **14:**4509–4521.

141. Cantley, L. C., Auger, K. R., Carpenter, C., Duckworth, B., Graziani, A., Kapeller, R., and Soltoff, S. (1991) Oncogenes and signal transduction. *Cell* **64:**281–302.

142. Li, W., Hu, P., Skolnik, E. Y., Ullrich, A., and Schlessinger, J. (1992) The SH2 and SH3 domain-containing Nck protein is oncogenic and a common target for phosphorylation by different surface receptors. *Mol. Cell. Biol.* **12:**5824–5833.

143. Chou, M. M., Fajardo, J. E., and Hanafusa, H. (1992) The SH2- and SH3-containing Nck protein transforms mammalian fibroblasts in the absence of elevated phosphotyrosine levels. *Mol. Cell. Biol.* **12:**5834–5842.

144. Meisenhelder, J. and Hunter, T. (1992) The SH2/SH3 domain-containing protein Nck is recognized by certain anti-phospholipase C-gamma1 monoclonal antibodies and its phosphorylation on tyrosine is stimulated by platelet-derived growth factor and epidermal growth factor treatment. *Mol. Cell. Biol.* **12:**5843–5856.

145. Pelicci, G., Lanfrancone, L., Grignani, F., McGlade, J., Cavallo, F., Forni, G., Nicoletti, I., Grignani, F., Pawson, T., and Pelicci, P. G. (1992) A novel transforming protein (SHC) with an SH2 domain is implicated in mitogenic signal transduction. *Cell* **70:**93–104.

146. McGlade, J., Cheng, A., Pelicci, G., Pelicci, P. G., and Pawson, T. (1992) Shc proteins are phosphorylated and regulated by the v-Src and v-Fps protein-tyrosine kinases. *Proc. Natl. Acad. Sci. USA* **89:**8869–8873.

147. Della Rocca, G. J., van Biessen, T., Daaka, Y., Luttrell, D. K., Luttrell, L. M., and Lefkowitz, R. J. (1997) Ras-dependent mitogen-activated protein kinase activation by G protein-coupled receptors. *J. Biol. Chem.* **272,** 19,125–19,132.

148. Feng, G.-S., Hui, C.-C., and Pawson, T. (1993) SH2-containing phosphotyrosine phosphatase as a target of protein-tyrosine kinases. *Science* **259:**1607–1611.

149. Ridley, A. J., Paterson, H. F., Johnston, C. L., Diekmann, D., and Hall, A. (1992) The small GTP-binding protein rac regulates growth factor-induced membrane ruffling. *Cell* **70**:401–410.

150. Ridley, A. J. and Hall, A. (1992) The small GTP-binding protein rho regulates the assembly of focal adhesions and actin stress fibers in response to growth factors. *Cell* **70**:389–399.

151. Settleman, J., Albright, C. F., Foster, L. C., and Weinberg, R. A. (1992) Association between GTPase activators for Rho and Ras families. *Nature* **359**:153,154.

152. Ridley, A. J. and Hall, A. (1994) Signal transduction pathways regulating Rho-mediated stress fibre formation: requirement for a tyrosine kinase. *EMBO J.* **13**:2600–2610.

153. Schaller, M. D., Borgman, C. A., Cobb, B. S., Vines, R. R., Reynolds, A. B., and Parsons, J. T. (1992) pp125[FAK], a structurally distinctive protein-tyrosine kinase associated with focal adhesions. *Proc. Natl. Acad. Sci. USA* **89**:5192–5196.

154. Hanks, S. K., Calalb, M. B., Harper, M. C., and Patel, S. K. (1992) Focal adhesion protein-tyrosine kinase phosphorylated in response to cell attachment to fibronectin. *Proc. Natl. Acad. Sci. USA* **89**:8487–8491.

155. Seufferlein, T. and Rozengurt, E. (1994) Lysophosphatidic acid stimulates tyrosine phosphorylation of focal adhesion kinase, paxillin, and p130. *J. Biol. Chem.* **269**:9345–9351.

156. Zachary, I. and Rozengurt, E. (1992) Focal adhesion kinase (p125[FAK]): a point of convergence in the action of neuropeptides, integrins, and oncogenes. *Cell* **71**:891–894.

157. Hamaguchi, M. and Hanafusa, H. (1987) Association of p60[src] with Triton X-100-resistant cellular structures correlates with morphological transformation. *Proc. Natl. Acad. Sci. USA* **84**:2312–2316.

158. Clark, E. A. and Brugge, J. S. (1993) Redistribution of activated pp60[c-src] to integrin-dependent cytoskeletal complexes in thrombin-stimulated platelets. *Mol. Cell. Biol.* **13**:1863–1871.

159. Clark, E. A. and Brugge, J. S. (1995) Integrins and signal transduction pathways: the road taken. *Science* **268**:233–239.

160. Kaplan, K. B., Bibbins, K. B., Swedlow, J. R., Arnaud, M., Morgan, D. O., and Varmus, H. E. (1994) Association of the amino-terminal half of c-Src with focal adhesions alters their properties and is regulated by phosphorylation of tyrosine 527. *EMBO J.* **13**:4745–4756.

161. Cobb, B., Schaller, M., Leu, T., and Parsons, J. (1994) Stable Association of pp60[src] and pp59[fyn] with the focal adhesion-associated protein tyrosine kinase, pp125[FAK]. *Mol. Cell. Biol.* **14**:147–155.

162. Schaller, M., Hildebrand, J., Shannon, J., Fox, J., Vines, R., and Parsons, J. (1994) Autophosphorylation of the focal adhesion kinase, pp125[FAK], directs SH2-dependent binding of pp60[src]. *Mol. Cell. Biol.* **14**:1680–1688.

163. Calalb, M., Polte, T., and Hanks, S. (1995) Tyrosine phosphorylation of focal adhesion kinase at sites in the catalytic domain regulates kinase activity: a role for Src family kinases. *Mol. Cell. Biol.* **15**:954–963.

164. Sinnett-Smith, J., Zachary, I., Valverde, A. M., and Rozengurt, E. (1993) Bombesin stimulation of p125 focal adhesion kinase tyrosine phosphorylation. *J. Biol. Chem.* **268:**14,261–14,268.

165. Seckl, M. and Rozengurt, E. (1993) Tyrphostin inhibits bombesin stimulation of tyrosine phosphorlation, c-fos expression, and DNA synthesis in Swiss 3T3 cells. *J. Biol. Chem.* **268:**9548–9554.

166. Burridge, K., Turner, C. E., and Romer, L. H. (1992) Tyrosine phosphorylation of paxillin and pp125FAK accompanies cell adhesion to extracellular matrix: a role in cytoskeletal assembly. *J. Cell Biol.* **119:**893–903.

167. Taniguchi, T. (1995) Cytokine signalling through nonreceptor protein tyrosine kinases. *Science* **268:**251–255.

168. Marrero, M., Scheffer, B., Paxton, W., Heerdt, L., Berk, B., Delafontaine, P., and Bernstein, K. (1995) Direct stimulation of JAK/STAT pathway by the angiotensin II AT1 receptor. *Nature* **375:**247–250.

169. Freshney, N. W., Rawlinson, L., Guesdon, F., Jones, E., Cowley, S., Hsuan, J., and Saklatvala, J. (1994) Interleukin-1 activates a novel protein kinase cascade that results in the phosphorylation of Hsp27. *Cell* **71:**1039–1049.

170. Rouse, J., Cohen, P., Trigon, S., Morange, M., Alonso-Llamazares, A., Zamanillo, D., Hunt, T., and Nebreda, A. R. (1994) A novel kinase cascade triggered by stress and heat shock that stimulates MAPKAP kinase-2 and phosphorylation of the small heat shock proteins. *Cell* **78:**1027–1037.

171. Zhou, G., Bao, Z. Q., and Dixon, J. E. (1995) Components of a new human protein kinase signal transduction pathway. *J. Biol. Chem.* **270:**12,665–12,669.

172. Pombo, C. P., Bonventre, J. V., Avruch, J., Woodgett, J. R., Kyriakis, J. M., and Force, T. (1994) The stress-activated protein kinases (SAPKs) are major c-Jun amino-terminal kinases activated by ischemia and reperfusion. *J. Biol. Chem.* **269:**26,546-26,551.

173. van Dam, H., Wilhelm, D., Herr, I., Steffen, A., Herrlich, P., and Angel, P. (1995) ATF-2 is preferentially activated by stress-activated protein kinases to mediate c-jun induction in response to genotoxic agents. *EMBO J.* **14:**1798–1811.

174. Livingstone, C., Patel, G., and Jones, N. (1995) ATF2 contains a phosphorylation dependent transcriptional activation domain. *EMBO J.* **14:**1785–1797.

175. Gupta, S., Campbell, D., Derijard, B., and Davis, R. (1995) Transcription factor ATF2 regulation by the JNK signal transduction pathway. *Science* **267:**389–393.

176. Derijard, B., Raingeaud, J., Barrett, T., Wu, I.-H., Han, J., Ulevitch, R., and Davis, R. (1995) Independent human MAP kinase signal transduction pathways defined by MEK and MKK isoforms. *Science* **267:**682–685.

177. Coso, O. A., Chiariello, M., Kalinec, G., Kyriakis, J. M., Woodgett, J., and Gutkind, J. S. (1995) Transforming G protein-coupled receptors potently activate JNK (SAPK). *J. Biol. Chem.* **270:**5620–5624.

178. Heasley, L. E., Storey, B., Fanger, G., Butterfield, L., Zamarripa, J., Blumberg, D., and Maue, R. A. (1996) GTPase-deficient Ga16 and Gaq induce PC12 cell differentiation and persistent activation of cJun Nh2-terminal kinases. *Mol. Cell. Biol.* **16:**648–656.

179. Zohn, I. E., Yu, H., Li, X., Cox, A. D., and Earp, H. S. (1995) Angiotensin II stimulates calcium-dependent activation of c-Jun N-terminal kinase. *Mol. Cell. Biol.* **15:**6160–6168.

180. Xia, Z., Dickens, M., Raingeaud, J., Davis, R. J., and Greenberg, M. E. (1995) Opposing effects of ERK and JNK-p38 MAP kinases on apoptosis. *Science* **270:**1326–1331.

181. Johnson, N. L., Gardner, A. M., Diener, K. M., Lange-Carter, C. A., Gleavy, J., Jarpe, M. B., Minden, A., Karin, M., Zon, L. I., and Johnson, G. L. (1996) Signal transduction pathways regulated by mitogen-activated/extracellular response kinase kinase kinase induce cell death. *J. Biol. Chem.* **271:**3229–3237.

182. Verheij, M., Bose, R., Hua Lin, X., Yao, B., Jarvis, W. D., Grant, S., Birrer, M. J., Szabo, E., Zon, L. I., Kyriakis, J. M., Haimovitz-Friedman, A., Fuks, Z., and Kolesnick, R. N. (1996) Requirement for ceramide-initiated in stress-induced apoptosis. *Nature* **380:**75–79.

183. Kapeller, R. and Cantley, L. C. (1994) Phosphatidylinositol 3-kinase. *Bioessays* **16:**565–576.

184. Rodriquez-Viciana, P., Waren, P. H., Dhand, R., Vanhaesebroeck, B., Gout, I., Fry, M. J., Waterfield, M. D., and Downward, J. (1994) Phosphatidylinositol-3-OH kinase as a direct target of Ras. *Nature* **370:**527–532.

185. Stephens, L., Smrcka, A., Cooke, F. T., Jackson, T. R., Sternweis, C., and Hawkins, P. T. (1994) A novel phosphoinositide 3 kinase activity in myeloid-derived cells is activated by G protein by subunits. *Cell* **77:**83–93.

186. Pombo, C., Kehrl, J., Sanchez, I., Katz, P., Avruch, J., Zon, L., Woodgett, J., Force, T., and Kyriakis, J. (1995) Activation of the SAPK pathway by the human STE20 homolog germinal centre kinase. *Nature* **377:**750–754.

Chapter 6

The Renal and Systemic Hemodynamic Actions of Endothelin

Robert O. Banks, David M. Pollock, and Jacqueline Novak

1. Introduction

The family of biologically active peptides known as the endothelins (ETs) has been the focus of considerable research since the isolation of an endothelial cell constricting factor (EDCF) by Hickey et al. in 1985 *(1)* and the subsequent cloning of endothelin-1 (ET-1) by Yanagisawa et al., in 1988 *(2)*. Endothelin and endothelin-related peptides (ET-1, ET-2, and ET-3) have profound effects on a number of hemodynamic variables relating to cardiovascular and renal function. ET-1 is one of the most potent vasoconstrictor agents that has been isolated. Systemic actions of the peptide require concentrations similar to those of angiotensin II and vasopressin *(3)*, whereas the renal hemodynamic potency exceeds other vasoconstrictors by approximately one order of magnitude. In addition, a number of studies have demonstrated that ET-1 possesses significant vasodilator properties, demonstrating that the molecule has rather unique properties among the long list of vasoactive, biologically important molecules.

The processing of ET-1 is the result of a series of proteolytic cleavages of the initial gene product with the final step converting Big ET-1 to ET-1, a step that is facilitated by a unique ET-converting enzyme. The biological effects of ET-1 result from binding to several

From: *Endothelin: Molecular Biology, Physiology, and Pathology*
Edited by R. F. Highsmith © Humana Press Inc., Totowa, NJ

receptor subtypes, two of which have been cloned from mammalian cells, ET_A and ET_B. The focus of this chapter is to review and evaluate hemodynamic actions of the endothelin peptides with a particular emphasis on the renal circulation.

2. Plasma Concentrations of Endothelin

Many groups have measured the concentration of endothelin in plasma and, based only on those analyses, have attempted to draw conclusions concerning the functional role of the peptide. Because many investigators believe that endothelin functions as an autocrine or paracrine factor, the interpretation and significance of circulating endothelin levels is uncertain at best. Biologically active agents can function as

1. traditional hormones, i.e., elements that are released into the circulation with target sites remote to the parent gland,
2. agents that act in a paracrine fashion, i.e., molecules that affect other cells within the organ or gland,
3. autocrine elements, i.e., agents that alter the biological function of the parent cell itself, or
4. agents that utilize some combination of these three paradigms.

It has yet to be resolved which of these events predominates in the biological scheme for endothelin. Endothelin appears somewhat unique in that it circulates in plasma, yet may be released in a highly localized manner. The concentration of endothelin in plasma is relatively low, in the 1–5 pM range, especially when compared with the K_D for the ET-1 receptor which is in the 0.05–1 nM range (*see* ref. *5* for review). Thus, the relatively low plasma concentration of the peptide has important implications, not only with regard to the question of local vs hormonal mechanisms of action of the peptide, but also with regard to the interpretation of published results that have utilized either bolus or constant infusion methods to deliver what is often a relatively large amount of the peptide to the experimental animal.

Frelin and Guedin *(5)* discussed evidence that suggests that ET-1/ET receptor interactions are characterized by stoichiometric binding. When the concentration of the receptor is much greater than the K_D of the receptor for the ligand, the binding of the ligand to the receptor conforms to a linear rather than a curvilinear relationship between the amount of ligand bound and the concentration of the ligand. Stoichiometric binding can also occur when the binding of the ligand to the receptor is irreversible, which appears to be the case for ET-1 and its receptor. Under conditions of stoichiometric binding, virtually all of the ligand is bound to the receptor at relatively low concentrations of the ligand. Thus, the free concentration of the ligand does not necessarily reflect the biological activity of the system. Therefore, significant biological actions may occur despite the fact that the concentration of ET is below that value which would be predicted for initiating significant physiological effects.

3. Renal Actions of Endothelin

3.1. Hemodynamic Effects of ET-1

Many of the biological effects of ET-1 are characterized by rather long time delays between the application or infusion of the peptide and the resultant steady-state response. A relatively long period of time is also required following removal of the peptide and the corresponding return to the basal state. These facts were observed in the original description of the EDCF-induced contraction of the porcine coronary artery by Hickey et al. *(1)* and are illustrated in Fig. 1. ET-1-induced increases in vascular smooth-muscle tone in vitro require 10–15 min to attain a steady state and are very slow to be reversed. Responses within intact animals or isolated organ systems are similarly associated with a slowly developing, intense vasoconstriction *(3,6–11)*. Figure 2A contains data from a study by Banks *(11)* and illustrates the renal hemodynamic profiles observed during constant infusions of ET-1 into the renal artery of anesthetized dogs. For comparative purposes, the temporal changes in renal blood flow (RBF) during intrarenal infusions of norepinephrine, angiotensin II, and vasopressin are illustrated in Figs. 2B, 2C, and 2D, respectively (the latter data are from Banks, ref. *12*). Compared with the other vasoconstrictor agents, the renal vasoconstriction observed during infusion of ET-1 develops slowly and renal blood flow remains significantly reduced for a prolonged period of time following termination of the ET-1 infusion (up to 4 h are required before renal blood flow returns to baseline following termination of a 20 min, intrarenal infusion of ET-1 at 10 ng/kg/min). Furthermore, renal blood flow during infusion of endothelin is not characterized by an "escape" phenomenon, i.e., there is no gradual return towards baseline during continued infusion of the peptide.

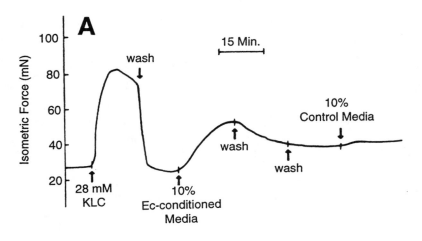

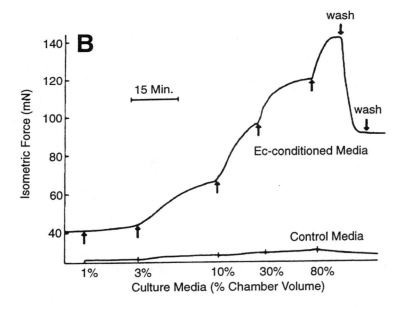

Fig. 1. A representative endothelial cell constricting factor (EDCF)-induced contraction of an of isolated ring of porcine coronary artery **(A)** and a cumulative tension recording of a porcine coronary artery during addition of increasing volumes of media containing EDCF **(B)**; data are from Hickey et al. *(1)*. Reprinted with the permission of the *American Journal of Physiology*.

The data summarized in Fig. 2 indicate that the renal circulation is approximately one order of magnitude more sensitive to endothelin than angiotensin II. Thus, to attain the degree of renal vasoconstriction observed with 10 ng/1 kg/min ET-1 infused directly into the renal artery (approx 5 pmol/kg/min), an intrarenal infusion of 50 ng/kg/min angiotensin II (approx 50 pmol/kg/min) is required.

Although ET-1 is one of the most potent endogenous vasoconstrictor agents, iv infusion of the peptide is often associated with a transient fall in blood pressure which is followed by a dose-dependent increase in arterial pressure *(2,7)*. In dogs, intravenous infusion of ET-1 increases arterial pressure by increasing peripheral vascular resistance; the peptide is also associated with an increase in coronary vascular resistance and a decrease in cardiac output *(3,6)*. ET-1 administration has also been reported to induce the release of atrial natriuretic factor (ANF), vasopressin, and aldosterone as well as renin, norepinephrine, and epinephrine *(see* ref. *13* for review). Some of the ET-1 induced changes in hormone secretion observed in vivo differ from those reported in vitro. For example, ET-1 invariably reduces renin secretion from isolated glomeruli, isolated kidney preparations and slices of the renal cortex *(see* ref. *14* for review).

As illustrated in Fig. 2, intrarenal infusion of ET-1 into the dog is characterized by a small transient renal vasodilation, which is then followed by vasoconstriction. The extent to which other vasoactive agents modulate or contribute to the renal vasodilation and/or vasoconstriction of ET-1 has been evaluated. Inhibitors of the α adrenergic system have no effect on the response to ET-1 in the rat, indicating that this system does not play a role in the cardiorenal responses to ET-1 *(15)*. Similarly, the prostaglandin-synthesis inhibitor, meclofenamate, has no effect on the cardiorenal actions of ET-1 in the rat *(16)*. In the dog, however, prostaglandin synthesis inhibition with indomethacin partially reduces the transient renal vasodilation associated with intrarenal infusion of ET-1 and augments the subsequent renal vasoconstriction *(17)*. The renin-angiotensin system does not appear to influence the actions of ET-1. Angiotensin II receptor blockade with saralasin has no effect on the decrease in renal blood flow prompted by an intrarenal infusion of ET-1 in the dog *(11)* or on the increase in mean arterial pressure in response to an intravenous infusion of ET-1 in the rat *(11)*. However, inhibition of the angiotensin II converting enzyme (kininase II) attenuates the ET-1 induced changes in renal function but has no effect on the blood-pressure response *(11,18,19)*.

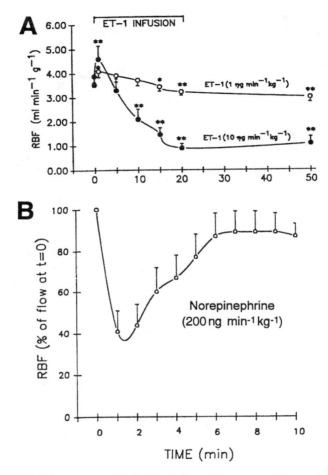

Fig. 2. (A) illustrates endothelin induced decreases in renal blood flow
(RBF), expressed in mL/kg/min, during a constant infusion of the peptide
for 20 min at 1 and at 10 ng/kg/min into the renal artery of two groups of
pentobarbital-anesthetized dogs. Similar experiments with norepinephrine (200 ng/kg/min; **B**), angiotensin II (50 ng/kg/min; **C**) and
vasopressin (10 mU/kg/min; **D**) infused for 10 min are also illustrated. In
the latter experiments, renal blood flow is plotted as percent of the baseline
values. Data are from Banks *(11,12)* and are reprinted with the permission of
the *American Journal of Physiology*.

Overall, these data indicate that the mechanism by inhibition of
angiotensin-converting enzyme attenuates the renal actions of ET-1
is owing to reduced kinin degradation.

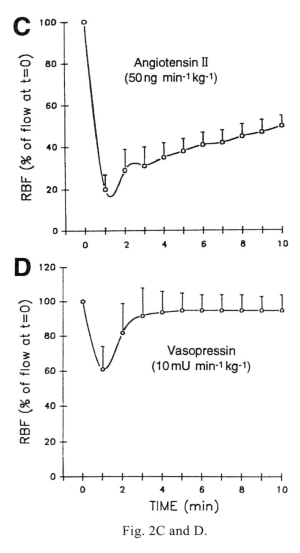

Fig. 2C and D.

The effect of chronic infusions of ET-1 into experimental animals has also been evaluated. In a study by Wilkins et al. *(20)*, ET-1 was infused for 8 d in amounts sufficient to produce circulating concentrations of the peptide similar to those reported in hypertensive states associated with arteriosclerosis, renal vascular disease and toxemia of pregnancy. Under these conditions, ET-1 induced significant increases in mean arterial pressure and total peripheral resistance coupled with a significant decrease in cardiac output. These results indicate that endothelin may be involved in the chronic hypertension in pathophysiological states associated with ET-cell dysfunction.

3.2. ET-1 and the Renal Microcirculation

Both afferent and efferent arterioles contract in response to exogenously administered endothelin. Although Edwards et al. *(21)* reported similar dose response curves for ET-1 in the two vascular segments isolated from the rabbit kidney, Lanese et al. *(22)* found ET-1 to be slightly more potent in the efferent arteriole of the rat. The latter observation is supported by the results of King et al. *(7)* using micropuncture techniques in intact rat kidneys to reveal that ET-1 increased efferent more than afferent arteriolar resistance. However, Loutenheizer et al. *(23)* found only a "modest" effect of ET-1 on the efferent arteriole when visualized in the hydonephrotic kidney of the rat. Nonetheless, using clearance techniques, a number of other investigators have observed that ET-1 has a more pronounced effect on renal blood flow as compared to glomerular filtration rate (GFR) in several species, again consistent with preferential efferent arteriolar constriction.

3.3. Glomerular Actions of Endothelin

It is well established that intravenous and or renal arterial infusions of endothelin are associated with dose dependent decreases in the GFR. In contrast to the rat, ET-1 produces a transient increase in renal blood flow during the first 5 min of a 30 min intrarenal infusion of 1 ng/kg/min in the dog *(11)*. This renal vasodilation is also associated with a transient increase in the GFR *(11)*.

As noted earlier, renal plasma flow and blood flow are more sensitive to ET-1 than is the GFR, i.e., ET-1 decreases renal plasma flow at doses that are lower than those required to reduce the GFR, thus significantly increasing the filtration fraction. ET-1 also increases glomerular-capillary pressure, proximal-tubular pressure and glomerular-transcapillary hydraulic pressure *(7)*. In addition to these changes in vascular resistance, endothelin-induced decreases in the glomerular ultrafiltration coefficient (K_f) also contribute to the decline in the GFR *(7)*. The effect of endothelin on K_f is likely caused by ET-1 induced contractions of mesangial cells. Badr et al. *(24)* demonstrated that ET-1 stimulates mesangial cell contraction via increases the cytoplasmic calcium concentration in mesangial cells.

3.4. Role of Extracellular Calcium

The ET-1 signal transduction pathway has been extensively investigated in vitro and is known to involve the influx of extracellular calcium (*see* ref. *25* for review). The role of extracellular calcium in mediating the cardiorenal actions of the peptide has also been evaluated in vivo. Both verapamil and manganese block ET-1 induced increases in mean arterial pressure but have no effect on ET-1 induced decreases in GFR in the euvolemic rat *(26)*. Verapamil also has no effect on ET-1 induced decreases in renal blood flow in the euvolemic dog during intrarenal infusions of the peptide *(26)*. On the other hand, in mannitol expanded rats, verapamil attenuates both the systemic and renal actions of ET-1 *(27)*. Similarly, lead, an agent known to block both L and T-type calcium channels, markedly attenuates both the increase in mean arterial blood pressure and the decrease in GFR; nickel, known to block primarily T-type calcium channels, has its most profound effect on the renal actions of ET-1 *(28)*. Montanes et al. *(29)* have reported that a new dihydropyridine derivative, pranedipine, blunts the effect of the ET-1 on renal vascular resistance and Takahashi et al. *(30)* found that manidipine, another newly developed dihydropyridine derivative, effectively reverses the renal actions of ET-1. Differences in the results of these studies may be related to a variety of factors, such as the dose of ET-1, the species of the experimental model, the dose and specificity of the calcium channel antagonist, the fluid volume state of the animal and/or to other factors. The dose of ET-1 may be a critical factor in determining which renal vascular-resistance segment is affected and, therefore, which type of calcium channel is involved in the response. ET-1 induced contractions of the afferent arteriole are reduced by L-type calcium-channel antagonists, indicating a significant peptide-induced mobilization of extracellular calcium in this segment of the renal vasculature *(21)*. By contrast, calcium channel antagonists have little effect on ET-induced contractions of the efferent arteriole *(21)*, an observation that is similar to that generally observed with most other vasoconstrictor agents in this resistance element. Consequently, at higher doses of ET-1, the effect of the peptide on the efferent arteriole may predominate, and thus would not be altered by an L-type calcium-channel antagonist. Other agents, such as nickel and lead, may attenuate the contractile events in both the pre- and post-glomerular segments. Also of interest, both enalapril and nifedipine can counteract the hypertensive effect of ET-1 in the human, but nifedipine is more effective in antagonizing the renal actions of the peptide *(31)*. These data further support the growing body of evidence that there are significant species-related differences in the biology of endothelin receptors and signal transduction mechanisms.

3.5. Other Endothelin Peptides

A number of investigators have evaluated the biological actions of Big ET-1. In rats, the pressor responses to Big ET-1 have been evaluated in vivo and in vitro (in isolated perfused kidneys) and both were reported to be dependent on the conversion of Big ET-1 to ET-1 by a phosphoramidon-sensitive converting enzyme *(32–36)*. In addition, Pollock et al. *(37)* have reported that iv administration of Big ET-1 in the rat induces significant decreases in RBF which are inhibited by phosphoramidon. Big ET-3 is not as potent as ET-1 as a pressor agent, but its activity is also inhibited by phosphoramidon *(38)*. Along these lines, Telemaque et al. *(36)*, using isolated, perfused rabbit kidneys, demonstrated that Big ET-1 and Big ET-2 produce a dose-dependent increase in renal-perfusion pressure and induce the release of prostacyclins. By contrast, Big ET-3 was inactive in their preparation. The effects of Big ET-1 and Big ET-2 on the isolated kidney were inhibited by phosphoramidon; therefore, in the rabbit kidney, the phosphoramidon-sensitive ET-converting enzyme can convert Big ET-1 and Big ET-2 but not Big ET-3.

Big ET-1 has direct vascular actions independent of conversion to ET-1 *(39,40)*. For example, Big ET-1 induces a concentration-dependent contraction in the rabbit saphenous vein and artery *(39)*. However, the actions in the artery, but not the vein, were sensitive to phosphoramidon; these data indicate that Big ET-1 can directly stimulate an endothelin receptor in the vein. It is also possible that there is a unique ET-converting enzyme that is not sensitive to phosphoramidon *(41)*.

Because the endothelin system is most likely autocrine and/or paracrine in nature, it can be hypothesized that sites where exogenous Big ET-1 has its most profound effects are probably also the sites where endothelin plays an important functional role. Furthermore, it is presumed that these are the sites rich with ET-converting enzyme. These ideas are supported by results indicating that ET-1 release from cultured endothelial cells is predominantly in the basal direction rather than luminally directed *(42)* and that ET-1 binding to its receptor is irreversible *(43,44)*. The latter observation provides a reasonable explanation for the fact that Big ET-1 infusion results in only modest elevations in circulating ET-1 levels yet produces dramatic hemodynamic effects *(45)*. Such findings also suggest that the amount of ET-1 circulating in plasma is not necessarily indicative of the activity of the local endothelin system. It appears that the sites where Big ET-1 is converted are also sites rich in ET_A receptors, because the ET_A receptor antagonist, BQ-123, completely prevents the systemic hypertensive response as well as the decrease in RBF and GFR induced by Big ET-1 *(46)*.

3.6. Endothelin Receptor Subtypes in the Kidney

Early pharmacological studies of endothelin receptors indicated that the vasoconstrictor actions of ET-1 were mediated exclusively by ET_A receptors with ET_B receptors responsible for the vasodilatory actions of the peptide. However, with the development of specific ET_A receptor antagonists, it became apparent that non-ET_A receptors mediate at least some of the vasoconstrictor actions of ET-1. In the rabbit and dog kidney, the vascular responses induced by ET-1 appear to be mediated by ET_A receptors *(47,48)*. However, there appears to be a species difference between the receptor subtypes present within the renal circulation. In the rat, Pollock and Opgenorth *(38,46)* demonstrated that there is a dose-dependent difference in the activation of ET-receptor subtypes. These investigators reported that BQ-123 blocks the renal response at low but not at high doses of ET-1 indicating that non-ET_A receptors mediate the response to a higher dose of the peptide. Binding studies suggest a mixed population of both ET_A and ET_B receptors in all species although the relative quantities of each subtype are not necessarily correlated to functional responses *(49–51)*.

More recently, Novak and Banks reported *(52)* that, in the rat, the ET_B receptor agonist, Ala[1,3,11,15]endothelin-1, causes only transient decreases in renal blood flow and glomerular-filtration rate, actions that are not affected by inhibition of prostaglandin or nitric oxide synthesis. These actions were also unaffected by the ET_A receptor antagonist, FR139317. Similarly, Wellings et al. *(53)* reported evidence of an important role for ET_B receptors in mediating the effects of ET-1 in the rat kidney. It is clear that ET_B receptors are present in the renal and several other arterial and venous circulations *(54–60)*. In addition, binding studies have confirmed the existence of ET_B receptors on vascular smooth muscle *(39,61)*.

Although only a single gene product has been cloned for ET_B receptors from mammalian cells, there is increasing evidence that there are subtypes of the ET_B receptor, i.e., the receptor subtype responsible for vasoconstriction has a different pharmacological profile from the receptor subtype responsible for vasodilation. Although the renal circulation contains both ET_A and ET_B receptors, ET_A receptor blockade completely prevents the decrease in RBF prompted by low doses of ET-1 in the rat *(46)*. If this decrease in renal blood flow was mediated by both ET_A and ET_B receptors, it would not be expected that ET_A receptor antagonists would completely prevent ET-1-induced renal vasoconstriction because ET-1 has a similar high affinity for both ET_A and ET_B receptors. In addition, Warner et al. *(59)* have demonstrated, in vitro, that the ET_B receptor present on vascular endothelium is responsible for the release of nitric oxide (termed ET_{B1}) and has a unique pharmacological profile compared to the ET_B receptor that mediates vasoconstriction (termed ET_{B2}). Nonetheless, at the present time there is no clear biochemical or molecular evidence for subtypes of the ET_B receptor.

3.7. Tubular and Excretion Variables Affected by Endothelin

Using doses of ET-1 that do not significantly decrease the GFR, King et al. *(7)* reported that there is a significant increase in urine flow and fractional sodium excretion. These investigators also showed that the excretory effects were abolished when renal perfusion pressure was controlled with an aortic snare, indicating that these may be pressure-related phenomena. These results were confirmed and extended by Uzuner and Banks *(62)*, who reported that ET-1-induced natriuresis and diuresis were abolished by removing the renal capsule or by preventing increases in renal arterial pressure. In addition, these authors reported that the site of tubular inhibition of sodium reabsorption is prior to the thick ascending limb. These data suggest that ET-induced natriuresis is primarily a pressure-related event. However, there is a growing body of evidence that endothelin indeed has direct tubular actions. ET-1 has been reported to inhibit arginine vasopressin-stimulated water and chloride absorption in vitro via ET_B receptors located on cortical collecting duct cells *(63–65)*. Furthermore, ET-1 inhibits sodium-potassium ATPase in the inner medullary-collecting duct *(66)*. These effects are consistent with the observation that endothelin often causes a natriuresis and diuresis in the isolated kidney wherein renal-perfusion pressure is held constant and extrarenal factors have been eliminated *(67,68)*. Other investigators have observed that ET-1 has potent diuretic and natriuretic effects when administered at doses that do not produce significant decreases in GFR *(69,70)*. Furthermore, Clavell et al. *(71)* reported that, in the dog, ET-induced diuresis is a tubular event related to the activation of ET_B receptors and that the natriuresis associated with low doses of endothelin is owing to a non-ET_A, non-ET_B receptor mediated decrease in proximal sodium reabsorption.

The renal excretory response to ET-1 and Big ET-1 again appears to be different between the two peptides. As noted by Hoffman et al. *(72)* and Pollock and Opgenorth *(35)*, Big ET-1 infusion results in a significant increase in both absolute and fractional sodium and water excretion not observed with ET-1. Even at doses that produce equivalent decreases in GFR, the diuretic and natriuretic properties of Big ET-1 are more prominent *(46)*. Blockade of the pressor response to Big ET-1 with an ET_A receptor antagonist does not prevent the increase in sodium and water excretion *(46)*. These results provide evidence for a direct action on tubular reabsorption that is mediated via non-ET_A receptors and are consistent with the observations that ET_B receptors are the predominant subtype located in the inner medullary collecting duct *(49,51,63,64)*. A direct action of Big ET-1 independent of conversion to ET-1 is unlikely because phosphoramidon inhibits the diuretic and natriuretic responses *(35)*. It is possible that Big ET-1 better survives metabolism in the brush border of the proximal tubule relative to ET-1 and thus can reach distal nephron sites in higher concentrations. This idea is supported by the observations that Big ET-1 has a much longer half-life in vivo and is less susceptible to the degrading effects of NEP 24.11 *(45,73)*, the enzyme capable of ET-1 metabolism found in high concentrations in the proximal tubule.

4. Systemic Actions of ET-1

The systemic actions of ET-1 are most commonly characterized by dose-dependent increases in arterial blood pressure and peripheral vascular resistance in both anesthetized and conscious animals *(3,6,74,75)*. In addition, others have reported that there is a transient decrease in arterial blood pressure and total peripheral resistance that precedes the sustained increases in these physiological variables *(74)*. MacLean et al. *(76)* have shown that the overall increase in total peripheral resistance is owing to a vasoconstriction in the spleen, stomach, large intestine, small intestine, kidney and pancreas and that cardiac output is redistributed to the heart, lung, liver, fat, and skin.

ET-1 has profound effects on the heart and the coronary circulation. The direct effects of ET-1 on the heart are different in vitro and in vivo. In isolated hearts, ET-1 has positive ionotropic and chronotropic effects *(77,78)*. In vivo, progressively higher doses of ET-1 are associated with a decrease in heart rate and cardiac output *(79,80)*. The opposing effects of ET-1, in vitro and in vivo, are likely related to a peptide-induced increase in coronary vasculature resistance. Within the coronary circulation, resistance vessels are more sensitive than conductive arteries to the vasoconstrictive effect of ET *(81)*. In anesthetized dogs, an intracoronary injection of ET-1 reduces coronary blood flow by 90% *(82)*. In fact, the endothelins have been shown to cause total coronary occlusion in several species *(44,83,84,85)*. It is also of interest to note that Cocks et al. *(86)* reported that coronary veins are more sensitive to ET than are coronary arteries.

The respiratory system is another system that produces ET peptides. This organ system is an important physiological component when considering the biological actions of the endothelin because the lungs may also play a role in the clearance of circulating endothelin peptides *(87)*. ET-1 causes a transient relaxation of tracheal smooth muscle, which is followed by a sustained contraction *(87,88)*; eicosanoids mediate at least some of these airway responses to the peptide. ET-1 induced contraction is attenuated by removing the epithelium or treating with the prostaglandin synthesis inhibitor, indomethacin *(89)*. ET-1 is also a potent bronchoconstrictor, in vivo *(90)*. This effect of ET can be potentiated by the β adrenergic blocker, propranolol *(91)*. This potentiation indicates that the sympathetic nervous system may antagonize the effects of ET-1.

The endothelin peptides are also produced within the gastrointestinal tract and so it is not surprising that the endothelins also affect this organ system. Intravenous infusion of ET-1 produces gastric vasoconstriction in the rat *(92)*. In addition, ET-1 induces constriction of the guinea pig ileum *(93)*. In the superior mesenteric arterial circulation maximal vasoconstriction to ET-1 is increased by pretreatment with indomethacin, suggesting that prostaglandins may modulate the actions of endothelin in this vascular bed.

ET-1 binding sites are present in the nonpregnant and pregnant uteri from several species including humans. All the endothelin peptides have been shown to cause contraction of the rat *(93–95)*, rabbit *(96)*, guinea pig *(97)*, sheep *(98)*, and human uterus *(99)*. In the rat uterus ET-1 causes two types of contractions; ET-1 induces both a phasic (rhythmic) and a tonic contraction. The phasic contractions can be inhibited by calcium channel antagonists whereas the tonic contractions are not dependent on extracellular calcium. In addition, there is evidence to suggest that the phasic contractions may be mediated by the ET_A receptor because the EC_{50} was not significantly different for ET-1, ET-2, and Sarafotoxin S6b, but was significantly higher for ET-3 *(95)*. In the latter study, Sakata and Karaki have also reported that ET-induced constriction of the uterine smooth muscle is highly dependent on the entry of extracellular calcium. In the nonpregnant uterus, this calcium influx is sensitive to verapamil and is therefore likely to involve L-type calciumchannels. In the pregnant uterus the ET response involves non-L-type calcium channels but does not appear to be dependent on the release of calcium from intracellular stores.

5. Summary and Conclusions

At the present time, the endothelins, and more specifically ET-1, are the most potent of the known vasoconstrictor agents that have been isolated. Endothelins produce a uniquely long-lasting vasoconstriction that is difficult and slow to reverse. Furthermore, the time required to attain a steady state is among the slowest of the known vasoactive agents. Given these characteristics, it seems likely that as the specific role(s) of these peptides in the regulation of regional hemodynamics is defined, the endothelins will be involved in more long-term regulation of the circulation, perhaps establishing or contributing to the basal state, rather than being involved in the short term regulation that occurs on a minute to minute scale.

References

1. Hickey, K. A., Rubanyi, G. M., Paul, R. J., and Highsmith, R. F. (1985) Characterization of a coronary vasoconstrictor produced by cultured endothelial cells. *Am. J. Physiol.* 248:C550–C556.
2. Yanagisawa, M., Kurihara, H., Kimura, S., Tomobe, Y., Kobayashi, M., Mitsui, Y., Yazaki, K., Goto, Y., and Masaki, T. (1988) A novel potent vasoconstrictor peptide produced by vascular endothelial cells. *Nature (London)* 332:411–415.
3. Goetz, K. L., Wang, B. C., Madwed, J. B., Zhu, J. L., and Leadley, R. J., Jr. (1988) Cardiovascular, renal, and endocrine responses to intravenous endothelin in conscious dogs. *Am. J. Phyiol.* 255:R1064–R1068.
4. Simonson, M. S. and Dunn, M. J. (1993) Endothelin peptides and the kidney. *Annu. Rev. Physiol.* 55:249–265.

5. Frelin, C. and Guedin, D. (1994) Why are circulating concentrations of endothelin-1 so low? *Cardiovas. Res.* **28:**1613–1622.
6. Miller, W. L., Redfield, M. M., and Burnett, J. C., Jr. (1989) Integrated cardiac, renal, and endocrine actions of endothelin. *J. Clin. Invest.* **83:**317–320.
7. King, A. J., Brenner, B. M., and Anderson, S. (1989) Endothelin: a potent renal and systemic vasoconstrictor peptide. *Am. J. Physiol.* **256:**F1051–F1058.
8. Kon, V., Yoshioka, T., Fogo, A., and Ichikawa, I. (1989) Glomerular actions of endothelin *in vivo. J. Clin. Invest.* **83:**1762–1767.
9. Lopez-Farre, A., Montanes, I., Mellas, I., and Lopez-Novoa, J. (1989) Effect of endothelin on renal function in rats. *Eur. J. Pharmacol.* **163:**187–189.
10. Tsuchiya, K., Naruse, M., Sanaka, T., Nitta, K., Demura, H., and Sugino, N. (1989) Effects of endothelin on renal regional blood flow in dogs. *Eur. J. Pharmacol.* **166:**541–543.
11. Banks, R. O. (1990) Effects of endothelin on renal function in dogs and rats. *Am. J. Physiol.* **258:**F775–F780.
12. Banks, R. O. (1988) Vasoconstrictor-induced changes in renal blood flow: role of prostaglandins and histamine. *Am. J. Physiol.* **254:**F470–F476
13. Takuwa, Y. (1993) Endothelin in vascular and endocrine systems: biological activities and its mechanism of action. *Endocrine J.* **40:**489–506.
14. Rubanyi, G. and Polokoff, M. (1994) Endothelins: molecular biology, biochemistry, pharmacology, physiology and pathophysiology. *Pharm. Rev.* **46(3):**325–415.
15. Cao, L. and Banks R. O. (1990) Effect of nephrectomy and of adrenergic receptor blockers on the cardiorenal actions of endothelin. *Proc. Soc. Exptl. Biol. Med.* **194:**119–124.
16. Cao, L. and Banks, R. O. (1990) Cardiorenal actions of endothelin, part II: effects of cyclooxygenase inhibitors. *Life Sci.* **46:**585–590.
17. Chou, S. Y., Dahhan, A., and Porush, J. G. (1990) Renal actions of endothelin: interaction with prostacyclin. *Am. J. Physiol.* **259:**F645–F652.
18. Cao, L. and Banks, R. O. (1990) Cardiorenal actions of endothelin, part I: effects of converting enzyme inhibition. *Life Sci.* **46:**577–583.
19. Chan, D. P., Clavell, A., Keiser, J., and Burnett, J. C., Jr. (1994) Effects of renin-angiotensin system in mediating endothelin-induced renal vasoconstriction: therapeutic implications. *J. Hypertens.* **12(Suppl. 4):**S43–S49.
20. Wilkins, F. C., Jr., Alberola, A., Mizelle, H. L., Opgenorth, T. J., and Granger, J. P. (1995) Systemic hemodynamics and renal function during long-term pathophysiological increases in circulating endothelin. *Am. J. Physiol.* **268:**R375–R381.
21. Edwards, R. M., Trizna, W., and Ohlstein, E. H. (1990) Renal microvascular effects of endothelin. *Am. J. Physiol.* **259:**F217–F221.
22. Lanese, D. M., Yuan, B. H., McMurtry, I., and Conger, J. D. (1992) Comparative sensitivities of isolated rat renal arterioles to endothelin. *Am. J. Physiol.* **263:**F894–F899.
23. Loutzenhiser, R., Epstein, M., Hayashi, K., and Horton, C. (1990) Direct visualization of effects of endothelin on the renal microvasculature. *Am. J. Physiol.* **258:**F61–F68.

24. Badr, K. F., Murray, J. J., Breyer, M. D., Takahashi, K., Inagami, T., and Harris, R. C. (1989) Mesangial cell, glomerular and renal vascular responses to endothelin in the rat kidney. *J. Clin. Invest.* **83:**336–342.
25. Highsmith, R. F., Blackburn, K., and Schmidt, D. J. (1992) Endothelin and calcium dynamics in vascular smooth muscle. *Annu. Rev. Physiol.* **54:**257–277.
26. Cao, L. and Banks, R. O. (1990) Cardiovascular and renal actions of endothelin: effects of calcium channel blockers. *Am. J. Physiol.* **258:**F254–F258.
27. Folzenlogen, S. L., Novak, J., and Banks, R. O. (1992) Renal actions of endothelin during mannitol and saline expansion. *Proc. Soc. Biol. Med.* **200:**378–382.
28. Novak, J. and Banks, R. O. (1995) Lead and nickel alter the cardiorenal actions of endothelin in the rat. *Proc. Soc. Exptl. Biol. Med.* **208:**191–198.
29. Montanes, I., Flores, O., Eleno, N., and Lopez-Novoa, J. M. (1994) Effects of a new dihydropyridine derivative, S12968 (pranedipine), and its stereoisomer, S12967, on renal effects of endothelin-1. *Can. J. Physiol. Pharmacol.* **72:**1294–1298.
30. Takahashi, K., Katoh, T., Fukunaga, M., and Badr, K. F. (1993) Studies on the glomerular microcirculatiory actions of manidipine and its modulation of the systemic and renal effects of endothelin. *Am. Heart J.* **125:**609–619.
31. Kaasjager, K. A., Koomans, H. A., and Rabelink, T. J. (1995) Effectiveness of enalapril versus nifedipine to antagonize blood pressure and the renal response to endothelin in humans. *Hypertension* **25:**620–625.
32. Gardiner, S. M., Compton, A. M., Kemp, P. A., and Bennett, T. (1991) The effects of phosphoramidon on the regional haemodynamic responses to human proendothelin [1–38] in conscious rats. *Br. J. Pharmacol.* **103:**2009–2015.
33. Matsumura, Y., Hisaki, K., Takaoka, M., and Morimoto, S. (1990) Phosphoramidon, a metalloprotease inhibitor, suppresses the hypertensive effect of big endothelin-1. *Eur. J. Pharmacol.* **185:**103–106.
34. McMahon, E. G., Palomo, M. A., Moore, W. M., McDonald, J. F., and Stern, M. K. (1991) Phosphoramidon blocks the pressor activity of porcine big endothelin-1-(1–39) *in vivo* and conversion of big endothelin-1-(1–39) to endothelin-1-(1–21) *in vitro. Proc. Natl. Acad. Sci. USA* **88:**703-707.
35. Pollock, D. M. and Opgenorth, T. J. (1991) Evidence for metalloprotease involvement in the in vivo effects of big endothelin 1. *Am. J. Physiol.* **261:**R257–R263.
36. Telemaque, S., Lamaire, D., Claing, A., and D'Orleans-Juste, P. (1992) Phosphoramidon-sensitive effects of big endothelins in the perfused rabbit kidney. *Hypertension* **20:**518–523.
37. Pollock, D. M., Divish, B. J., Milicic, I., Novosad, E. I., Burres, N. S., and Opgenorth, T. J. (1993) In vivo characterization of a phosphoramidon-sensitive endothelin-converting enzyme in the rat. *Eur. J. Pharmacol.* **231:**459–464.

38. Pollock, D. M. and Opgenorth, T. J. (1993) Evidence for endothelin-induced renal vasoconstriction independent of ET$_A$ receptor activation. *Am. J. Physiol.* **264**:R222–R226.

39. Auguet, M., Delaflotte, S., Chabrier, P. E., and Braquet, P. (1992) The vasoconstrictor action of big endothelin-1 is phosphoramidon-sensitive in rabbit saphenous artery but not in saphenous vein. *Eur. J. Pharmacol.* **224**:101,102.

40. Salvati, P., Dho, L., Calabresi, M., Rosa, B., and Patrono, C. (1992) Evidence for a direct vasoconstrictor effect of big endothelin-1 in the rat kidney. *Eur. J. Pharmacol.* **221**:267–273.

41. Opgenorth, T., Wu-Wong, J. R., and Shiosaki, K. (1992) Endothelin-converting enzymes. *FASEB J.* **6**:2653–2659.

42. Wagner, O. F., Christ, G., Wojta, J., Vierhapper, H., Parzer, S., Nowotny, P. J., Schneider, B., Waldhausl, W., and Binder, B. R. (1992) Polar secretion of endothelin-1 by cultured endothelial cells. *J. Biol. Chem.* **267**:16,066–16,068.

43. Hirata, Y., Yoshimi, H., Takaichi, S., Yanagisawa, M., and Masaki, T. (1988) Binding and receptor down-regulation of a novel vasoconstrictor endothelin in cultured rat vascular smooth muscle cells. *FEBS Lett.* **239**:13–17.

44. Clozel, M., Fischli, W., and Guilli, C. (1989) Specific binding of endothelin on human vascular smooth muscle cells in culture. *J. Clin. Invest.* **83**:1758–1761.

45. Hemsen, A., Pernow, J., and Lundberg, J. M. (1991) Regional extraction of endothelins and conversion of big endothelin to endothelin-1 in the pig. *Acta Physiol. Scand.* **141**:325–334.

46. Pollock, D. M. and Opgenorth, T. J. (1994) ET$_A$ receptor-mediated responses to endothelin-1 and big endothelin-1 in the rat kidney. *Br. J. Pharmacol.* **111**:729–732.

47. Yamashita, Y., Yukimura, T., Miura, K., Okumura, M., and Yamamoto, K. (1991) Effects of endothelin-3 on renal functions. *J. Pharmacol. Exp. Ther.* **259**:1256–1260.

48. Telemaque, S., Gratton, J. P., Claing, A., and D'Orleans-Juste, P. (1993) Endothelin-1 induces vasoconstriction and prostacyclin release via the activation of endothelin ET$_A$ receptors in the perfused rabbit kidney. *Eur. J. Pharmacol.* **237**:275–281.

49. Karet, F. E., Kuc, R. E., and Davenport, A. P. (1993) Novel ligands BQ123 and BQ3020 characterize endothelin receptor subtypes ET$_A$ and ET$_B$ in human kidney. *Kidney Internat.* **44**:36–42.

50. Nambi, P., Pullen, M., Wu, H. L., Aiyar, N., and Ohlstein, E. H. (1992) Identification of endothelin receptor subtypes in human renal cortex and medulla using subtype-selective ligands. *Endocrinology* **131**: 1081–1086.

51. Nambi, P., Wu, H. L., Pullen, M., Aiyar, N., Bryan, H., and Elliott, J. (1992) Identification of endothelin receptor subtypes in rat kidney cortex using subtype-selective ligands. *Mol. Pharmacol.* **42**:336–339.

52. Novak, J. and Banks, R. O. (1994). The cardiorenal response to the ET_B agonist, [Ala$^{1-3-11-15}$]ET-1. *FASEB J.* **8**:A580.
53. Wellings, R. P., Corder, R., Warner, T. D., Cristol, J. P., Thiemermann, C., and Vane, J. R. (1994) Evidence from receptor antagonists of an important role for ET_B receptor-mediated vasoconstrictor effects of endothelin-1 in the rat kidney. *Br. J. Pharmacol.* **111**:515–520.
54. Battistini, B., Warner, T. D., Fournier, A., and Vane, J. R. (1994) Characterization of ET_B receptors mediating contractions induced by endothelin-1 or IRL 1620 in guinea pig isolated airways: effects of BQ-123, FR 139317 or PD 145065. *Br. J. Pharmacol.* **111**:1009–1016.
55. Bigaud, M. and Pelton, J. T. (1992) Discrimination between ET_A- and ET_B-receptor-mediated effects of endothelin-1 and [Ala 1,3,11,15] endothelin-1 by BQ-123 in the anesthetized rat. *Br. J. Pharmacol.* **107**:912–918.
56. Clozel, M., Gray, G. A., Breu, V., Loffler, B. M., and Osterwalder, R. (1992) The endothelin ET_B receptor mediates both vasodilation and vasoconstriction in vivo. *Biochem. Biophys. Res. Comm.* **186**:867–873.
57. Cristol, J. P., Warner, T. D., Thiemermann, C., and Vane, J. R. (1993) Mediation via different receptors of the vasoconstrictor effects of endothelins and sarafotoxins in the systemic circulation and renal vasculature of the anaesthetized rat. *Br. J. Pharmacol.* **108**:776–779.
58. McMurdo, L., Corder, R., Thiemermann, C., and Vane, J. (1993) Incomplete inhibition of the pressor effects of endothelin-1 and related peptides in the anesthetized rat with BQ-123 provides evidence for more than one vasoconstrictor receptor. *Br. J. Pharmacol.* **108**:557–561.
59. Warner, T. D., Mitchell, J. A., de Nucci, G., and Vane, J. R. (1989) Endothelin-1 and endothelin-3 release EDRF from isolated perfused arterial vessels of the rat and rabbit. *J. Cardiovasc. Pharmacol.* **13**:S85–S88.
60. Warner, T. D., Battistini, B., Allcock, G. H., and Vane, J. R. (1993) Endothelin ET_A and ET_B receptors mediate vasoconstriction and prostanoid release in the isolated kidney of the rat. *Eur. J. Pharmacol.* **250**:447–453.
61. Webb, M. L., Liu, E. C. K., Monshizadegan, H., Chao, C. C., Lynch, J., Fisher, S. M., and Rose, P. M. (1993) Expression of endothelin receptor subtypes in rabbit saphenous vein. *Mol. Pharmacol.* **44**:959–965.
62. Uzuner, K. and Banks, R. O. (1993) Endothelin-induced natriuresis and diuresis are pressure-dependent events in the rat. *Am. J. Physiol.* **265**:R90–R96.
63. Edwards, R. M., Stack, E. J., Pullen, M., and Nambi, P. (1993) Endothelin inhibits vasopressin action in rat inner medullary collecting duct via the ET_B receptor. *J. Pharmacol. Exp. Ther.* **267**:1028–1033.
64. Kohan, D. E., Padilla, E., and Hughes, A. K. (1993) Endothelin B receptor mediates ET-1 effects on cAMP and PGE2 accumulation in rat IMCD. *Am. J. Physiol.* **265**:F670–F676.
65. Nadler, S. P., Zimpelmann, J. A, and Hebert, R. L. (1992) Endothelin inhibits vasopressin-stimulated water permeability in rat terminal inner medullary collecting duct. *J. Clin. Invest.* **90**:1458–1466.

66. Zeidel, M. L., Brady, H. R., Kone, B. C., Gullans, S. R., and Brenner, B. M. (1989) Endothelin, a peptide inhibitor of Na+-K+-ATPase in intact renal tubular epithelial cells. *Am. J. Physiol.* **257**:C1101–C1107.
67. Ferrario, R. G., Foulkes, R., Salvati, P., and Patrono, C. (1989) Hemodynamic and tubular effects of endothelin and thromboxane in isolated perfused rat kidney. *Eur. J. Pharmacol.* **171**:127–134.
68. Perico, N., Cornejo, R. P., Benigni, A., Malachini, B., Ladny, J. R., and Remuzzi, G. (1991) Endothelin induces diuresis and natriuresis in the rat by acting on proximal tubular cells through a mechanism mediated by lipoxygenase products. *J. Am. Soc. Nephol.* **2**:57–69.
69. Harris, P. J., Zhou, J., Mendelsohn, F. A. O., and Skinner, S. L. (1991) Haemodynamic and renal tubular effects of low doses of endothelin in anaesthetized rats. *J. Physiol.* **433**:25–39.
70. Schnermann, J., Lorenz, J. N., Briggs, J. P., and Keiser, J. A. (1992) Induction of water diuresis by endothelin in rats. *Am. J. Physiol.* **263**:F516–F526.
71. Clavell, A. L., Stingo, A. J., Margulies, K. B., Brandt, R. R., and Burnett, J. C. (1995) Role of endothelin receptor subtypes in the in vivo regulation of renal function. *Am. J. Physiol.* **37**:F455–F460.
72. Hoffman, A., Grossman, E., and Keiser, H. R. (1990) Opposite effects of endothelin-1 and Big endothelin-1(1–39) on renal function in rats. *Eur. J. Pharmacol.* **182**:603–606.
73. Abassi, Z. A., Golomb, E., Bridenbaugh, R., and Keiser, H. R. (1993) Metabolism of endothelin-1 and big endothelin-1 by recombinant neutral endopeptidase EC.3.4.24.11. *Br. J. Pharmacol.* **109**:1024–1028.
74. Hoffman, A., Grossman, E., Ohman, K. P., Marks, E., and Keiser, H. R. (1989) Endothelin induces an initial increase in cardiac output associated with selective vasodilation in rats. *Life Sci.* **45**:249–255.
75. Mortensen, L. H. and Fink, G. D. (1990) Hemodynamic effect of human and rat endothlein administration into conscious rats. *Am. J. Physiol.* **258**:H362–H368.
76. MacLean, M., Randall, M., and Hiley, C. (1989) Effects of moderate hypoxia, hypercapnia and acidosis on hemodynamic changes induced by endothelin-1 in the pithed rat. *Br. J. Pharmacol.* **98**:1055–1065.
77. Baydoun, A., Peers, S., Cirino, G., and Woodward, B. (1989) Effects of endothelin-1 on the rat isolated heart. *J. Cardiovasc. Pharmacol.* **13(Suppl. 5)**:S193–S196.
78. Firth, J., Roberts, A., and Raine, A. (1990) Effect of endothelin on the function of the isolated perfused working heart. *Clin. Sci.* **79**:221–226.
79. Lerman, A., Kubo, S., Tschumperlin, L., and Burnett, J. (1992) Plasma endothelin concentrations in humans with end stage heart failure and after heart transplantation. *J. Am. Coll. Cardiol.* **20**:849–853.
80. Lerman, A., Sandok, E., Hildebrand, J., and Burnett, J. (1992) Inhibition of endothelium derived relasing factor enhances endothelin mediated vasoconstriction. *Circulation* **85**:1894,1895.

81. Tippins, J. R., Antoniw, J. W., and Maseri, A. (1989) Endothelin-1 is a potent constrictor in conductive and resistive coronary arteries. *J. Cardiovasc. Pharmacol.* **13(Suppl. 5):**S177–S179.

82. Kurihara, H., Yamaoki, K., Nagai, R., Yoshizumi, M., Takaku, F., Satoh, H,. Inui, J., and Yazaki, Y. (1989) Endothelin: a potent vasoconstrictor associated with coronary vasospasm. *Life Sci.* **44:**1937–1943.

83. Chester, A. H., Dashwood, M. R., Clarke, J. G., Larken, S. W., Davies, G. J., Tadjkarimi, S., Maseri, A., and Yacoub, M. H. (1989) Influence of endothelin on human coronary arteries and localization of its binding. *Am. J. Cardiol.* **63:**1395–1398.

84. Kasuya, Y., Takuwa, Y., Yanagisawa, M., Kimura, S., Goto, K., and Masaki, T. (1989) Endothelin-1 induces vasoconstriction through two functionally distinct pathways in porcine coronary artery: contribution of phosphoinositide turnover. *Biochem. Biophys. Res. Commun.* **161:**1049–1055.

85. Hom, G. J., Touhey, B., and Rubanyi, G. M. (1992) Effects of intracoronary administration of endothelin in anesthetized dogs: comparison with Bay K 8644 and U46619. *J. Cardiovasc. Pharmacol.* **19:**194–200.

86. Cocks, T., Faulkner, N., Sudhir, K., and Angus, J. (1989) Reactivity of endothelin-1 on human and canine large veins compared with large arteries in vitro. *Eur. J. Pharmacol.* **171:**17–24.

87. DeNucci, G., Thomas, R., D'Orleans-Juste, P., Antunes, E., Walder, C., Warner, T., and Vane, J. (1988) Pressor effects of circulating endothelin are limited by its removal in the pulmonary circulation and by the release of prostacyclin and endotheium derived relaxing factor. *Proc. Natl. Acad. Sci. USA* **85:**9797–9800.

88. Filep, J. G., Battistini, B., and Sirois, P. (1990) Endothelin induces thromboxane release and contraction of isolated guinea pig airways. *Life Sci.* **47:**1845–1850.

89. White, S., Hathaway, D., Umans, J., Tallet, J., Abrahams, C., and Leff, A. (1991) Epithelial modulation of airway smooth muscle response to endothelin. *Am. Rev. Respir. Di.* **144:**373–378.

90. Uchida, Y., Ninomiya, H., Saotome, M., Nomura, A., Ohtsucka, M., Yanagisawa, M., Goto, K., Masaki, T., and Hasegawa, S. (1988) Endothelin, a novel vasoconstrictor peptide, as a potent bronchoconstrictor. *Eur. J. Pharmacol.* **154:**227,228.

91. Macquin-Mavier, I., Levame, M., Istin, N., and Harf, A. (1989) Mechanisms of endothelin mediated bronchoconstriction in the guinea pig. *J. Pharmacol. Exp. Ther.* **250:**740–745.

92. Wallace, J., Keenan, C., MacNaughton, W., and McKnight, G. (1989) Comparison of the effects endothelin-1 and endothelin-3 on the rat stomach. *Eur. J. Pharmacol.* **167:**41–47.

93. Borges, R., Von Grafenstein, H., and Knight, D. (1989) Tissue selectivity of endothelin. *Eur. J. Pharmacol.* **165:**223–230.

94. Kozuka, M., Ito, T., Hirose, S., Takahashi, K., and Hagiwara, H. (1989) Endothelin induces two types of contractions of rat uterus: phasic con-

tractions by way of voltage dependent calcium channels and developing contraction through a second type calcium channels. *Biochem. Biophys. Res. Comm.* **159**:317–323.

95. Sakata, K. and Karaki, H. (1992) Effects of endothelin on cytosolic calcium level and mechanical activity in rat uterine smooth muscle. *Eur. J. Pharmacol.* **221**:9–15.

96. Suzuki, Y. (1990) Properties of endothelin induced contractions in the rabbit non-pregnant and pregnant myometria. *Fukushima J. Med. Sci.* **36**:29–40.

97. Eglen, R., Michel, A., Sharif, N., Swank, S., and Whiting, R. (1989) The pharmacological properties of the peptide, endothelin. *Br. J. Pharmacol.* **97**:1297–1307.

98. Yang, D. and Clark, K. (1992) Effect of endothelin-1 on the uterine vasculature of the pregnant and estrogen treated nonpregnant sheep. *Am. J. Obstet. Gynecol.* **167**:1642–1650.

99. Svane, D., Larsson, B., Alm, P., Andersson, K., and Forman, A. (1993) Endothelin-1: immunocytochemistry, localization of binding sites and contractile effects in human uteroplacental smooth muscle. *Am. J. Obstet. Gynecol.* **168**:233–241.

Chapter 7

The Development of Specific Endothelin-Receptor Antagonists

Timothy D. Warner

1. Introduction

The endothelins (ETs) *(1,2)* are produced and active in almost all tissues. However, they are best known for their effects within the cardiovascular system, where they are potent vasoconstrictors and pressor agents, although there may also be accompanying vasodilatation, particularly at low concentrations *(2,3)*. The ETs also have numerous other effects, such as stimulating the release of autacoids and hormones, contracting nonvascular smooth muscle, potentiating and reducing neurotransmitter release, decreasing glomerular filtration, acting as cardiac inotropes and chronotropes, and increasing cell growth and division *(3–11)*. Despite this wide variety of effects, much endothelin research has examined the regulatory effects of the endothelins in the cardiovascular system, and the production of ET-receptor antagonists has principally been aimed at generating compounds that will reduce the deleterious effects of the endothelins in vascular pathologies ranging from hypertension to renal failure and stroke.

2. Involvement of Endothelin in Disease: Rationale for Producing Endothelin Receptor Antagonists

Healthy subjects have a low circulating level of immunoreactive-endothelin, approx 1.5 pmol/L, which is about one-tenth of that of circulating human atrial natriuretic peptide and several times less

From: *Endothelin: Molecular Biology, Physiology, and Pathology*
Edited by R. F. Highsmith © Humana Press Inc., Totowa, NJ

than that of angiotensin II (*see* ref. *12*). In a wide number of disease states such as acute myocardial infarction, cardiogenic shock, acute and chronic renal failure, hypertension, atherosclerosis, congestive heart failure, Raynaud's phenomenon, and surgery (*6*, *see* ref. *13*) this level is elevated. It is not clear, however, whether there is any causal relationship between these increases, which are almost without exception in the order of two- to threefold, and the disease states. However, the facts that ET-1 appears to be principally released abluminally *(14)* and has a particularly short half-life within the circulation *(15)* suggest that measurements of the plasma concentrations of ET-1 may not be particularly indicative of increases in its production within the vasculature. Further experiments using lung tissue from patients suffering from pulmonary hypertension do show, however, that increases in circulating endothelin are associated with an increase in ET-1-like immunoreactivity in endothelial cells and increased messenger RNA (mRNA) for ET-1 *(16)*.

Data from animal models of disease also suggest that endothelin is involved in numerous pathological states. For instance, increased circulating levels of immunoreactive endothelin are found in models of both experimental heart failure *(17)* and pulmonary hypertension *(18)*, and alterations in the expression of endothelin receptors are seen after local vascular insults *(19,20)*. Finally, before ET-receptor antagonists became available, infusion of endothelin antibodies was found to reduce both coronary infarct size in the rat and rabbit *(21–23)*, the deleterious effects of renal ischaemia and reperfusion in the rat *(24,25)*, the renal damaging effects of cyclosporine *(26,27)*, the increases in blood urea nitrogen and plasma creatinine and the falls in urine production and urinary sodium excretion following lipopolysaccharide injection to rats *(28)*, the ulcerogenic effects of alcohol *(29,30)* or indomethacin *(31)* applied to the inner surface of the stomach, the intestinal hypoperfusion associated with iv administration of live *Escherichia coli* *(32)*, and the damaging effects of ischemia and reperfusion in the liver *(33)*. Together these observations strongly encouraged the production of ET-receptor antagonists.

3. Endothelin Receptors

Soon after the characterization of the endothelin family of peptides, it became apparent that there was more than one endothelin receptor. For instance, although in vivo and in many vascular beds and isolated vascular tissues, ET-3 is less potent than ET-1 at producing vasoconstriction, these two peptides are equipotent at producing vasodilatation and the release of nitric oxide *(1,34,35)*. From this it appeared that there could be two different endothelin receptors: an isopeptide selective receptor (ET-1 > ET-3) that mediated the pressor effects of the endothelins and a nonselective receptor (ET-1 = ET-3) present on the endothelium. Similarly, receptor-binding assays indicated the presence of heterogeneous populations of endothelin receptors in a variety of tissues (*see* ref. *10*). Molecular biology soon confirmed these suggestions with the cloning and expression of two endothelin receptors, the ET_A receptor, that is selective for ET-1, ET-2 or SX6b over ET-3 or SX6c *(36)*, and the ET_B receptor that does not discriminate among the endothelin/sarafotoxin peptides *(37)*. These receptors have very similar predicted molecular weights of approx 47 kDa and contain seven transmembrane domains of 20–27 hydrophobic amino-acid residues, typical of the rhodopsin-type superfamily of G protein-coupled receptors. As may be expected, the genes encoding these receptors have been suggested to be expressed in a wide variety of tissues and species (*see* ref. *4*).

Within the vasculature, it appeared initially that the contractile effects of the endothelins were mediated by the isopeptide selective (ET_A) receptor present on smooth muscle and that endothelial cells expressed the ET_B receptor, activation of which led to the production of nitric oxide and vasodilatation. This was not a very long-lived idea because it quickly became clear that within the vasculature either ET_A or ET_B receptors may mediate vasoconstriction *(38–46)*. Although it still appears to be the rule that only ET_B receptors mediate vasodilatation.

3.1. Additional Endothelin Receptors

Despite the cloning of only two mammalian endothelin receptors, functional evidence suggests the presence of additional subtypes. The most widely proposed of these is the ET_C receptor *(47)*, classified as being selective for ET-3 over ET-1. This may be present on some bovine endothelial cells and its activation appears to lead to the release of nitric oxide *(48,49)*. It may also be expressed elsewhere, as receptor-binding assays have identified high affinity receptors selective for ET-3 in rat brain and atria *(20,50)* and similar receptors have been detected in anterior pituitary cells *(51)*. However, to date such a receptor has only been cloned from nonmammalian species *(52)*. There is also accumulating data suggesting that the ET_B receptor present on the endothelium, which mediates the release of nitric oxide in response to the endothelins, is functionally different from the ET_B receptor mediating the vasoconstrictor effects of the endothelins (44,45,53). These have tentatively been classified as ET_{B1} (present on the endothelium) and ET_{B2} (present on vascular and nonvascular smooth muscle) (45). Similarly, it has also been suggested that there may exist ET_{A1} and ET_{A2} receptors, where the former are BQ-123-sensitive and the latter BQ-123-insensitive (54). In addition, other functional studies have suggested non ET_A/ET_B receptors to mediate responses to the endothelins in smooth-muscle preparations from the rat, guinea pig, and rabbit (see ref. 4). It must, however, also be noted that experiments with novel antagonists of the ET_A and ET_B receptors (respectively BQ-123 and BQ-788, see Sections 4.1. and 4.2.) have led to the suggestion (see ref. 55) that the two cloned mammalian receptors may account for all the responses reported, but variations in the relative populations of these receptors in different tissues may confound receptor characterization (56). The answers to these questions will become more clear as it becomes possible to study the activities of tissues derived from ET-receptor deficient animals (57), as long as such animals prove to be viable (see ref. 58).

4. Endothelin Antagonists

There are strong indications that an increase in the production of endothelin is a promoting factor in a number of disease states. Taken together with the characterization of endothelin receptors, there is therefore a clear rationale and a good scientific background for the development of ET-receptor antagonists. However, an alternative approach to antagonizing the effects of ET-1, second to its production, is to limit its synthesis, most obviously by inhibiting endothelin-converting enzyme (ECE). This has attractions as a therapeutic route because it would be effective irrespective of any alterations in the population of endothelin receptors that may occur with pathological changes (19). Experiments to produce inhibitors of ECE have been complicated by a lack of purified enzyme, but fortunately this problem has recently been overcome by the purification of ECE (59–65). Indeed, this research has revealed a group of related proteins named ECE-1a, ECE-1b and ECE-2 (see ref. 58). With this background it is interesting to speculate on the effects of blockade of ECE. If this is the enzyme responsible for the "physiological" formation of ET-1 from big ET-1, would its blockade lead to an increase in circulating levels of big ET-1, as would appear to be the case in cultured endothelial cells *(66)*? If so, this would present more substrate to other enzymes that can convert big ET-1 to ET-1 such as elastase, released from neutrophils *(67)*, or chymase released from mast cells *(68)*, both of which are more active converters of big ET-1 than the "physiological" ECE. These systems could become important in pathological states when these enzymes may be released from cells. It is also interesting to speculate whether the final step in conversion of big ET-1 to ET-1 does indeed take place outside the cell responsible for the synthesis of big ET-1 as the circulating levels of big ET-1 are two- to threefold higher than the circulating levels of ET-1 (*see* ref. *13*). Thus, it may be that conversion of big ET-1 outside the endothelial cell, either by other endothelial cells or alternative cell types such as vascular smooth muscle *(69)*, is of more importance in the body than intracellular conversion followed by release. Inhibitors of ECE could therefore regulate the activities of endothelin both in health and disease. These questions may possibly be answered by the development of selective ECE inhibitors and data from animals in which the ECE gene(s) has been deleted.

Many substances have been reported as being endothelin receptor antagonists (*see* Table 1). However, this chapter will concentrate on those that have been used most widely, and those, particularly non-peptidic antagonists, which will probably be of the greatest future interest.

4.1. ET_A Receptor-Selective Antagonists

The most well known of the ET_A receptor-selective antagonists, in particular BQ-123 and BQ-153, were developed from peptides discovered in the broth from the mycelium of *Streptomyces misakiensis* *(70–72, see ref. 73)*. These are cyclic pentapeptides that have a high affinity for ET_A receptors in porcine and rat vascular smooth muscle *(19,71,72,74)*, whereas they are ineffective at displacing binding from ET_B receptors, e.g., in cerebellar membranes. Related to these are two linear tripeptidic, selective ET_A receptor antagonists, FR 139317 *(75–78)* and BQ-610 *(79)* that were developed from the same natural product. A number of other ET_A selective antagonists have also been reported including TTA-101 (*t*-Bu OCO-Leu-Trp-Ala), TTA-386 *(80)*, myriceron caffeoyl ester (50-235), a nonpeptide isolated from the bayberry *Myrica cerifera (81)*, and asterric acid *(82)*. However, in contrast to BQ-123 and FR 139317, which are the compounds that have been mainly used, very few studies have been published using

Table 1
Notable Endothelin Receptor Antagonists

Compound	Type	Selectivity	In vivo activity	Ref.
[D-Arg[1], D-Phe[5], D-Trp[7,9],Leu[11]]-SP	Peptidic	ET_A?		*183*
[Dpr[1],Asp[15]]-ET-1	Peptidic	ET_A?		*184*
BE-18257B	Peptidic	ET_A		*70*
BQ-123	Peptidic	ET_A	iv	*71*
BQ-153	Peptidic	ET_A	iv	*71*
BQ-485	Peptidic	ET_A	iv	*172*
FR 139317	Peptidic	ET_A	iv	*78*
50-235	Nonpeptidic (myricerone)	ET_A		*81*
TTA-386	peptidic	ET_A		*80*
Asterric acid	Nonpeptidic	ET_A?		*82*
BMS-182874	Nonpeptidic (sulfonamide)	ET_A	iv, po	*83*
PD 155080	Nonpeptidic	ET_A		*58*
PD 155719	Nonpeptidic	ET_A		*58*
PD 156707	Nonpeptidic	ET_A	iv, po	*84*
IRL 1038	Peptidic	ET_B	iv	*85*
IRL 2500	Peptidic	ET_B	iv	*58*
IRL 2659	Peptidic	ET_B		*58*
IRL 2796	Peptidic	ET_B		*58*
RES-701-1	Peptidic	ET_B	iv	*90*
BQ-788	Peptidic	ET_B	iv	*88*
Ro 46-8443	Nonpeptidic (sulfonamide)	ET_B		*58*
TAK-044	Peptidic	ET_A/ET_B	iv	*96*
PD 142893	Peptidic	ET_A/ET_B	iv	*91*
PD 145065	Peptidic	ET_A/ET_B	iv	*92*
Cochinmicins	Cyclodepsipeptides	ET_A/ET_B		*104*
Ro 46-2005	Nonpeptidic (sulfonamide)	ET_A/ET_B	iv, po	*98*
Ro 47-0203	Nonpeptidic (sulfonamide)	ET_A/ET_B	iv, po	*99*
SB 209670	Nonpeptidic	ET_A/ET_B	iv, id[a]	*100*
SB 217242	Nonpeptidic	ET_A/ET_B		*58*
L751281	Nonpeptidic (sulfonamide)	ET_A/ET_B		*58*
CGS 27830	Nonpeptidic (dihydropyridine)	ET_A/ET_B	iv	*103*

[a]id = intraduodenally.

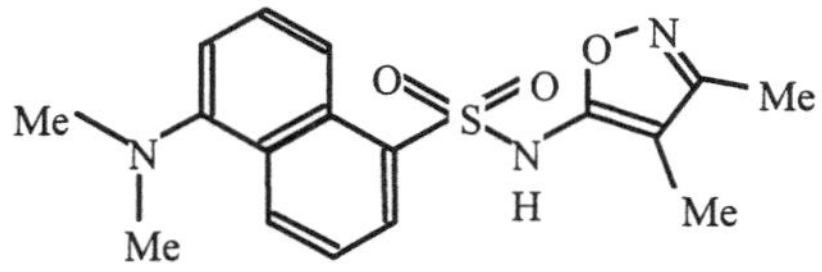

Fig. 1. Structure of the nonpeptide, selective ET_A receptor antagonist BMS-182874 *(83)*.

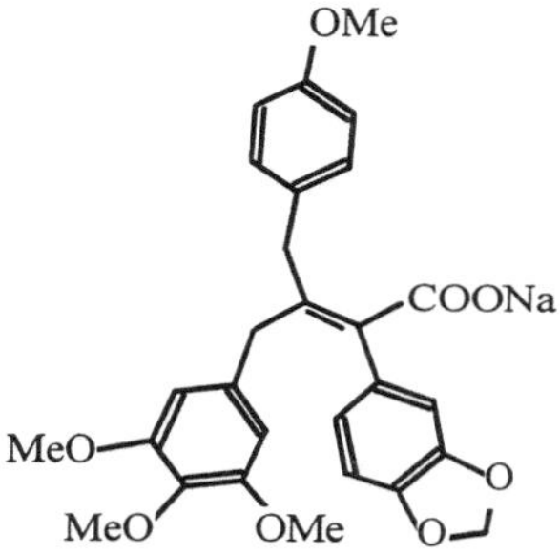

Fig. 2. Structure of the nonpeptide, selective ET_A receptor antagonist PD 156707 *(84)*.

these latter antagonists and as such it is difficult to discuss their selectivity or possible utility.

There have only been a few reports of the production of nonpeptide antagonists of which the most notable is a sulfonamide, BMS-182874 (5-(dimethylamino)-N-(3,4-dimethyl-5-isoxazolyl)-1-napthalene-sulfonamide) (Fig. 1), that is also orally active *(83)*. This agent inhibits the binding of ET-1 to ET_A receptors with an IC_{50} value of 55 nM whereas it has little activity on ET_B receptors, such that overall it has a 3600-fold selectivity for the ET_A receptor. Most recently PD 155080, PD 155719 and PD 156707 (Fig. 2) have also been reported to be potent nonpeptide ET_A receptor antagonists *(see refs. 58,84)*. Little has currently been disclosed about the activities of these new compounds, but it has been reported that PD 156707 inhibits the binding of ET-1 to cloned human ET_A and ET_B receptors with K_i values of 0.17 and 133.8 nM, and the vasoconstrictions induced by ET-1 in rabbit blood vessels, with pA_2 values of 7.5 and 4.7, respectively *(84)*.

4.2. ET_B Receptor-Selective Antagonists

Currently there is less information with regard to ET_B receptor selective antagonists than other classes of ET-receptor antagonists.

In particular, almost all of these have peptidic structures. IRL 1038, ([Cys^{11}–Cys^{15}]–ET–1$_{(11-21)}$), was one of the first reported of these peptide antagonists, and was stated to have a much higher affinity for ET$_B$ receptors (K_i = 6–11 nM) than for ET$_A$ receptors (K_i = 400–700 nM) and to antagonize functional responses mediated by ET$_B$ receptors *(85)*. However, it has subsequently appeared that conclusions drawn from experiments using this compound should be regarded very cautiously *(86)*. BQ-788 has also been disclosed as a selective ET$_B$ receptor antagonist. This is a linear peptide that inhibits binding to ET$_B$ receptors with an IC$_{50}$ value of 1.2 nM and to ET$_A$ receptors with an IC$_{50}$ value of 280 nM *(87)*. In isolated rabbit pulmonary arteries, BQ-788 competitively antagonises the vasoconstrictions induced by an ET$_B$-selective agonist BQ-3020 with a pA$_2$ of 8.4 *(88)*. Interestingly, when administered in vivo it abolishes the initial transient depressor response induced by bolus injection of ET-1 and reveals an initial pressor effect. When given to the anesthetized rat as an infusion together with ET-1, BQ-788 also increases the regional vasoconstrictor effects of ET-1, reinforcing the notion that ET$_B$ receptors are particularly important in limiting the vasoconstrictor and pressor effects of endothelin *(89)*. The cyclic-peptide antagonist RES-701-1, isolated from *Streptomyces sp.*, has also been reported to be a selective ET$_B$ receptor antagonist *(90,54)* and to inhibit the binding of ET-1 to ET$_B$ receptors with an IC$_{50}$ value of 10 nM. This compound does not affect binding of ET-1 to ET$_A$ receptors, even when used at concentrations up to 5 µM. Like BQ-788, RES-701-1 also attenuates the depressor and enhances the pressor effects of intravenously applied ET-1 in anaesthetized rats.

4.3. ET$_{A/B}$ Receptor Nonselective Antagonists

As both ET$_A$ and ET$_B$ receptors mediate the contractile effects of the endothelins in the vasculature, both have been implicated as mediating the deleterious effects of the endothelins. ET$_{A/B}$ receptor nonselective antagonists may, therefore, be the most effective in a range of disease states. The first well known of these nonselective antagonists were those produced by Parke-Davis. These peptide antagonists were developed by a rational approach starting with ET$_{(16-21)}$, which is known to interact with ET receptors *(91–94)*. Modification of the C-terminal hexapeptide portion of ET-1 by substituting His^{16} with (β-Phenyl)-D-Phe produced PD 142893, and incorporation of D-Bhg (5H-dibenzyl[a,d]cycloheptene-10,11-dihydroglycine) in

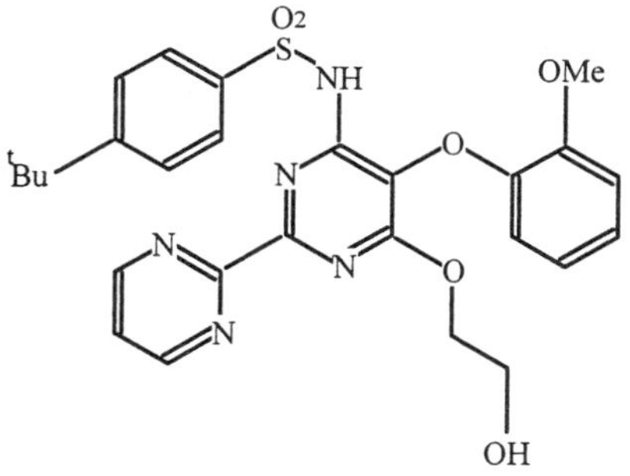

Fig. 3. Structure of the nonpeptide, nonselective ET receptor antagonist bosentan (Ro 47-0203) *(99)*.

position 16, produced PD 145065 (*see* Table 1). This latter compound had a greater binding affinity to both ET_A and ET_B receptors than did PD 142893. Other much larger ET-1-derivatives, such as [Thr^{18}, γ methyl Leu^{19}]ET-1, have also been shown to bind with high affinities to both ET_A and ET_B receptors. However, there is little information as to the usefulness of this latter compound as a functional antagonist of endothelin responses *(95)*. Compounds related to BQ-123 have also been developed as nonselective ET-receptor antagonists *(96)*. The most active of these is TAK-044 (cyclo(-D-Asp-AlaPhp-Asp-D-Thg-Leu-D-Trp-) where Php=3-[(4-phenylpiperazin-1-yl)carbonyl] and Thg = 2-(2-thienyl)glycine), which has an IC_{50} to inhibit binding of ET-1 to ET_A receptors of 0.08 n*M* and to ET_B receptors of 120 n*M*. TAK-044 also antagonizes ET_A receptor mediated constrictions of isolated porcine coronary arteries and ET_B receptor mediated constrictions of isolated porcine coronary vein. As may be expected when tested in vivo, this compound blocks both the pressor and the depressor responses to bolus injection of ET-1 *(97)*.

Product library screening has led to the discovery of the orally active nonpeptide ET-receptor antagonist, Ro 46-2005 *(98)*. Ro 46-2005 inhibits binding to both ET_A and ET_B receptors, although with considerably less affinity than the nonselective peptidic antagonist, PD 145065. On the other hand, Ro 46-2005 has the advantage of being orally active (30% bioavailability), which peptide antagonists rarely are. Ro 46-2005 has been superseded by Ro 47-0203 (bosentan) (Fig. 3), which is a more potent receptor nonselective antagonist *(99)*. Bosentan inhibits binding of ET-1 to ET_A receptors with a K_i of 4.7 n*M* and to ET_B receptors with a K_i of 95 n*M*. Predict-

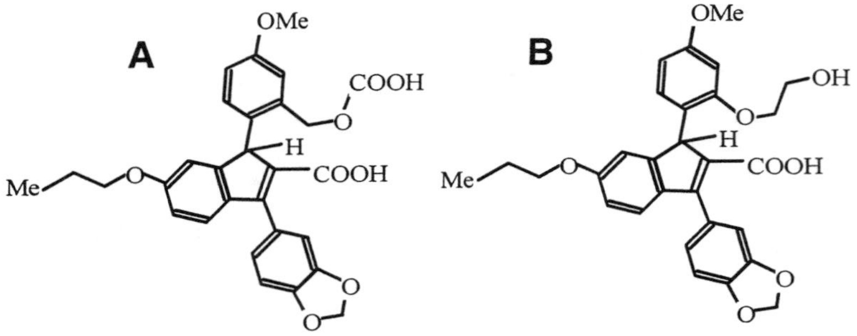

Fig. 4. Structure of the nonpeptide, nonselective ET receptor antagonists **(A)** SB 209670 *(100)* and **(B)** SB 217242 *(58)*.

ably, it inhibits the pressor effects of big ET-1, when both antagonist and peptide are administered intravenously to pithed rats. Of great interest, it is also active when administered orally.

SB 209670 is another nonpeptide, nonselective ET-receptor antagonist, which was rationally designed using conformational models of ET-1 (Fig. 4; *100*). This agent inhibits binding to ET_A and ET_B receptors, and, for instance, has K_d values for binding to human ET_A and ET_B receptors of 1 and 10 nM *(101)*. In vitro, it inhibits contractions of the rat thoracic aorta induced by ET-1, an ET_A receptor-mediated response, with a K_B value of 0.4 nM and ET_B receptor mediated contractions of rabbit pulmonary artery with a K_B value of 88 nM *(102)*. This agent inhibits both the pressor and depressor effects of intravenously applied ET-1 *(102)*. Finally, within the sulfonamide derivatives, L751281 (Fig. 5) has also been reported as a nonselective antagonist, but little further information is currently available *(see ref. 58)*.

CGS 27830 (Fig. 6), which is derived from the quite structurally different dihydropyridine class of calcium ion modulators, potently inhibits binding to ET_A receptors (IC_{50} value 16 nM), but has less activity at ET_B receptors (IC_{50} value 295 nM) *(103)*. This agent also inhibits contractions of the rabbit aorta induced by ET-1 and the increases in inositol phosphate turnover stimulated by ET_A receptor activation. In vivo, CGS 27830 abolishes the pressor effect and reduces the depressor effect of a bolus injection of ET-1. In a fashion analogous to the discovery of BQ-123 and related compounds, the cochinmicins I, II, and III, which are products of *Microspora sp.* ATCC55140, have also been reported to be nonselective $ET_{A/B}$ antagonists *(104,105)*.

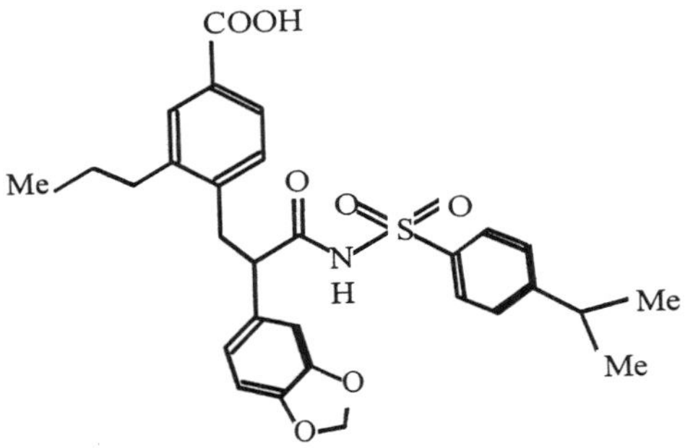

Fig. 5. Structure of the nonpeptide, nonselective ET receptor antagonist L751281 *(58)*.

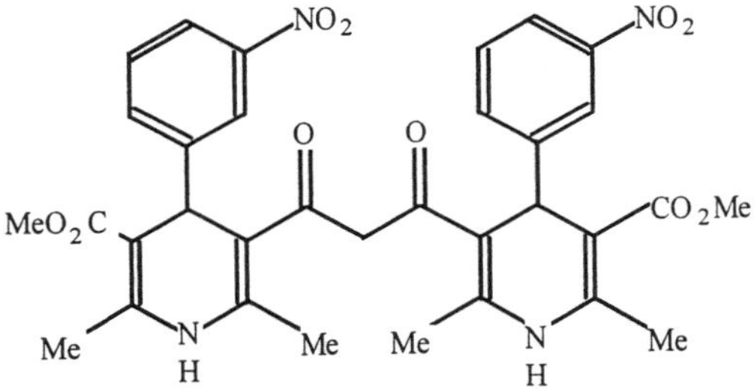

Fig. 6. Structure of the nonpeptide, nonselective ET receptor antagonist CGS 27830 *(103)*.

5. Effects of ET-Receptor Antagonists

The ET_A receptor selective antagonists are the compounds that have been most widely studied. As might be expected, BQ-123 antagonizes constrictions of the isolated porcine coronary artery induced by ET-1, inhibits binding to ET_A receptors on vascular smooth-muscle cells, and blunts, but does not ablate, the pressor effects of ET-1 in anesthetized rats *(71)*. The incomplete suppression of the pressor effects of ET-1 is owing to the presence of non-ET_A constrictor receptors within the rat circulation, most notably within the mesenteric and renal beds *(106–109)*. Thus, PD 145065 or TAK-044 block the renal constrictor effects of ET-1 in the anesthetized rat, illustrating the importance of ET_B vasoconstrictor receptors *(97)*. However, the other side of their potency on ET_B receptors is that PD 142893, PD 145065, or TAK-044 block the depressor effects of intravenously administered ET-1 *(91,92,97,109)*, as does the selective ET_B receptor antagonist, BQ-788 *(88)*. This action is in contrast to BQ-123 or FR 139317, which either do not affect or tend to potentiate this portion of the ET-1 response *(78,110)*. From these experiments it therefore appears that in the rat, both ET_A and ET_B receptors mediate the vasoconstrictor effects of the endothelins and that ET_B receptors, most probably present on the endothelium *(34,35,44,45)*, mediate the transient-depressor response to the endothelins. In addition, these nonselective antagonists have been suggested to increase the circulating levels of ET-1 by displacing it from ET_B receptors *(111)*.

In all other species so far tested it also appears that although both ET_A and ET_B receptors mediate vasoconstriction, only ET_B receptors mediate vasodilatation. However, the relative importance of different endothelin receptors in various tissues differs among species. For instance, in the rat, the renal vasoconstrictor effects of the endothelins are mediated by a mixed population of ET_A and ET_B receptors. However, in the pig, these responses are more dependent on ET_A receptors *(112),* and in the rabbit, they are entirely blocked by BQ-123 *(113)*. Similarly, contractions of the pulmonary artery from the rabbit are mediated mainly by ET_B receptors and not sensitive to BQ-123 *(44,45,56,114,115)*, whereas in porcine, guinea-pig, and human vessels, ET_A receptors predominate *(40,53,116)*. Furthermore, there are variations in the endothelin receptors mediating the effects of the endothelins in nonvascular tissue. For instance, BQ-123 or FR 139317 are not effective against ET-1 induced contractions of the trachea or upper bronchi from the guinea-pig *(12)* or bronchi from the human *(41)*, whereas they may reduce contractions induced by ET-1 in the rat trachea *(117)*.

In most species, e.g., dog *(118,119)*, application of ET-receptor antagonists does not generally affect the basal blood pressure. However, there are exceptions to this rule. For instance, in either anesthetized or conscious guinea pigs, both bosentan and BQ-123 lower blood pressure *(120)*. Interestingly, in the rat, removal of nitric oxide vasodilator tone by application of inhibitors of nitric oxide synthase, causes an increase in blood pressure that is reduced by either BQ-123 or bosentan *(121)*. Most importantly, preliminary observations suggest that ET-1 maintains vascular tone in humans, as infusion of phosphoramidon or BQ-123 into the brachial artery increases forearm blood flow *(122)*. Furthermore, in healthy humans, iv application of TAK-044 (10–100 mg, iv) has been reported to lower blood pressure by approx 10%, an effect that is sustained for at least 4 h *(123)*.

Table 2
Disease Models in Which Endothelin-Receptor Antagonists Are Effective

Model	Species	Reference
Atherosclerosis	Hamster	*162*
Subarachnoid hemorrhage	Dog	*170,171,173*
	Rabbit	*55,174*
	Rat	*55,98*
Pulmonary hypertension	Dog	*158,159*
	Rat	*154,155*
	Sheep	*156,175*
Hypertension	Rat	*55,83,142,146–151*
	Dog	*118*
	Monkey	*98*
Malignant hypertension	Rat	*152*
Myocardial ischemia/reperfusion	Rat	*126–128*
	Rabbit	*129*
	Pig	*130*
	Dog	*124*
Chronic heart failure	Rat	*133*
Vascular restenosis	Rat	*163,166,167*
Renal ischemia/reperfusion	Rat	*98,126,134–139*
	Dog	*140, 185*
Cyclosporine nephrotoxicity	Rat	*26,141*
Radiocontrast dye nephrotoxicity	Dog	*143*
	Rat	*144*
Lupus nephritis	Mouse	*145*
Diabetic neuropathy	Rat	*178,179*

6. ET-Receptor Antagonists in Disease Models

ET-receptor antagonists have been tested for their efficacy in a number of disease models (*see* Table 2), as suggested by earlier experiments using antiendothelin antibodies or by measurements of the circulating levels of endothelin in disease states. It is true, however, that the most widely studied pathologies have been those characterized by cardiovascular dysfunction, as is evident from the following sections.

6.1. Myocardial Infarction and Heart Disease

In the dog, BQ-123 decreases the size of the infarction following 90 min of ischemia and 5 h of reperfusion *(124)*, although not following 90 min of ischemia and 4 h of reperfusion *(125)*. TAK-044 has been reported to decrease infarct size in a rat model of coronary ischemia and reperfusion *(126,127)* For instance, administration of TAK-044 (3 mg/kg) 10 min prior to the period of ischemia (1 h) and reperfusion (24 h) reduced the infarct size by 54% *(127)*. Similarly, in both rabbit and rat models of myocardial ischemia and reperfusion, FR 139317 has been associated with a reduction in infarct size over the acute period of a 90–180 min reperfusion *(128,129)*. In the pig, following ligation of the left anterior descending coronary artery for 45 min and 4 h of reperfusion, bosentan significantly reduces infarct size, by about 50% and greatly enhances the recovery of coronary-blood flow *(130)*. These data clearly imply a role for endothelin in ischemia/reperfusion injury. However, this conclusion must be weighted by other observations suggesting that endothelin only plays a minor role under these conditions. In the rat, for instance, although bosentan increases coronary flow in paced hearts, it does not influence the recovery of cardiac function after 20 min of global ischemia *(131)*, nor does it affect heart rate, arterial pressure or the rate pressure product before or during ischemia or during 2 h of reperfusion *(132)*. There is some evidence supportive of a role for endothelin in chronic heart failure. In a conscious rat model, chronic administration of bosentan significantly reduces arterial blood pressure even in the presence of cilazapril, an angiotensin-converting enzyme inhibitor *(133)*.

6.2. Renal Disease

ET-1 is expressed throughout the kidney, in the glomeruli, small cortical vessels, early proximal tubules, collecting ducts, and vasa recta, and ET-binding sites are similarly found in the glomeruli, early proximal tubules, inner medullary-collecting ducts and vasa recta. These binding sites represent both ET_A receptors, particularly in the vascular portion of the kidney, and ET_B receptors, particularly in the tubular portion.

A high dose (0.5 mg/kg/min) of BQ-123 is necessary to show a very small protective effect in a model of ischemic acute renal failure in the rat *(134)*. However, more positive data have been shown in a model of severe post-ischemic acute renal failure *(135)*. In uninephrectomized rats, 45 min of renal occlusion and then reperfusion was associated with a 98% fall in glomerular-filtration rate and a very marked increase in the fractional excretion of sodium. All animals died within 4 d. Treatment with BQ-123 for 3 h 1 d after ischemia resulted in an improved survival rate (75%) and an improved reabsorption of sodium. In a similar model, 10-min pretreatment with the nonselective antagonist TAK-044 prior to artery occlusion was associated with an attenuation of the increase in plasma creatinine seen at 24 h *(136)*. In rats, BMS-182874 gives weak protection of glomerular-filtration rate 2 h after a 30-min ischemic period in the kidney, but not after 24 h *(137)*. PD 145065 treatment for 60 min either side of a 60 min renal ischemia is also associated with a reduction in mortality at 2–3 d *(138)*, and iv infusion of SB 209670 1 d after 45-min renal artery occlusion in uninephrectomised rats reduces the mortality such that at d 4 in control animals there is 100% mortality and in treated animals 75% recovery *(139)*. Similarly, the nonselective antagonist Ro 46-2005 partially restores the initial (20–30 min) fall in renal-blood flow that follows ischemia and reperfusion *(98)*. In acute experiments examining the effects of 60 min of renal ischemia in uninephrectomized dogs, the reduction in inulin clearance and creatinine clearance and the increase in fractional sodium excretion were all attenuated by treatment with SB 209670, but not by BQ-123 *(140)*. This suggests that in the dog, the ET receptor mechanisms involved in acute renal failure may include ET_B-receptor-induced sodium transport. In vivo and in vitro models of acute cyclosporine nephrotoxicity do reveal a better protective effect of BQ-123 *(26,141)* as well as of SB 209670. The reason for this difference is not clear, but may be because in these latter models, endothelin produces deleterious effects at nonvascular sites, such as the mesangial cell, where BQ-123 might act *(80)*. Interestingly, in a model of hypertension driven by renal-mass reduction, the increase in blood pressure over 60 d is greatly attenuated by the daily ip injection of FR 139317 *(142)*. In one other model of renal dysfunction, SB 209670 is also found to prevent the renal vasoconstriction caused by the intrarenal infusion of the radiocontrast medium Hypaque to indomethacin-treated anesthetized dogs *(143)*. Similarly, the fall in renal perfusate flow and glomerular-filtration rate caused by ioversol in the isolated perfused kidney of the rat are greatly reduced in the presence of BQ-123 *(144)*. Finally, it has also been suggested that ET-1 may be involved in murine lupus nephritis because chronic treatment (28 d) with FR 139317 suppresses the appearance of indicators of this condition, such as histological lesions, proteinuria, and hypertension *(145)*.

6.3. Hypertension

BQ-123 has been shown to lower blood pressure in stroke-prone spontaneously hypertensive rats *(146)* and blood pressure and peripheral resistance in spontaneously hypertensive rats (SHRs, *147*) and BMS-182874 to reduce the blood pressure of SHRs, but not sodium-depleted SHRs. These data suggest that ET_A receptor activation may play a role in volume-dependent or low-renin hypertension but is unlikely to be important in all hypertensive states *(148)*. However, this whole question is unclear because the $ET_{A/B}$ receptor nonselective antagonist, Ro 46-2005, lowers the blood pressures of normotensive, but sodium-depleted, squirrel monkeys *(98)*, which are more likely to be in a high-renin state, and SB 209670 reduces the blood pressures of renin-hypertensive rats *(149)*. Intravenous or intraduodenally applied SB 209670 also lowers the blood pressure of SHR but not WKY rats *(149,150)*, and bosentan reduces the blood pressures, as does BMS-182874 *(151)*, and the resistances of the iliac, renal, and mesenteric vascular beds of deoxycorticosterone acetate (DOCA) salt-treated rats, without any effect on cardiac output or heart rate *(see ref. 126)*. Bosentan also reduces the blood pressure of DOCA-salt SHRs, a model of malignant hypertension *(152)*, although this same group report it to be without effect on the blood pressures of SHR *(153)*. Finally, in nonrat models, endothelin antagonists have also been reported to be antihypertensive. For example, in a canine model of renal hypertension, bosentan reduces blood pressure in hypertensive animals to a much greater extent than in their matched normotensive controls *(118)*.

6.4. Pulmonary Hypoxic Constriction and Pulmonary Hypertension

As discussed previously, there is evidence for an involvement of endothelin in the development of pulmonary hypertension in the human. Studies from animal models also support this connection. For instance, in anesthetized rats, acute hypoxia-induced pulmonary hypertension is markedly attenuated by BQ-123 *(154)*, and in conscious rats exposed to hypoxia for 15 d, there is an increase in pulmonary artery pressure and a right-ventricular hypertrophy that is reduced by bosentan given orally *(155)*. Similarly, in the conscious lamb, bolus administration of BQ-123 into the pulmonary artery causes a reduction in the rise in pulmonary-vascular resistance that results from alveolar hypoxia *(156)*, and ET-1 may contribute to the high pulmonary-vascular resistance in the normal foetus, for intrapulmonary infusions of BQ-123 increases left pulmonary-artery flow in late-gestation fetal lambs *(157)*. Finally, in the dog, pulmonary hypertension caused by injection of dehydromonocrotaline is reduced by FR 139317, but increased by RES-701-1, suggesting that ET-1 production is elevated in this model, but also partly mitigates the pulmonary hypertension by acting on ET_B receptors *(158,159)*.

6.5. Atherosclerosis

In diseases of the vascular wall, such as atherosclerosis, there may be a reduction in the release of ET-derived nitric oxide (NO) and an increase in ET-1 production. Thus, an imbalance in the production of NO and ET-1 may contribute to the alteration in vascular tone characteristic of cardiovascular disease. Evidence also suggests that an increase in the production of ET-1 by the endothelium may be one of the pathological changes underlying atherosclerosis. In atherosclerotic human subjects, for instance, an increase in the circulating levels of ET-1 as well as an increase in immunoreactive ET-1 within the blood-vessel wall is seen *(see refs. 160,161)*. Similarly, cholesterol feeding of pigs is associated with an increase in the circulating levels of ET-1 and a great increase in circulating ET-1 following intra-coronary infusion of acetylcholine. This may well correlate with the observation that intra-coronary infusion of acetylcholine to these cholesterol-fed animals also produces coronary vasoconstriction, instead of the vasodilatation seen in normal animals, supporting the idea of an imbalance in ET-mediator production. Returning to human subjects, there is also a very marked correlation between ET-1 concentrations in the coronary sinus and the vasoconstriction that follows infusion of acetylcholine. There exists, therefore, circumstantial evidence of a role for endothelin in the vascular dysfunction associated with atherosclerosis *(see ref. 160)*. This appears supported by the first data on the effects of endothelin antagonists in animal models of atherosclerosis. Thus, in cholesterol-fed hamsters, BMS-182874 decreases the area of the fatty streak by reducing the number and size of macrophage-foam cells *(162)*.

6.6. Vascular Restenosis

In humans the effectiveness of percutaneous transluminal coronary angioplasty (PTCA) is limited by the high incidence of neointimal formation and subsequent vascular restenosis. The changes after PTCA are characterized by an initial phase of platelet deposition and cellular infiltration followed by medial proliferation and cellular migration and matrix formation. In vitro, ET-1 will produce many of these effects. For instance, ET-1 is pro-mitogenic in vascular smooth-muscle cells, a response that is inhibited by BQ-123 (IC_{50} approx 30 nM), SB 209670 (IC_{50} approx 6 nM) or TAK-044 (IC_{50} approx 60 nM), probably indicating mediation by ET_A receptors *(163,164)*. In addition, ET-1 is also a chemotactic agent for vascular smooth-muscle cells, although it only weakly produces this effect compared to PDGF, and increases the formation of matrix by vascular smooth-muscle cells in culture *(see ref. 164)*. In vivo experiments also suggest a role for ET-1 in the changes within blood vessels that follow PTCA. For instance, intra-arterial administration of ET-1 over a 30-min period following balloon angioplasty of the rat carotid artery dose-dependently increases the degree of neointima formation (by up to 150% after 14 d) *(165)*. Finally, and most interestingly, ip administration of SB 209670 (2.5 mg/kg, ip, twice a day) for 3 d before and 14 d after balloon angioplasty of the rat carotid artery reduces neointimal formation by approx 50% *(163)*. Similarly, TAK-044 gives some protection against neointimal lesion in the same model *(166)*, as does BMS-182874 *(167)*. ET-1 therefore has some of the properties expected of a mediator of vascular restenosis. There is therefore increasing support for the idea that endogenous ET-1 is involved in the pathogenesis of angioplasty-induced lesion formation in the rat. However, at the same time it must be remembered that there may be particular species variations. For instance, in the rabbit, although it appears that ET-1 may be involved in neointima formation following balloon denudation of the carotid artery, chronic iv administration of BQ-123 does not affect the progression of the intimal hyperplasia *(168)*.

6.7. Subarachnoid Hemorrhage and Cerebrovascular Disease

Much evidence points to a role for endothelin in states associated with cerebral vasospasm. For instance, cerebral vessels in general are very sensitive to the effects of the endothelins with the canine basilar artery being about 100 times more sensitive to the contractile effects of ET-1 than the canine saphenous artery *(see ref. 169)*. Animal models have therefore been used to assess the possible involvement of endothelin in ischemic pathologies within the brain. Thus, in a 7-d canine model of subarachnoid hemorrhage (injection on d 1 of autologous blood to cause clotting around the basilar and spinal arteries) SB 209670 was continually applied to the subarachnoid space by minipump. On d 7, the cross-sectional areas of the basilar artery in SB 209670-treated dogs was 68% of control (i.e., 68% of the pretreatment diameter on d 1), whereas it was 27% of control in vehicle-treated animals. Similarly, SB 209670 was protective in the spinal arteries in which the blood vessel diameters on d 7 were 78% of control in drug-treated animals and 38% of control in those given vehicle *(170)*. In both the dog and rat, FR 139317 *(171)*, BQ-485 (an ET_A-receptor selective antagonist, *172*) and Ro 46-2005 *(98)* also attenuate the reductions in basilar-artery diameter that follow the local injection of autologous blood. Similarly, bosentan given twice daily for up to 7 d to dogs significantly lessens the reduction in basilar artery diameter that follows the injection of autologous blood *(173)*, and in rabbits exposed to similar manipulations, bosentan produces a reversal of basilar-artery vasospasm similar to that following an intraverterbral injection of sodium nitroprusside *(174)*.

6.8. Shock

There has been some examination of the efficacy of ET-receptor antagonists in models of shock: BMS-182874, for instance, has been found to greatly decrease the pulmonary hypertension caused by endotoxin administration *(175)*. On the other hand, an elevation in circulating ET-1 levels suggests that an increase in ET-1 helps to maintain systemic vascular resistance following hemorrhagic shock in the rat *(176)*. Indeed, in this model, infusion of BQ-123 causes a lowering of systemic vascular resistance. Similarly, BQ-123 reduces the gastric-mucosal injury following hemorrhagic shock, suggesting that this condition increases ET-1 production, and indicating that endogenous ET-1 plays an important role in the pathogenesis of hemorrhagic shock-induced gastric-mucosal damage *(177)*.

6.9. Diabetes

Abnormal vascular-endothelium function may contribute to the reduced nerve perfusion implicated in the etiology of neuropathy in diabetes mellitus. Evidence from antagonist studies suggest that this could, at least in part, be owing to an increased production of ET-1. Thus, in rats, oral administration of bosentan *(178)* or prolonged iv infusion of BQ-123 *(179)* attenuates both the reduction in sciatic-nerve conduction velocity and blood flow that follows the induction of a diabetic state.

7. Summary

As the endothelin system is defined and the newer orally active ET-receptor antagonists are tested, it is becoming increasingly clear that endothelin does have roles to play in some forms of hypertension, in the events following ischemia and reperfusion, and possibly in pathologies associated with inappropriate vascular-cell proliferation. Studies with endothelin antagonists suggest that these compounds may be able to reverse these effects, although we should bear in mind that established responses to the endothelins are only very slowly overcome owing to the almost-irreversible binding of ET-1 to its receptors *(36,180–182)*. This caveat aside, we may still hope that the development of drugs that modulate the activities of endothelin will yield new therapies in a number of diseases associated with vascular dysfunction.

Acknowledgments

The author holds a British Heart Foundation Lectureship (BS/95003).

References

1. Inoue, A., Yanagisawa, M., Kimura, S., Kasuya, Y., Miyauchi, T., Goto, K., and Masaki, T. (1989) The human endothelin family: three structurally and pharmacologically distinct isopeptides predicted by three separate genes. *Proc. Natl. Acad. Sci. USA* **86:**2863–2867.
2. Yangisawa, M., Kurihara, H., Kimura, S., Tomobe, Y., Kobayishi, Y., Mistui, Y., Yazaki, Y., Goto, K., and Masaki, T. (1988) A novel potent vasoconstrictor peptide produced by vascular endothelial cells. *Nature* **332:**411–415.
3. Masaki, T. and Yanagisawa, M. (1990) Cardiovascular effects of the endothelins. *Cardiovasc. Drug Rev.* **8:**373–385.
4. Gray, G. A. and Webb, D. J. (1996) The endothelin system and its potential as a therapeutic target in cardiovascular disease. *Pharmacol. Ther.* **72:**109–148.
5. De Nucci, G., Thomas, R., D'Orleans-Juste, P., Antunes, E., Walder, C., and Warner, T. D., and Vane, J. R. (1988) Pressor effects of circulating endothelin are limited by its removal in the pulmonary circulation and by the release of prostacyclin and endothelium-derived relaxing factor. *Proc. Natl. Acad. Sci. USA* **85:**9797–9800.
6. Huggins, J. P., Pelton, J. T., and Miller, R. C. (1993) The structure and specificity of endothelin receptors: their importance in physiology and medicine. *Pharmacol. Ther.* **59:**55–123.

7. Masaki, T., Kimura, S., Yanagisawa, M., and Goto, K. (1991) Molecular and cellular mechanism of endothelin regulation. Implications for vascular function. *Circulation* **84:**1457–1468.

8. Rubanyi, G. M. and Parker Botelho, L. H. (1991) Endothelins. *FASEB J.* **5:**2713–2720.

9. Simonson, M. S. and Dunn, M. J. (1990) Endothelin. Pathways of transmembrane signaling. *Hypertension* **15:**I-5–I-11.

10. Sokolovsky, M. (1992) Endothelins and sarafotoxins: physiological regulation; receptor subtypes and transmembrane signaling. *Pharmacol. Ther.* **54:**129–149.

11. Yanagisawa, M. and Masaki, T. (1989) Endothelin, a novel endothelium-derived peptide. Pharmacological activities, regulation and possible roles in cardiovascular control. *Biochem. Pharmacol.* **38:**1877–1883.

12. Battistini, B., Warner, T. D., Fournier, A., and Vane, J. R. (1994) Characterization of ET_B receptors mediating contractions induced by endothelin-1 or IRL 1620 in guinea-pig isolated airways: effects of BQ-123, FR 139317 or PD 145065. *Br. J. Pharmacol.* **111:**1009–1016.

13. Battistini, B., D'Orleans-Juste, P., and Sirois, P. (1993) Endothelins: circulating plasma levels and presence in other biologic fluids. *Lab. Invest.* **68:**600–628.

14. Wagner, O. F., Vierhapper, H., Gasic, S., Nowotny, P., and Waldhausl, W. (1992) Regional effects and clearance of endothelin-1 across pulmonary and splanchnic circulation. *Eur. J. Clin. Invest.* **22:**277–282.

15. Anggård, E. E., Galton, S., Rae, G., Thomas, R., McLoughlin, L., de Nucci, G., and Vane, J. R. (1989) The fate of radioiodinated endothelin-1 and endothelin-3 in the rat. *J. Cardiovasc. Pharmacol.* **13(Suppl. 5):**S46–S49.

16. Giaid, A., Yanagisawa, M., Langleben, D., Michel, R. P., Levy, R., Shennib, H., Kimura, S., Masaki, T., Duguid, W. P., and Stewart, D. J. (1993) Expression of endothelin-1 in the lungs of patients with pulmonary hypertension. *N. Engl. J. Med.* **328:**1732–1739.

17. Margulies, K. B., Hildebrand, F. L., Lerman, A., Perella, M. A., and Burnett, J. C., Jr. (1990) Increased endothelin in experimental heart failure. *Circulation* **82:**2226–2230.

18. Stelzner, T. J., O'Brien, R. F., Yanagisawa, M., Sakurai, T., Sato, K., Webb, S., Zamora, M., McMurtry, I. F., and Fisher, J. H. (1992) Increased lung endothelin-1 production in rats with idiopathic pulmonary hypertension. *Am. J. Physiol.* **262:**L614–L620.

19. Nambi, P., Pullen, M., Contino, L. C., and Brooks, D. P. (1990) Upregulation of renal endothelin receptors in rats with cyclosporine A-induced nephrotoxicity. *Eur. J. Pharmacol.* **187:**113–116.

20. Nambi, P., Pullen, M., and Feuerstein, G. (1990) Identification of endothelin receptors in various regions of rat brain. *Neuropeptides* **16:**195–199.

21. Kusumoto, K., Fujiwara, S., Awane, Y., and Watanabe, T. (1993) The role of endogenous endothelin in extension of rabbit myocardial infarction. *J. Cardiovasc. Pharmacol.* **22(Suppl. 8):**S339–S342.

22. Watanabe, T., Suzuki, N., Shimamoto, N., Fujino, M., and Imada, A. (1990) Endothelin in myocardial infarction. *Nature* **344:**114.

23. Watanabe, T., Suzuki, N., Shimamoto, N., Fujino, M., and Imada, A. (1991) Contribution of endogenous endothelin to the extension of myocardial infarct size in rats. *Circ. Res.* **69:**370–377.

24. Kon, V., Yoshioka, T., Fogo, A., and Ichikawa, I. (1989) Glomerular actions of endothelin in vivo. *J. Clin. Invest.* **83:**1762–1767.

25. Shibuota, Y., Suzuki, N., Shino, A., Matsumoto, H., Terashita, Z. I., Kondo, K., and Nishikawa, K. (1990) Pathophysiological role of endothelin in acute renal failure. *Life Sci.* **46:**1611–1618.

26. Bloom, I. T. M., Bentley, F. R., and Garrison, R. N. (1993) Acute cyclosporine-induced renal vasoconstriction is mediated by endothelin-1. *Surgery* **114:**480–488.

27. Kon, V., Sugiura, M., Inagami, T., Harvie, B. R., Ichikawa, I., and Hoover, R. L. (1990) Role of endothelin in cyclosporine-induced glomerular dysfunction. *Kidney Int.* **37:**1487–1491.

28. Morise, Z., Ueda, M., Aiura, K., Endo, M., and Kitajima, M. (1994) Pathophysiological role of endothelin-1 in renal function in rats with endotoxin shock. *Surgery* **115:**199–204.

29. Kitajima, T., Tani, K., Yamaguchi, T., Kubota, Y., Okuhira, M., Fujimura, K., Hiramatsu, A., Mizuno, T., and Inoue, K. (1993) Role of endogenous endothelin in gastric hemodynamic disturbance induced by haemorrhagic shock in rats. *Gastroenterology* **104:**A119.

30. Morales, R. E., Johnson, B. R., and Szabo, S. (1992) Endothelin induces vascular and mucosal lesions, enhances the injury by HCl/ethanol, and the antibody exerts gastroprotection. *FASEB J.* **6:**2354–2360.

31. Kitajima, T., Yamaguchi, T., Tani, K., Fujimara, K., Okuhira, M., Kubota, Y., Hiramatsu, A., Mizuno, T., Inoue, K., and Yamada, H. (1992) Role of vasoactive substances on indomethacin-induced gastric mucosal lesions—evaluation of endothelin and platelet activating-factor. *Gastroenterology* **102:**A97.

32. Wilson, M. A., Steeb, G. D., and Garrison, R. N. (1993) Endothelins mediate intestinal hypoperfusion during bacteremia. *J. Surg. Res.* **55:**168–175.

33. Goto, M., Takei, Y., Kawano, S., Nagano, K., Tsuji, S., Masuda, E., Nishimura, Y., Okumura, S., Kashigawa Fusamoto, H., and Kamada, T. (1994) Endothelin-1 is involved in the pathogenesis of ischaemia/reperfusion liver injury by hepatic microcirculatory disturbances. *Hepatology* **19:**675–681.

34. Warner, T. D., de Nucci, G., and Vane, J. R. (1989) Rat endothelin is a vasodilator in the isolated perfused mesentery of the rat. *Eur. J. Pharmacol.* **159:**325, 326.

35. Warner, T. D., Mitchell, J. A., de Nucci, G., and Vane, J. R. (1989) Endothelin-1 and endothelin-3 release EDRF from isolated perfused arterial vessels of the rat and rabbit. *J. Cardiovasc. Pharmacol.* **13(Suppl. 5):**S85–S88.

36. Arai, H., Hori, S., Aramori, I., Ohkubo, H., and Nakanishi, S. (1990) Cloning and expression of a cDNA encoding an endothelin receptor. *Nature* **348:**730–732.

37. Sakurai, T., Yanagisawa, M., Takuwa, Y., Miyazaki, H., Kimura, S., Goto, K., and Masaki, T. (1990) Cloning of a cDNA encoding a non-isopeptide-selective subtype of the endothelin receptor. *Nature* **348:**732–735.
38. Clozel, M., Gray, G. A., Breu, W., Löffler, B. M., and Osterwalder, R. (1992) The endothelin ET_B receptor mediates both vasodilatation and vasoconstriction in vivo. *Biochem. Biophys. Res. Comm.* **186:**867–873.
39. Harrison, V. J., Randriantsoa, A., and Schoeffer, P. (1992) Heterogeneity of endothelin-sarafotoxin receptors mediating contraction of pig coronary artery. *Br. J. Pharmacol.* **105:**511–513.
40. Hay, D. W. P. (1992) Pharmacological evidence for distinct endothelin receptors in guinea-pig bronchus and aorta. *Br. J. Pharmacol.* **106:** 759–761.
41. Hay, D. W. P., Luttman, M. A., Hubbard, W. C., and Undem, B. J. (1993) Endothelin receptor subtypes in human and guinea-pig pulmonary tissues. *Br. J. Pharmacol.* **110:**1175–1183.
42. Moreland, S., McMullen, D. M., Delaney, C. L., Lee, V. G., and Hunt, J. T. (1992) Venous smooth muscle contains vasoconstrictor ET_B-like receptors. *Biochem. Biophys. Res. Commun.* **184:**100–106.
43. Sumner, M. J., Cannon, T. R., Mundin, J. W., White, D. G., and Watts, I. S. (1992) Endothelin ET_A and ET_B receptors mediate vascular smooth muscle contraction. *Br. J. Pharmacol.* **107:**858–860.
44. Warner, T. D., Allcock, G. H., Corder, R., and Vane, J. R. (1993) Use of the endothelin receptor antagonists BQ-123 and PD 142893 to reveal three endothelin receptors mediating smooth muscle contraction and the release of EDRF. *Br. J. Pharmacol.* **110:**777–782.
45. Warner, T. D., Allcock, G. H., Mickley, E. J., Corder, R., and Vane, J. R. (1993) Comparative studies with the endothelin-receptor antagonists BQ-123 and PD 142893 indicate at least three endothelin-receptors. *J. Cardiovasc. Pharmacol.* **22(Suppl. 8):**S117–S120.
46. Warner, T. D., Battistini, B., Allcock, G. H., and Vane, J. R. (1993) Endothelin ET_A and ET_B receptors mediate vasoconstriction and prostanoid release in the isolated kidney of the rat. *Eur. J. Pharmacol.* **250:**447–453.
47. Sakurai, T., Yanagisawa, M., and Masaki, T. (1992) Molecular characterization of endothelin receptors. *Trends Pharmacol. Sci.* **13:**103–108.
48. Emori, T., Hirata, Y., and Marumo, F. (1990) Specific receptors for endothelin-3 in cultured bovine endothelial cells and its cellular mechanism of action. *FEBS Lett.* **263:**261–264.
49. Warner, T. D., Schmidt, H. H. H. W., and Murad, F. (1992) Interactions of endothelins and EDRF in bovine native endothelial cells: selective effects of endothelin-3. *Am. J. Physiol.* **262:**H1600–H1605.
50. Sokolovsky, M., Ambar, I., and Galron, R. (1992) A novel subtype of endothelin receptors. *J. Biol. Chem.* **267:**20,551–20,554.
51. Samson, W. K., Skala, D., Alexander, B. D., and Huang, F. L. S. (1990) Pituitary site of action of endothelin: selective inhibition of prolactin release *in vitro*. *Biochem. Biophys. Res. Commun.* **169:**737–743.

52. Karne, S., Jayawickreme, C. K., and Lerner, M. R. (1993) Cloning and characterization of an endothelin-3 specific receptor (ET_C receptor) from *Xenopus laevis* dermal melanophores. *J. Biol. Chem.* **268**:19,126–19,133.

53. Sudjarwo, S. A., Hori, M., Takai, M., Urade, Y., Okada, T., and Karaki, H. (1993) A novel subtype of endothelin B receptor mediating contraction in swine pulmonary vein. *Life Sci.* **53**:431–437.

54. Sudjarwo, S. A., Hori, M., Tanaka, T., Matsuda, Y., Okada, T., and Karaki, H. (1994) Subtypes of endothelin ET_A and ET_B receptors mediating venous smooth muscle contraction. *Biochem. Biophys. Res. Commun.* **200**:627–633.

55. Warner, T. D. and Battistini, B. (1994) IBC Conference. Endothelin inhibitors—advances in therapeutic application and development. *Drug News Persp.* **7**:249–253.

56. Fukuroda, T., Ozaki, S., Nakajima, A., Fujikawa, T., Ihara, M., Ishikawa, K., Yano, M., and Nishikibe, M. (1994) Analysis of non-ET_A-mediated lung tissue responses using BQ-788, a novel selective ET_B receptor ligand. *Can. J. Pharmacol. Physiol.* **72(Suppl. I)**:173.

57. Baynash, A. G., Hosoda, K., Giaid, A., Richardson, J. A., Emoto, N., Hammer, R. E., and Yanagisawa, M. (1994) Interaction of endothelin-3 with endothelin-B receptor is essential for development of epidermal melanocytes and enteric neurons. *Cell* **79**:1277–1285.

58. Battistini, B., Botting, R., and Warner, T. D. (1995) Endothelin: a knockout in London. *Trends Pharmacol. Sci.* **16**:217–222.

59. Takahashi, M., Matsushita, Y., Iijima, Y., and Tanzawa, K. (1993) Purification and chacterization of endothelin converting enzyme from rat lung. *J. Biochem.* **268**:21,394–21,398.

60. Ikura, T., Sawamura, T., Shiraki, T., Hosokawa, H., Kido, T., Hoshikawa, H., Shimada, K., Tanzawa, K., Kobayishi, S., and Miwa, S. (1994) cDNA cloning and expression of bovine endothelin converting enzyme. *Biochem. Biophys. Res. Commun.* **203**:1417–1422.

61. Schmidt, M., Kroger, B., Jacob, E., Seulberger, H., Subkowski, T., Otter, R., Meyer, T., Schmalzing, G., and Hillen, H. (1994) Molecular characterization of human and bovine endothelin converting enzyme (ECE-1). *FEBS Letts.* **356**:238–243.

62. Shimada, K., Takahashi, M., and Tanzawa, K. (1994) Cloning and functional expression of endothelin-converting enzyme from rat endothelial cells. *J. Biol. Chem.* **269**:18,275–18,278.

63. Xu, D., Emoto, N., Giaid, A., Slaughter, C., Kaw, S., deWit, D., and Yanagisawa, M. (1994) ECE-1: a membrane bound metalloprotease that catalyzes the proteolytic activation of big endothelin-1. *Cell* **78**:473–485.

64. Shimada, K., Matsushita, Y., Wakabayashi, K., Takahashi, M., Matsubara, A., Iijima, Y., and Tanzawa, K. (1995) Cloning and functional expression of human endothelin-converting enzyme cDNA. *Biochem. Biophys. Res. Commun.* **207**:807–812.

65. Yorimitsu, K., Moroi, K., Inagaki, N., Saito, T., Masuda, Y., Masaki, T., Seino, S., and Kimura, S. (1995) Cloning and sequencing of a

human endothelin converting enzyme in renal adenocarcinoma (ACHN) cells producing endothelin-2. *Biochem. Biophys. Res. Commun.* **208:** 721–727.

66. Sawamura, T., Kasuya, Y., Matsushita, Y., Suzuki, N., Shinmi, O., Kishi, N., Sugita, Y., Yanagisawa, M., Goto, K., Masaki, T., and Kimura, S. (1988) Phosphoramidon inhibits the intracellular conversion of big endothelin-1 to endothelin-1 in cultured endothelial cells. *Biochem. Biophys. Res. Commun.* **174:**779–784.

67. Kaw, S., Hecker, M., Southan, G. J., Warner, T. D., and Vane, J. R. (1992) Characterization of serine protease-derived metabolites of big endothelin in the cytosolic fraction from human polymorphonuclear leukocytes. *J. Cardiovasc. Pharmacol.* **20(Suppl. 12):**S22–S24.

68. Wypij, D. M., Nichols, J. S., Novak, P. J., Stacy, D. L., Berman, J., and Wisemam, J. S. (1992) Role of mast cell chymase in the extracellular processing of big-endothelin-1 to endothelin-1 in the perfused rat lung. *Biochem. Pharmacol.* **43:**845–853.

69. Ikegawa, R., Matsumura, Y., Tsukahara, Y., Takaoka, M., and Morimoto, S. (1991) Phosphoramidon inhibits the generation of endothelin-1 from exogenously applied big endothelin-1 in cultured vascular endothelial cells and smooth muscle cells. *FEBS Lett.* **293:**45–48.

70. Ihara, M., Fukuroda, T., Saeki, T., Nishikibe, M., Kojiri, K., Suda, H., and Yano, M. (1991) An endothelin receptor (ET$_A$) antagonist isolated from *streptomyces misakiensis*. *Biochem. Biophys. Res. Commun.* **178:**132–137.

71. Ihara, M., Noguchi, K., Saeki, T., Fukuroda, T., Tsuchida, S., Kimura, S., Fukami, T., Ishikawa, K., Nishikibe, M., and Yano, M. (1992) Biological profiles of highly potent novel endothelin antagonists selective for the ET$_A$ receptor. *Life Sci.* **50:**247–255.

72. Ihara, M., Ishikawa, K., Fukuroda, T., Saeki, T., Funabashi, K., Fukami, T., Suda, H., and Yano, M. (1992) *In vitro* biological profile of a highly potent novel endothelin (ET) antagonist BQ-123 selective for the ET$_A$ receptor. *J. Cardiovasc. Pharmacol.* **20(Suppl. 12):**S11–S14.

73. Moreland, S. (1994) BQ-123, a selective endothelin ETA receptor antagonist. *Cardiovasc. Drug Rev.* **12:**48–69.

74. Ishikawa, K., Fukami, T., Nagase, T., Fujita, K., Hayama, T., Niiyama, K., et al. (1992) Cyclic pentapeptide endothelin antagonists with high ET$_A$ selectivity. Potency- and solubility-enhancing modifications. *J. Med. Chem.* **35:**2139–2142.

75. Aramori, A., Nirei, H., Shoubo, M., Sogabe, K., Nakamura, K., Kojo, H., Notsu, Y., Ono, T., and Nakanishi, S. (1993) Subtype selectivity of a novel endothelin antagonist, FR 139317, for the two endothelin receptors in transfected chinese hamster ovary cells. *Mol. Pharmacol.* **43:**127–131.

76. Hemmi, K., Neya, M., Fukami, N., Hashimoto, M., Tanaka, H., and Kayakiri, N. (1992) Peptides having endothelin antagonist activity, a process for preparation thereof and pharmaceutical compositions comprising the same. *Eur. Pat. Appl. No.* 0457195A2.

77. Sogabe, K., Nirei, H., Shoubo, M., Hamada, K., Nomoto, A., Henmi, K., Notsu, Y., and Ono, T. (1992) A novel endothelial receptor antagonist: studies with FR 139317. *J. Vasc. Res.* **29**:201.

78. Sogabe, K., Nirei, H., Shoubo, M., Nomoto, A., Ao, S., Notsu, Y., and Ono, T. (1993) Pharmacological profile of FR 139317, a novel, potent endothelin ET_A receptor antagonist. *J. Pharmacol. Exp. Ther.* **264**:1040–1046.

79. Ishikawa, K., Fukami, T., Nagase, T., Mase, T., Hayama, T., Niiyama, K., et al. (1993) Endothelin antagonistic peptide derivatives with high selectivity for ET_A receptors, in: *Peptides 1992 (XXII EPS)* (Schneider, C. H. and Eberle, A. N., eds.), ESCOM, Leiden, The Netherlands, pp. 685,686.

80. Takeda, M., Breyer, M. D., Noland, T. D., Homma, T., Hoover, R. L., Inagami, T., and Kon, V. (1992) Endothelin-1 receptor antagonist: effects on endothelin- and cyclosporine-treated mesangial cells. *Kid. Int.* **42**:1713–1719.

81. Fujimoto, M., Mihara, S.-I., Nakajima, S., Ueda, M., Nakamura, M., and Sakurai, K.-S. (1992) A novel non-peptide endothelin antagonist isolated from bayberry, *Myrica cerifera*. *FEBS Lett.* **305**:41–44.

82. Ohashi, H., Akiyama, H., Nishikori, K., and Mochizuki, J.-I. (1992) Asterric acid, a new endothelin binding inhibitor. *J. Antibiotics* **45**:1684,1685.

83. Stein, P. D., Hunt, J. T., Floyd, D. M., Moreland, S., Dickinson, K. E. J., Mitchell, C., Liu, E. C.-K., Webb, M. L., Murguresan, N., Dickey, J., McMullen, D., Zhang, R., Lee, V. G., Serafino, R., Delaney, C., Schaeffer, T. R., and Kozlowski, M. (1994) The discovery of sulfonamide endothelin antagonists and the development of the orally active ET_A antagonist 5-(dimethylamino)-N-(3,4-dimethyl-5-isoxazolyl)-1-napthalene-sulfonamide (BMS-182874). *J. Med. Chem.* **37**:329–331.

84. Reynolds, E. E., Keiser, J. A., Haleen, S. J., Walker, D. M., Olszewski, B., Schroeder, R. L., Taylor, D. G., Hwang, O., Welch, K. M., Flynn, M. A., Thompson, D. M., Edmunds, J. J., Berryman, K. A., Plummer, M., Cheng, X. M., Patt, W. C., and Doherty, A. M. (1995) Pharmacological characterization of PD-156707, an orally-active ET_A receptor antagonist. *J. Pharmacol. Exp. Ther.* **273**:1410–1417.

85. Urade, Y., Fujitani, Y., Oda, K., Watakabe, T., Umemura, I., Takai, M., Okada, T., Sakata, K., and Karaki, H. (1992) An endothelin B receptor-selective antagonist: IRL 1038, [Cys[11]-Cys[15]]-endothelin-1 (11–21). *FEBS Lett.* **311**:12–16.

86. Urade, Y., Fujitani, Y., Oda, K., Watakabe, T., Umemura, I., Takai, M., Okada, T., Sakata, K., and Karaki, H. (1994) Retraction concerning an endothelin B receptor-selective antagonist: IRL 1038, [Cys[11]-Cys[15]]-endothelin-1 (11–21). *FEBS Lett.* **342**:103.

87. Mase, T., Fukami, T., Nagase, T., Yamakawa, T., Takahashi, H., Naya, A., Amano, Y., Katsuki, K., Noguchi, K., Fukuroda, T., Nishikibe, M., Saeki, T., Ihara, M., Yano, M., and Ishikawa, K. (1993) Structure activity relationships of endothelin B receptor-selective antagonists. *14th Symp. Med. Chem.*, Pharmaceutical Society of Japan, p. 28.

88. Ishikawa, K., Ihara, M., Noguchi, K., Mase, T., Mino, N., Saeki, T., Fukuroda, T., Fukami, T., Ozaki. S., Nagase, T., Nishikibe, M., and Yano, M. (1994) Biochemical and pharmacological profile of a potent and selective endothelin B-receptor antagonist, BQ-788. *Proc. Natl. Acad. Sci. USA* **91:**4892–4896.

89. Allcock, G. H., Warner, T. D., and Vane, J. R. (1995) Roles of endothelin A and B receptors in the regional and systemic vascular responses to ET-1 in the anaesthetised ganglion-blocked rat: use of the antagonists, BQ-123, BQ-788 and PD145065. *Br. J. Pharmacol.* **116:**2482–2486.

90. Matsuda, Y., Tanaka, T., Morishita, Y., Nozasa, M., Ohno, T., and Yamada, K. (1993) Pharmacological profile of RES-701-1, a novel, potent endothelin subtype B receptor antagonist of microbial origin. *Circulation* **88:**I-281.

91. Cody, W. L., Doherty, A. M., He, J. X., DePue, P. L., Rapundalo, S. T., Hingorani, G. A., Major, T. C., Panek, R. L., Dudley, D. T., Haleen, S. J., LaDouceur, D., Hill, K. E., Flynn, M. E., and Reynolds, E. E. (1992) Design of a functional hexapeptide antagonist of endothelin. *J. Med. Chem.* **35:**3301–3303.

92. Cody, W. L., Doherty, A. M., He, J. X., DePue, P. L., Waite, L. A., Topliss, J. G., Haleen, S. J., Ladouceur, D., Flynn, M. A., Hill, K. E., and Reynolds, E. E. (1993) The rational design of a highly potent combined ET_A and ET_B receptor antagonist (PD 145065) and related analogues. *Med. Chem. Res.* **3:**154–162.

93. Doherty, A. M., Cody, W. L., He, J. X., Depue, P. L., Cheng, X. M., Welch, K. M., et al. (1993) *In vitro* and *in vivo* studies with a series of hexapeptide endothelin antagonists. *J. Cardiovasc. Pharmacol.* **22:**S98–102.

94. Doherty, A. M., Cody, W. L., He, X., DePue, P. L., Leonard, D. M., Dunbar, J. B., Jr., Hill, K. E., Flynn, M. A., and Reynolds, E. E. (1993) Design of C-terminal peptide antagonists of endothelin: structure-activity relationships of ET-1[16–21, D-His[16]]. *Bioorg. Med. Chem. Lett.* **3:**497–502.

95. Shimamoto, N., Kubo, K., Watanabe, T., Suzuki, N., Abe, M., Kikuchi, T., et al. (1993) Pharmacological profile of $ET_{A/B}$ antagonist [Thr[18], g Methyl Leu[19]]- endothelin-1. *J. Cardiovasc. Pharmacol.* **22:**S107–S110.

96. Kikuchi, T., Ohtaki, T., Kawata, A., Imada, T., Asami, T., Masuda, Y., Sugo, T., Kusumoto, K., Kubo, K., Watanabe, T., Wakimasu, M., and Fujino, M. (1994) Cyclic hexapeptide endothelin receptor antagonists highly potent for both receptor subtypes ET_A and ET_B. *Biochem. Biophys. Res. Commun.* **200:**1708–1712.

97. Ikeda, S., Awane, Y., Kusumoto, K., Wakimasu, M., Watanabe, T., and Fujino, M. (1994) A new endothelin receptor antagonist, TAK-044, shows long-lasting inhibition of both ET_A- and ET_B-mediated blood pressure responses in rats. *J. Pharmacol. Exp. Ther.* **270:**728–733.

98. Clozel, M., Breu, V., Burri, K., Cassal, J. M., Fischli, W., Gray, G. A., Hirth, G., Löffler, B.-M., Müller, M., Neidhart, W., and Ramuz, H. (1993) Pathophysiological role of endothelin revealed by the first orally active endothelin receptor antagonist. *Nature* **365:**759–761.

99. Clozel, M., Breu, V., Gray, G. A., Kalina, B., Löffler, B.-M., Burri, K., Cassal, J.-M., Hirth, G., Müller, M., Neidhart, W., and Ramuz, H. (1994) Pharmacological characterization of bosentan, a new potent orally active non-peptide endothelin receptor antagonist. *J. Pharmacol. Exp. Ther.* **270:**228–235.

100. Ohlstein, E. H., Nambi, P., Douglas, S. A., Beck, G., Gleason, J., Ruffolo, R. R., Jr., Feuerstein, G., Elliott, J. D. (1994) *In vitro* characterization of the nonpeptide endothelin receptor antagonist SB 209670. *FASEB J.* **8:**A803.

101. Nambi, P., Wu, H.-L., Pullen, M., Slater, C., Saunder, D., Heys, R., Leber, J., Elliott, J. D., Ohlstein, E. H., Brooks, D. P., Gleason, J., and Ruffolo, R. R., Jr. (1994) Identification and characterization of endothelin (ET) receptors using [³H] (±)-SB 209670, a novel nonpeptide ET receptor antagonist. *FASEB J.* **8:**A102.

102. Douglas, S. A., Elliott, J. D., and Ohlstein, E. H. (1994) SB 209670 inhibits the hemodynamic effects of endothelin-1 (ET-1) in the anesthetized rat. *FASEB J.* **8:**A42.

103. Mugrage, B., Moliterni, J., Robinson, L., Webb, R. L., Shetty, S. S., Lipson, K. E., Chin, M. H., Neale, R., and Cioffi, C. (1993) CGS 27830, a potent nonpeptide endothelin receptor antagonist. *Bioorganic. Med. Chem. Lett.* **3:**2099–2104.

104. Lam, Y. K. T., Williams, D. L., Sigmund, J. M., Sanchez, M., Genilloud, O., Kong, Y. L., Stevens-Miles, S., Huang, L., and Garrity, G. M. Cochinmicins, novel and potent cyclodepsipeptide endothelin antagonists from A Microbispora sp. *J. Antibiotic* **45:**1709–1716.

105. Zink, D., Hensens, O. D., Lam, Y. K. T., Reamer, R., and Liesch, J. M. Cochinmicins, novel and potent cyclodepsipeptide endothelin antagonists from a microspora sp.2. structure determination. *J. Antibiotic* **45:** 1717–1722.

106. Bigaud, M. and Pelton, J. T. (1992) Discrimination between ET_A- and ET_B-receptor-mediated effects of endothelin-1 and [Ala^{1,3,11,15}]endothelin-1 by BQ-123 in the anaesthetized rat. *Br. J. Pharmacol.* **107:**912–918.

107. Cristol, J. P., Warner, T. D., Thiemermann, C., and Vane, J. R. (1993) Mediation via different receptors of the vasoconstrictor effects of endothelins and sarafotoxins in the systemic circulation and renal vasculature of the anaesthetized rat. *Br. J. Pharmacol.* **108:**776–779.

108. Pollock, D. M. and Opgenorth, T. J. (1993) Evidence for endothelin-induced renal vasoconstriction independent of ET_A receptor activation. *Am. J. Physiol.* **264:**R222–R226.

109. Wellings, R. P., Warner, T. D., Thiemermann, C., Corder, R., and Vane, J. R. (1993) Vasoconstriction in the rat kidney induced by endothelin-1 is blocked by PD 145065. *J. Cardiovasc. Pharmacol.* **22(Suppl. 8):**S103–S106s.

110. McMurdo, L., Corder, R., Thiemermann, C., and Vane, J. R. (1993) Incomplete inhibition of the pressor effects of endothelin-1 and related peptides in the anaesthetised rat with BQ-123 provides evidence for more than one vasoconstrictor receptor. *Br. J. Pharmacol.* **108:**557–561.

111. Löffler, B.-M., Breu,, V., and Clozel, M. (1992) Effect of different endothelin receptor antagonists and of the novel non-peptide antagonist Ro 46-2005 on endothelin levels in rat plasma. *FEBS Lett.* **333:**108–110.

112. Cirino, M., Motz, C., Maw, J., Ford-Hutchinson, A. W., and Yano, M. (1992) BQ-153, a novel endothelin (ET)A antagonist, attenuates the renal vascular effects of endothelin-1. *J. Pharm. Pharmacol.* **44:**782–785.

113. Télémaque, S., Gratton, J.-P., Claing, A., and D'Orleans-Juste, P. (1993) Endothelin-1 induces vasoconstriction and prostacyclin release via the activation of endothelin ET_A receptors in the perfused rabbit kidney. *Eur. J. Pharmacol.* **237:**275–281.

114. Maggi, C. A., Giuliani, S., Patacchini, R., Santicioli, P., Giachetti, A., and Meli, A. (1990) Further studies on the response of the guinea-pig isolated bronchus to endothelins and sarafotoxin 6b. *Eur. J. Pharmacol.* **176:**1–9.

115. Panek, R. L., Major, T. C., Hingorani, G. P., Doherty, A. M., Taylor, D. G., and Rapundalo, S. T. (1992) Endothelin and structurally related analogs distinguish between endothelin receptor subtypes. *Biochem. Biophys. Res. Commun.* **183:**566–571.

116. Fukuroda, T., Nishikibe, M., Ohta, Y., Ihara, M., Yano, M., Ishikawa, K., Fukami, T., and Ikemoto, F. (1992) Analysis of responses to endothelins in isolated porcine blood vessels by using a novel endothelin antagonist, BQ-153. *Life Sci.* **50:**PL107–PL112.

117. Henry, P. J. (1993) Endothelin-1 (ET-1)-induced contraction in rat isolated trachea: involvement of ET_A and ET_B receptors and multiple signal transduction systems. *Br. J. Pharmacol.* **110:**435–441.

118. Donckier, J., Stoleru, L., Hayashida, W., Vanmechelen, H., Selvais, P., Galanti, L., Clozel, J. P., Ketelsegers, J. M., and Pouleur, H. (1995) Role of endogenous endothelin-1 in experimental renal hypertension in dogs. *Circulation* **92:**106–113.

119. Teerlink, J. R., Carteaux, J. P., Sprecher, U., Loffler, B. M., Clozel, M., and Clozel, J. P. (1995) Role of endogenous endothelin in normal hemodynamic status of anesthetized dogs. *Am. J. Physiol.* **268:**H432–440.

120. Veniant, M., Clozel, J. P., Hess, P., and Clozel, M. (1994) Endothelin plays a role in the maintenance of blood pressure in normotensive guinea-pigs. *Life Sci.* **55:**445–454.

121. Richard, V., Hogie, M., Clozel, M., Loffler, B. M., and Thuillez, C. (1995) In vivo evidence of an endothelin-induced vasopressor tone after inhibition of nitric oxide synthesis in rats. *Circulation* **91:**771–775.

122. Webb, D. J. (1995) Endogenous endothelin generation maintains vascular tone in humans. *J. Human Hypertens.* **9:**459–463.

123. Haynes, W. G., Ferro, C. J., O'Kane, K. P., Somerville, D., Lomax, C. C., and Webb, D. J. (1996) Systemic endothelin receptor blockade decreases peripheral vascular resistance and blood pressure in humans. *Circulation* **93:**1860–1872.

124. Grover, G. J., Dzwonczyk, S., and Parham, C. S. (1993) The endothelin-1 receptor antagonist BQ-123 reduces infarct size in a canine model of coronary occlusion and reperfusion. *Cardiovasc. Res.* **27:**1613–1618.

125. Krause, S. M., Lynch, J. J., Jr., Stabilito, I. I., and Woltmann, R. F. (1994) Intravenous administration of the endothelin-1 antagonist BQ-123 does not ameliorate myocardial ischaemic injury following acute coronary artery occlusion in the dog. *Cardiovasc. Res.* **28**:1672–1678.

126. Watanabe, T., Kusumoto, K., Awane, Y., Ikeda, S., Kikuchi, T., Wakimasu, M., and Fujino, M. (1994) Pharmacological profile of an endothelin receptor antagonist, TAK-044, and its effects in animal models of acute myocardial infarction and acute renal failure. *Can. J. Pharmacol. Physiol.* **72(Suppl. I)**:102.

127. Watanabe, T., Awane, Y., Ikeda, S., Fujiwara, S., Kubo, K., Kikuchi, K., Kusumoto, K., Wakimasu, M., and Fujino, M. (1995) Pharmacology of a non-selective ET_A and ET_B receptor antagonist, TAK-044 and the inhibition of myocardial infarct size in rats. *Br. J. Pharmacol.* **114**:949–954.

128. Lee, J. Y., Warner, R. B., Alder, A. L., and Opgenorth, T. J. (1994) Endothelin ET_A receptor antagonist reduces myocardial infarction induced by coronary artery occlusion and reperfusion in the rat. *Pharmacology* **49**:319–324.

129. Nelson, R. A., Burke, S. E., and Opgenorth, T. (1994) Endothelin receptor antagonist FR139317 reduces infarct size in a rabbit coronary occlusion model. *FASEB J.* **8**:A854.

130. Wang, Q. D., Li, X. S., Lundberg, J. M., and Pernow, J. (1995) Protective effects of nonpeptide endothelin receptor antagonist bosentan on myocardial ischemic and reperfusion injury in the pig. *Cardiovasc. Res.* **29**:805–812.

131. Dagassan, P. H., Breu, V., Clozel, M., and Clozel, J. P. (1994) Role of endothelin during reperfusion after ischemia in isolated perfused rat heart. *J. Cardiovasc. Pharmacol.* **24**:867–874.

132. Richard, V., Kaeffer, N., Hogie, M., Tron, C., Blanc, T., and Thuillez, C. (1994) Role of endogenous endothelin in myocardial and coronary endothelial injury after ischaemia and reperfusion in rats: studies with bosentan, a mixed ET_A-ET_B antagonist. *Br. J. Pharmacol.* **113**:869–876.

133. Teerlink, J. R., Loffler, B. M., Hess, P., Maire, J. P., Clozel, M., and Clozel, J. P. (1994) Role of endothelin in the maintenance of blood pressure in conscious rats with chronic heart failure. Acute effects of the endothelin receptor antagonist Ro 47-0203 (bosentan). *Circulation* **90**:2510–2518.

134. Mino, N., Kobayishi, M., Nakajima, A., Amano, J., Shimamoto, K., Ishikawa, K., Watanabe, K., Nishikibe, M., Yano, M., and Ikemoto, F. (1992) Protective effect of a selective endothelin receptor antagonist, BQ-123, in ischemic acute renal failure in rats. *Eur. J. Pharmacol.* **221**:77–83.

135. Gellai, M., Jugus, M., Fletcher, T., DeWolf, R., and Nambi, P. (1994) Reversal of postischemic acute renal failure with a selective endothelinA receptor antagonist in the rat. *J. Clin. Invest.* **93**:900–906.

136. Kusumoto, K., Kubo, K., Kandori, K., Kitayoshi, T., Sato, S., Wakimasu, M., Watanabe, T., and Fujino, M. (1994) Effects of a new endothelin

antagonist, TAK-044, on post-ischemic acute renal failure in rats. *Life Sci.* **55:**301–310.

137. Bird, J. E., Webb, M. L., Wasserman, A. J., Liu, E. C., Giancarli, M. R., and Durham, S. K. (1995) Comparison of a novel ET_A receptor antagonist and phosphoramidon in renal ischemia. *Pharmacology* **50:**9–23.

138. Haleen, S., Davis, L., Schroeder, R., and Keiser, J. (1994) PD 145065, a non-selective endothelin receptor antagonist, significantly reduces the incidence of mortality in rats subjected to ischaemia-induced acute renal failure. *FASEB J.* **8:**A103.

139. Gellai, M., Jugus, M., Fletcher, T. A., Nambi, P., Brooks, D. P., Ohlstein, E. H., Elliott, J. D., Gleason, J., and Ruffolo, R. R., Jr. (1994) The endothelin receptor antagonist, (±)-SB 209670, reverses ischaemia-induced acute renal failure (ARF) in the rat. *FASEB J.* **8:**A260.

140. Brooks, D. P., DePalma, P. D., Gellai, M., Nambi, P., Ohlstein, E. H., Elliott, J. D., Gleason, J. G., and Ruffolo, R. R., Jr. (1994) Nonpeptide endothelin receptor antagonists. III. Effect of SB 209670 and BQ123 on acute renal failure in the dog. *J. Pharmacol. Exp. Ther.* **271:**769–775.

141. Fogo, A., Hellings, S. E., Inagami, T., and Kon, V. (1992) Endothelin receptor antagonism is protective in *in vivo* acute cyclosporine toxicity. *Kidney Int.* **42:**770–774.

142. Benigni, A., Perico, N., Gaspari, F., Zoja, C., Bellizi, L., Gabanelli, M., and Remuzzi, G. (1991) Increased renal endothelin production in rats with reduced renal mass. *Am. J. Physiol.* **260:**F331–F339.

143. Brooks, D. P. and DePalma, P. D. (1997) Blockade of radiocontrast-induced nephrotoxicity by the endothelin receptor antagonist, SB 209670. *Nephron* **72:**629–636.

144. Oldroyd, S. D., Haylor, J. L., and Morcos, S. K. (1995) The acute effect of ioversol on kidney function—role of endothelin. *Eur. J. Radiol.* **19:**91–95.

145. Nakamura, T., Ebihara, I., Tomino, Y., and Koide, H. (1995) Effect of a specific endothelin A receptor antagonist on murine lupus nephritis. *Kidney Int.* **47:**481–489.

146. Nishikibe, M., Tsuchida, S., Okada, M., Fukuroda, T., Shimamoto, K., Yano, M., Ishikawa, K., and Ikemoto, F. (1993) Antihypertensive effect of a newly synthesized endothelin antagonist, BQ-123, in a genetic hypertensive model. *Life Sci.* **52:**717–724.

147. Ohlstein, E. H., Douglas, S. A., Ezekiel, M., and Gellai, M. (1993) Antihypertensive effects of the endothelin receptor antagonist BQ-123 in conscious spontaneously hypertensive rats. *J. Cardiovasc. Pharmacol.* **22(Suppl. 8):**S321–S324.

148. Bazil, M. K., Lappe, R. W., and Webb, R. L. (1992) Pharmacologic characterization of an endothelin$_A$ (ET_A) receptor antagonist in conscious rats. *J. Cardiovasc. Pharmacol.* **20:**940–948.

149. Douglas, S. A., Gellai, M., Ezekiel, M., Feuerstein, G. Z., Elliott, J. D., and Ohlstein, E. H. (1995) Antihypertensive actions of the novel nonpeptide endothelin receptor antagonist SB 209670. *Hypertension* **25:**818–822.

150. Elliott, J. D., Ezekiel, M., Gellai, M., Douglas, S. A., and Ohlstein, E. H. (1994) Antihypertensive effect of the endothelin receptor antagonist SB 209670 in conscious spontaneously hypertensive rats (SHR). *FASEB J.* **8:**A7.

151. Bird, J. E., Moreland, S., Waldron, T. L., and Powell, J. R. (1995) Antihypertensive effects of a novel endothelin-A receptor antagonist. *Hypertension* **25:**1191–1195.

152. Schiffrin, E. L., Sventek, P., Li, J.-S., Turgeon, A., and Reudelhuber, T. (1995) Antihypertensive effect of an endothelin receptor antagonist in DOCA-salt spontaneously hypertensive rats. *Br. J. Pharmacol.* **115:**1377–1381.

153. Li, J. S. and Schiffrin, E. L. (1995) Effect of chronic treatment of adult spontaneously hypertensive rats with an endothelin receptor antagonist. *Hypertension* **25:**495–500.

154. Oparil, S., Chen, S. J., Meng, Q. C., Elton, T. S., Yano, M., and Chen, Y. F. (1995) Endothelin-A receptor antagonist prevents acute hypoxia-induced pulmonary hypertension in the rat. *Am. J. Physiol.* **268:**L95–L100.

155. Eddahibi, S., Raffestin, B., Clozel, M., Levame, M., and Adnot, S. (1995) Protection from pulmonary hypertension with an orally active endothelin receptor antagonist in hypoxic rats. *Am. J. Physiol.* **268:**H828–H835.

156. Wang, Y., Coe, Y., Toyoda, O., and Coceani, F. (1995) Involvement of endothelin-1 in hypoxic pulmonary vasoconstriction in the lamb. *J. Physiol.* **482:**421–434.

157. Ivy, D. D., Kinsella, J. P., and Abman, S. H. (1994) Physiologic characterization of endothelin A and B receptor activity in the ovine fetal pulmonary circulation. *J. Clin. Invest.* **93:**2141–2148.

158. Okada, M., Yamashita, C., Okada, M., and Okada, K. (1995) Role of endothelin-1 in beagles with dehydromonocrotaline-induced pulmonary hypertension. *Circulation* **92:**114–119.

159. Okada, M., Yamashita, C., Okada, M., and Okada, K. (1995) Endothelin receptor antagonists in a beagle model of pulmonary-hypertension—contribution to possible potential therapy. *J. Amer. Coll. Cardiol.* **25:**1213–1217.

160. Lerman, A. and Burnett, J. C., Jr. (1992) Intact and altered endothelium in regulation of vasomotion. *Circulation* **86(Suppl. III):**III-12–III-19.

161. Winkles, J. A., Alberts, G. F., Brogi, E., and Libby, P. (1993) Endothelin-1 and endothelin receptor mRNA expression in normal and atherosclerotic human arteries. *Biochem. Biophys. Res. Commun.* **191:**1081–1088.

162. Kowala, M. C., Rose, P. M., Stein, P. D., Goller, N., Reece, R., Beyer, S., Valentine, M., Barton, D., and Durham, S. K. (1995) Selective blockade of the endothelin subtype A receptor decreases early atherosclerosis in hamsters fed cholesterol. *Am. J. Pathol.* **146:**819–826.

163. Douglas, S. A., Louden, C., Vickery-Clarke, L. M., Storer, B. L., Hart, T., Feuerstein, G. Z., Elliott, J. D., and Ohlstein, E. H. (1994) A role for endogenous endothelin-1 in neointimal formation after rat carotid artery balloon angioplasty. Protective effects of the novel nonpeptide endothelin receptor antagonist SB 209670. *Circ. Res.* **75:**190–197.

164. Ohlstein, E. H. and Douglas, S. A. (1993) Endothelin-1 modulates vascular smooth muscle structure and vasomotion: implications in cardiovascular pharmacology. *Drug Dev. Res.* **29**:108–128.

165. Douglas, S. A. and Ohlstein, E. H. (1993) Endothelin-1 promotes neointima formation after balloon angioplasty in the rat. *J. Cardiovasc. Pharmacol.* **22(Suppl. 8)**:S371–S373.

166. Tsujino, M., Hirata, Y., Eguchi, S., Watanabe, T., Chatani, F., and Marumo, F. (1995) Nonselective ET_A/ET_B receptor antagonist blocks proliferation of rat vascular smooth-muscle cells after balloon angioplasty. *Life Sci.* **56**:PL449–PL454.

167. Jenkins-West, T., Valentine, M., Moreland, S., and Ferrer, P. (1995) Intimal lesion development in balloon-injured rat carotid arteries is suppressed by the endothelin receptor antagonist BMS-182874. *FASEB J.* **9**:A343.

168. Azuma, H., Hamasaki, H., Niimi, Y., Terada, T., and Matsubara, O. (1994) Role of endothelin-1 in neointima formation after endothelial removal in rabbit carotid arteries. *Am. J. Physiol.* **267**:H2259–H2267.

169. Willette, R. N. and Ohlstein, E. H. (1994) Endothelin: cerebrovascular disease. *Drug News Persp.* **7**:75–81.

170. Willette, R. N., Zhang, H., Mitchell, M. P., Sauermelch, C. F., Ohlstein, E. H., and Sulpizio, A. C. (1994) Nonpeptide endothelin antagonist. Cerebrovascular characterization and effects on delayed cerebral vasospasm. *Stroke* **25**:2450–2455.

171. Nirei, H., Hamada, K., Shoubo, M., Sogabe, K., Notsu, Y., and Ono, T. (1993) An endothelin ET_A receptor antagonist, FR 139317, ameliorates cerebral vasospasm in dogs. *Life Sci.* **52**:1869–1874.

172. Itoh, S., Sasaki, T., Ide, K., Ishikawa, K., Nishikibe, M., and Yano, M. (1993) A novel endothelin ET_A receptor antagonist, BQ-485, and its preventive effect on experimental cerebral vasospasm in dogs. *Biochem. Biophys. Res. Commun.* **195**:969–975.

173. Shigeno, T., Clozel, M., Sakai, S., Saito, A., and Goto, K. (1995) The effect of bosentan, a new potent endothelin receptor antagonist, on the pathogenesis of cerebral vasospasm. *Neurosurgery* **37**:87–90.

174. Roux, S., Loffler, B. M., Gray, G. A., Sprecher, U., Clozel, M., and Clozel, J. P. (1995) The role of endothelin in experimental cerebral vasospasm. *Neurosurgery* **37**:78–85.

175. Thabes, J. S., Lefferts, P. L., Lu, W. X., and Snappe, J. R. (1994) An endothelin-A receptor antagonist (BMS-182874) attenuates endotoxin-induced pulmonary hypertension in sheep. *9th Int. Conf. Prostagl. Rel. Comp.* **1**:24.

176. Zimmerman, R. S., Maymind, M., and Barbee, R. W. (1994) Endothelin blockade lowers total peripheral resistance in hemorrhagic shock recovery. *Hypertension* **23**:205–210.

177. Michida, T., Kawano, S., Masuda, E., Kobayishi, I., Nishimura, Y., Tsuji, M., Hayashi, N., Takei, Y., Tsuji, S., and Nagano, K. (1994) Role of endothelin 1 in haemorrhagic shock-induced gastric mucosal injury in rats. *Gastroenterology* **106**:988–993.

178. Stevens, E. J. and Tomlinson, D. R. (1995) Effects of endothelin receptor antagonism with bosentan on peripheral nerve function in experimental diabetes. *Br. J. Pharmacol.* **115:**373–379.

179. Cameron, N. E., Dines, K. C., and Cotter, M. A. (1994) The potential contribution of endothelin-1 to neurovascular abnormalities in streptozotocin-diabetic rats. *Diabetologia* **37:**1209–1215.

180. Marsault, R., Feolde, E., and Frelin, C. (1993) Receptor externalization determines sustained contractile responses to endothelin-1 in the rat aorta. *Am. J. Physiol.* **264:**C687–C693.

181. Waggoner, W. G., Genova, S. L., and Rash, V. A. (1992) Kinetic analyses demonstrate that the equilibrium assumption does not apply to [^{125}I]endothelin-1 binding data. *Life Sci.* **51:**1869–1876.

182. Warner, T. D., Allcock, G. H., and Vane, J. R. (1994) Reversal of established responses to endothelin-1 *in vivo* and *in vitro* by the endothelin receptor antagonists BQ-123 and PD 145065. *Br. J. Pharmacol.* **112:**207–213.

183. Fabregat, I. and Rozengurt, E. (1990) [D-Arg^1, D-Phe^5, D-Trp^{7,9}, Leu^{11}] Substance P, a neuropeptide antagonist, blocks binding, Ca^{2+}-mobilizing, and mitogenic effects of endothelin and vasoactive intestinal contractor in mouse 3T3 cells. *J. Cell Physiol.* **145:**88–94.

184. Spinella, M. J., Malik, A. B., Everitt, J., and Andersen, T. T. (1991) Design and synthesis of a specific endothelin 1 antagonist: effects on pulmonary vasoconstriction. *Proc. Natl. Acad. Sci. USA* **88:**7443–7446.

185. Stingo, A. J., Clavell, A. L., Aarhus, L. L., and Burnett, J. C. (1993) Biological role of the ET$_A$ receptor in a model of increased endogenous endothelin. *3rd Int. Conf. on Endothelin*, Houston, TX. Feb. 14–17 abst. no 118.

Chapter 8

Pathophysiological Role of Endothelin and Potential Therapeutic Targets for Receptor Antagonists

David P. Brooks, Diane K. Jorkasky, Martin I. Freed, and Eliot H. Ohlstein

1. Introduction

In the decade following the discovery of endothelin (ET) by Yanagisawa and his colleagues *(1)*, there has been a prodigious number of studies on endothelin, its receptors, and their potential role in physiological and pathophysiological processes. There is an ever-increasing literature describing the importance of endothelin and the potential use of ET-receptor antagonists in a number of diverse diseases (Table 1). A detailed description of the evidence implicating endothelin in all the diseases listed as well as citing all the relevant papers cannot be conducted within the confines of one chapter. We have, on occasion, therefore, used review articles in place of multiple citations and have concentrated our discussion on four disease areas for which there is the most evidence and provide brief descriptions of some of the other areas for which reports have appeared. As ET-receptor antagonists enter clinical development and different clinical trials are conducted, it is likely that some of these "other diseases" take more prominent positions with regard to intervention with endothelin antagonists.

From: *Endothelin: Molecular Biology, Physiology, and Pathology*
Edited by R. F. Highsmith © Humana Press Inc., Totowa, NJ

Table 1
Endothelin and Disease

Cardiovascular disease	Renal disease
Hypertension	Ischemia-induced acute renal failure
Congestive heart failure	Cyclosporine A nephrotoxicity
Atherosclerosis	FK506 nephrotoxicity
Vascular restenosis	Cisplatin nephrotoxicity
Myocardial ischemia/infarction	Radiocontrast nephropathy
Pre-eclampsia	Amphotericin B nephrotoxicity
Cerebral vasospasm	Polycystic kidney disease
Stroke	Hepatorenal syndrome
Migraine	Ureteric obstruction
Raynaud's disease	Benign prostatic hypertrophy
Endotoxic shock	
	Other diseases
Pulmonary disease	Diabetes
Asthma	Diabetic retinopathy
Pulmonary hypertension	Glaucoma
Acute respiratory-distress syndrome	Cancer (various)
Cystic fibrosis	Systemic sclerosis
	Skin disease
	Peptic ulcers
	Inflammatory bowel disease
	Organ rejection

2. Cardiovascular Disease

2.1. Hypertension

Endothelin is the most potent vasoconstrictor yet identified and thus its potential role in the development and/or maintenance of hypertension has been studied extensively. Research has concentrated primarily on its effects on the systemic circulation and the kidney because the kidney plays a primary role in the long-term control of blood pressure.

When given exogenously, endothelin causes potent vasoconstriction in all animals studied, including humans (2–4). Chronic elevations of endogenous endothelin in man can also result in hypertension as observed in two patients with malignant hemangioendothelioma resulting in increased circulating endothelin. In these patients, the hypertension disappeared or recurred, depending on the presence of the tumor and elevated plasma endothelin (5). Long-term infusion of exogenous endothelin to dogs leads to a chronic increase in blood pressure (6) and overexpression of human prepro-ET-1 in rats (7) leads to sustained elevations in blood pressure. Studies evaluating the levels of circulating endothelin in patients with essential hypertension have produced variable results, however, evidence suggests that endothelin is indeed modestly elevated in hypertension *(8)*. Plasma endothelin also appears to be greater in obese individuals and particularly obese hypertensives. One group reported that, whereas no change in plasma endothelin levels between normotensives and borderline hypertensives was observed, there was a greater increase in circulating endothelin following a cold pressor stimulus in the hypertensive group *(9)*. There appear to be some racial differences in plasma ET-1 concentrations in individuals with hypertension. Thus, both male and female black hypertensives have nearly fourfold higher endothelin levels than male and female white hypertensives *(10)*. Studies measuring plasma endothelin in animal models of hypertension have also provided equivocal data with both increases and decreases being reported *(11)*.

Circulating or urinary endothelin may not necessarily reflect the true role of endothelin in maintaining blood pressure since endothelin may be having more local effects. Blood vessel endothelin expression has been shown to be increased in deoxycorticosterone acetate (DOCA)-salt hypertensive but not spontaneously hypertensive rats *(12)*, whereas there are increased cardiac levels of ET-1-like immunoreactivity in spontaneously hypertensive rats *(13)*. Renal prepro-ET-1 mRNA level is also increased in DOCA-salt hypertensive animals *(14)* and endothelin production from cultured endothelial cells is upregulated in hypertensive rats *(15)*.

Studies evaluating endothelin receptors in hypertension have provided inconsistent data. Both ET_A and ET_B receptors have been shown to be reduced in mesenteric vessels of spontaneously hypertensive rats *(16)*, however, augmented expression of ET_A receptor mRNA has been demonstrated in both glomeruli *(17)*, as well as mesangial cells *(18)* from spontaneously hypertensive and stroke-prone spontaneously hypertensive rats, respectively. One study demonstrated a significant decrease in ET_A receptors but an increase in ET_B receptors in the kidney cortex of spontaneously hypertensive rats, and this change paralleled alterations in the ability of endothelin to produce renal vasoconstriction, which is mediated via ET_B receptors in rats *(19)*.

In addition to possible changes in ET-receptor number in hypertension *(20)*, there is a change in endothelin sensitivity *(11)*. Compared to WKY rats, the ability of endothelin to contract aortic vascular smooth muscle is greater in DOCA-hypertensive rats and there is a greater sensitivity to the renal-vasoconstrictor effects of endothelin in isolated perfused kidneys from spontaneously hypertensive rats *(21)*. In addition, mesangial cells from prehypertensive DOCA-salt-sensitive rats appear to be more sensitive to the actions of endothelin *(22)*. Inhibition of endothelin with either antibodies *(23)* or interstitial infusion of ET-receptor antagonists *(24)* leads to improved renal perfusion and glomerular filtration.

There are a number of experimental studies demonstrating that blockade of endothelin can have beneficial effects in hypertension. Administration of the endothelin converting enzyme inhibitor, phosphoramidon *(25)*, or ET-receptor antagonists *(14,23,26–34)* have been shown to reduce blood pressure in a number of different hypertensive-rat models. There is one report, however, that chronic treatment of spontaneously hypertensive rats for 4 wk with bosentan was ineffective *(35)*. An interesting recent study demonstrated that an ET_B-selective receptor antagonist increased blood pressure in spontaneously hypertensive and DOCA-salt hypertensive animals, indicating the importance of blockade of vasorelaxant ET_B receptors *(36)*. In rats made hypertensive by overexpression of prepro-ET-1, intravenous infusion of the ET_A receptor antagonist FR 139317 reduced blood pressure to levels seen in the control group and intravenous infusion of the ET_B receptor antagonist BQ788 caused a small but significant increase in blood pressure in both groups *(7)*. The ability of ET-receptor antagonists to lower blood pressure in animal models has not been limited to rats because bosentan also lowers blood pressure in renal hypertensive dogs *(37)*.

Limited studies have been conducted in man, however, ET-receptor antagonists can lower blood pressure in patients with congestive heart failure *(38)* and endogenous ET-induced vasoconstriction has been demonstrated in man using phosphoramidon and BQ123, which alone resulted in forearm vasodilation *(39)*. Although endothelin may contribute to maintaining elevated blood pressure in hypertensives, it is not clear whether it is important in maintaining blood pressure in normotensives. One study has demonstrated that administration of TAK 044 lowered mean arterial pressure by 18 mm Hg *(40)*, whereas in another study, SB 217242 appeared to have a clinically insignificant effect on blood pressure *(41)*.

2.2. Congestive Heart Failure

Congestive heart failure (CHF) is a progressive disease whereby, following myocardial damage, attempts to maintain cardiac output are accompanied by increased peripheral vasoconstriction and neurohumoral activation. In addition, there is impaired relaxation of peripheral and coronary vasculatures and cardiac remodeling. There is growing evidence that endothelin may be involved in the pathogenesis of congestive heart failure. The majority of studies evaluating circulating endothelin in patients with heart failure have demonstrated an increase *(8)*. It has been reported that the increase in endothelin in patients with heart failure represents principally elevation of big endothelin and that this correlates with the magnitude of alterations in cardiac hemodynamics as well as functional class *(42)* and survival *(43)*. Another report indicates that circulating ET-1 levels are increased both in the acute phase of myocardial infarction and in CHF, where the levels are closely correlated with indices of disease severity, such as capillary-wedge pressure, left ventricular ejection fraction, New York Heart Association (NYHA) class, cardiac index, and, most notably, 12 mo survival *(44)*. Spontaneous endothelin production in circulating mononuclear cells from patients with heart failure has also been reported *(45)*.

Endothelin is also elevated in experimental models of heart failure *(46)* and a number of different animal studies have indicated that the increase in systemic endothelin correlates with ventricular mass *(46)*. In addition, left ventricular hypertrophy induced by chronic pressure overload is associated with enhanced prepro-ET-1 mRNA and endothelin immunoreactivity *(47)* as well as increased endothelin binding in cardiac tissue *(48)*. Evidence suggests that endothelin may have a direct effect to promote cardiac hypertrophy and may be involved in cardiomyocyte hypertrophy induced by mechanical stress *(49)*.

Various investigators have studied the effects of endothelin antagonists in rat models of heart failure and reported that it can reduce left-ventricular hypertrophy *(50)* and lower blood pressure *(51)*. Inhibition of endothelin with BQ123 in rats with myocardial infarction-induced heart failure resulted in increased survival and amelioration of left-ventricular dysfunction and ventricular remodeling *(52)* and ET-receptor antagonists have also been shown to have beneficial effects in dogs with heart failure *(53)*. Treatment of patients with heart failure with drugs such as ACE inhibitors have demonstrated conflicting results on plasma ET levels. Several reports with angiotensin-converting enzyme (ACE) inhibitors have shown that treatment of heart-failure patients produces a reduction in plasma endothelin levels *(54,55)*; however, Grenier et al. *(56)* reported that captopril had no significant effect on circulating endothelin levels in these patients. In another report, the novel-vasodilating β blocker, carvedilol, decreased circulating endothelin *(57)*. Furthermore, the change in endothelin was an independent, noninvasive predictor of the functional and hemodynamic responses to carvedilol *(57)*. When the ET-receptor antagonist, bosentan, was administered intravenously to patients with heart failure, it was shown to have beneficial effects, reducing mean arterial pressure, pulmonary-artery pressure, right-atrial pressure, and pulmonary artery wedge pressure and increasing cardiac index *(38)*.

2.3. Atherosclerosis and Vascular Restenosis

Vasospasm and vascular remodeling are important complications associated with atherosclerosis and vascular restenosis such as is observed following percutaneous transluminal balloon angioplasty. There is increasing evidence that endothelin may be involved in both pathologies. Oxidized low density lipoprotein (LDL), which is an important risk factor in atherosclerosis, stimulates endothelin synthesis in human and porcine macrophages and endothelial-cell cultures *(58)*. Atherosclerosis, hyperliproteinemia, and angioplasty are all associated with enhanced endothelin immunoreactivity *(8)*. Indeed, plasma endothelin concentration correlates with the severity and extent of coronary atherosclerosis *(59)* and ET-1 immunoreactivity is most prevalent in foamy macrophages and myofibroblasts in the vicinity of necrotic areas with signs of previous intraplaque hemorrhage *(60)*. A recent study has demonstrated a significant increase in patients with hypercholesterolemia without evidence of atherosclerosis *(61)*. In animal models of atherosclerosis, circulating endothelin is increased in hypercholesterolemic pigs *(62)* and tissue endothelin-like immunoreactivity is increased 4 wk following balloon injury to the carotid artery of rats *(63)*. Moreover, Wang et al. *(64)* reported a marked upregulation of mRNA for ET-converting enzyme, prepro-ET-1, ET_A and ET_B receptors following rat carotid balloon angioplasty.

Both atherosclerosis and balloon angioplasty enhance the vasoconstrictor activity of endothelin *(65)*. Systemic administration of radiolabeled endothelin accumulates within atherosclerotic plaques of hypercholesterolemic rabbits *(66)*, hyperplastic regions in pig femoral arteries *(67)* and atheromatous human saphenous veins and coronary arteries (68). Endothelin binding has also been characterized in the vaso vasorum and in regions of neovascularization *(67)* and increased endothelin binding has been demonstrated in hyperplastic arteries of rats and rabbits *(63,69)* and in atherosclerotic human arterial vessels *(70)*.

Both acute *(71)* and chronic *(72)* administration of endothelin augments the degree of neointima formation following carotid-artery balloon angioplasty in rats and studies with ET-receptor antagonists have demonstrated that SB 209670 *(73)* and BMS 182874 *(74)* but not BQ123 *(63,73)* are effective in suppressing neointimal development in this model. In addition, blockade of ET_A receptors with BMS 182874 decreased early atherosclerosis in cholesterol-fed hamsters *(75)*.

2.4. Myocardial Ischemia

Endothelin is a potent constrictor of coronary arteries and, as such, its involvement in the pathogenesis of angina pectoris, coronary-artery vasospasm, and myocardial infarction has been studied. Exogenous endothelin can induce myocardial ischemia in dogs *(76)* and coronary vasospasm in mice has been shown to be the primary cause of death owing to the venom of the burrowing asp, *Atractaspis Engaddensis*, *(77)*. The venom of this snake, of course, contains the endothelin isopeptide, sarafotoxin 6c, a potent agonist at the ET_B receptor.

There is good evidence that circulating endothelin is increased in patients with coronary vasospasm and myocardial infarction *(8)*. In one study in patients, arterial endothelin levels following myocardial infarction significantly correlated with mean pulmonary-artery pressure, central-venous pressure, and pulmonary-vascular resistance, and these levels also significantly correlated with peak-creatinine kinase and creatinine-kinase isozyme MB *(78)*. These investigators concluded that the increased plasma-endothelin concentration at the early stage of acute myocardial infarction reflected higher pulmonary-artery pressure and pulmonary-vascular resistance, whereas in the later stage, the plasma-endothelin elevation was related to infarct size *(78)*. When endothelin expression was measured in the hearts from pigs that had undergone myocardial ischemia, a twofold increase in expression was observed in ischemic myocardium compared to nonischemic myocardium and *in situ* hybridization demonstrated a considerable increase in endothelin mRNA in ischemic cardiomyocytes *(79)*.

Studies evaluating endothelin levels in non-infarct states such as angina pectoris have provided inconsistent data; however, there is evidence that endothelin is increased in acute unstable angina *(8)*. There is good evidence that endothelin levels are increased following coronary angioplasty; however, it is unclear whether the increased endothelin levels are related to myocardial injury *(80)* or endothelial-cell damage *(81)*.

Early studies using endothelin antibodies or phosphoramidon, an inhibitor of endothelin converting enzyme, demonstrated that blockade of endothelin could reduce left-ventricular infarct size following coronary-artery ligation/reperfusion in rats and rabbits *(8,11)*. Studies with ET-receptor antagonists have provided equivocal data with some reports failing to observe a protective effect, whereas others demonstrating reduction in infarct size in both rats and rabbits *(82–84)*. In rabbits, FR139317 had no effect on infarct size following coronary-artery occlusion *(85,86)*. Similar studies were observed with this antagonist in dogs with and without preconditioning *(87)* and with PD156707 in pigs *(88)*. In contrast, bosentan in rats *(84)* and pigs *(89)*, BQ123 in dogs *(90)*, PD 145065 in rabbits *(86)*, and TAK 044 in rats *(91,92)* have all been shown to reduce infarct size. In addition, BQ610 preserved mechanical function and energy metabolism during ischemia/reperfusion injury in isolated perfused rat hearts *(93)* and BQ123 prevented ET-induced exacerbation of ischemic arrhythmias in anesthetized rats *(94)*.

Experimental studies have not provided conclusive evidence for the importance of endothelin in myocardial ischemia and thus clinical trials may be required to provide a definitive answer. Certainly, the report that long-term mortality of patients following acute myocardial infarction appears to be related to plasma endothelin levels is intriguing *(95)*.

2.5. Cerebral Vasospasm

Initial evidence to suggest that endothelin may be involved in cerebral vasospasm, especially that induced by subarachnoid hemorrhage, was provided by observations that endothelin is a potent vasoconstrictor of the cerebrovasculature *(96)*, that hemoglobin is a potent stimulator of endothelin biosynthesis *(97)* and that both cerebrospinal fluid and plasma-endothelin levels are elevated following subarachnoid hemorrhage and cerebral-artery vasospasm *(98)*. In recent experimental studies, the time course of changes in endothelin levels in plasma and central nervous system (CNS) have been measured following subarachnoid hemorrhage and it appears that the levels in the cerebrospinal fluid increase earlier than levels in plasma *(99)*. Other studies have been able to show that increased endothelin in plasma or cerebrospinal fluid increased coincident with symptomatic vasospasm *(100)* and furthermore that the volume of hematoma in the basal cisterns, as detected by computerized tomography, was predictive of the concentrations of endothelin in the cerebral spinal fluid *(100)*. Some studies have failed to demonstrate increased endothelin levels following a cerebrovascular event *(101)*, however, the discrepancy in observations may be owing to reduced frequency of the monitoring of endothelin levels as well as the difficulty of measuring cerebral vasospasm clinically. In animal models of subarachnoid hemorrhage, endothelin levels in the cerebral spinal fluid have also been shown to be elevated *(102)*. Additionally, in one study measuring ET_A receptor mRNA from brain tissue following subarachnoid hemorrhage, a marked increase was observed 3 d following subarachnoid hemorrhage and this was sustained until d 7 *(103)*.

Evaluation of endothelin blockers in animal models of subarachnoid hemorrhage-induced cerebral vasospasm have provided variable results. Phosphoramidon and the ET_A receptor antagonist, BQ123, have been reported to be effective *(104–108)* as well as ineffective *(109)* in models of vasospasm. Other ET-enzyme converting inhibitors, such as C9526303 *(110)*, or ET-receptor antagonists, such as BQ485 *(103)*, Ro-46-2005 *(111)*, FR139317 *(112)*, bosentan *(102,113–115)*, and SB 209670 *(116)* administered by various routes have all been shown to be effective at preventing subarachnoid hemorrhage-induced cerebral vasospasm in animals. The ability of ET-receptor antagonists to prevent or reverse subarachnoid hemorrhage-induced cerebral vasospasm may be dependent on the route of administration, their ability to cross the blood–brain barrier, and the integrity of the blood–brain barrier itself. In one study in monkeys, systemic administration of BQ123, but not bosentan was effective, however, only BQ123 could be detected in the cerebral spinal fluid *(108)*. In other studies, systemic administration of bosentan to dogs has been shown to be effective *(113)*. Certainly, systemic rather than intracisternal administration of drug will be a requirement for the potential treatment of patients with this disorder.

2.6. Stroke

Endothelin and its receptors are widely distributed throughout the brain *(117,118)* and there is growing evidence that an ET-receptor antagonist may be therapeutic in this condition. Endothelin is a potent constrictor of cerebral arterioles (*see* Section 2.5.) and microinjections of endothelin-1 adjacent to the right middle-cerebral artery results in a reproducible pattern of focal-cerebral infarction *(119)*. In addition, intracerebral injection of ET-1 produces focal-brain ischemia and is the basis of a model of cerebral infarction *(120)*.

There have been a number of studies demonstrating increased plasma-endothelin levels in patients with cerebral infarction. Seventy-two hours following the onset of nonhemorrhagic cerebral infarction, plasma levels of ET-1 were significantly elevated *(121)* and similar observations were made by other investigators in patients following cerebral infarction *(122)*. Immunoreactive endothelin has also been reported to be increased in gerbils following transient forebrain ischemia *(123,124)* and in rats following permanent and transient focal ischemia *(125,126)*. Immunohistochemical staining for ET-1 in astrocytes was observed in the hippocampus following bilateral common carotid occlusion in the stroke-prone spontaneously hypertensive rat *(127)*.

Only a few studies have been performed looking at endothelin receptors following brain ischemia. In the gerbil, 10 min after forebrain ischemia, there appeared to be a decrease in ET-receptor density *(124)*, however, 4–7 d after brain ischemia in rats, there was a large increase in ET-binding sites in hippocampal CA1 and dentate gyrus, ventral thalamic nucleus, and cortical vessels *(128)*.

A number of studies have evaluated the effects of ET-receptor antagonists in animal models of nonhemorrhagic stroke and the preponderance of the data indicate beneficial effects. BQ123 *(129)* and SB 209670 *(29,118)* have been shown to be neuroprotective in the gerbil-stroke model, inhibiting the degree of CA1 neurodegeneration associated with focal-cerebral ischemia induced by cerebral-artery ligation. SB 217242 given orally for 7 d reduced cerebral focal-ischemic brain injury induced by middle cerebral artery occlusion in the spontaneously hypertensive rat *(130)*, however, bosentan had minimal effects on postischemic hyperperfusion in the 3 h following bilateral common carotid occlusion with concomitant hemorrhagic hypertension (transient global ischemia) in rats *(131)*. It was unclear whether bosentan crossed the blood-brain barrier in this study, however, it has been demonstrated that systemic administration of bosentan to cats can gain access to the adventitial surface of pial resistance arterioles *(132)*. Another study in cats demonstrated that the ET_A-selective antagonist, PD 156707, reduced the hemispheric volume of ischemic damage following middle cerebral artery occlusion *(133)*.

2.7. Pre-Eclampsia

Pre-eclampsia occurs in the latter half of pregnancy and is characterized by an acute elevation in blood pressure, edema, proteinuria, and reduced renal-blood flow. Evidence suggests that endothelin may play a role in this disease. Endothelin is widely distributed in the vascular endothelium of the human placenta *(134)*. There are numerous reports indicating that maternal plasma levels of endothelin are increased in pre-eclampsia *(8)*, however, there does not seem to be any correlation between plasma-endothelin levels and either systolic or diastolic blood pressure *(135)*. Others, however, have failed to observe an increase in patients with pre-eclampsia *(136)*. In addition, pre-eclampsia is associated with decreased release of endothelin from trophoblastic cells in vitro *(137)*.

There are conflicting reports on whether endothelin expression is altered in pre-eclampsia. One report indicated that ET-1 mRNA in placental villous tissue was significantly higher in pre-eclamptic women when compared to control subjects *(138)*, however, others have reported that placental preproendothelin gene expression and immunoreactive big ET-1, as well as ET-1, 2, and 3, were comparable in placental tissue from pre-eclamptic and normal pregnant women *(136)*. Furthermore, urinary endothelin excretion, which is likely to reflect the renal synthesis of the peptide, was significantly decreased in patients with pre-eclampsia when compared to normal pregnant women *(136)*.

The reports on endothelin binding in pre-eclampsia are similarly controversial. In one study, an increase in the density of endothelin receptors and placental membranes from pre-eclamptic women was reported *(139)*, whereas in another report, there was a decrease in endothelin binding to placental membranes but an increase in binding to trophoblastic cells *(140)*. In addition, when the ability of endothelin to contract omental arteries from menopausal women, normotensive pregnant women, and pre-eclamptic patients was evaluated, there were no significant differences in either the sensitivity or efficacy of endothelin *(141)*. It is unclear, therefore, whether an ET-receptor antagonist would be beneficial in pre-eclampsia.

2.8. Cardiovascular Summary

Endothelin is a potent vasoconstrictor and smooth muscle mitogen in a wide variety of species, including humans and may be involved in a number of different cardiovascular diseases. Indeed, in addition to the diseases previously described, it has been proposed that endothelin is involved in endotoxic shock *(142,143)*, Raynaud's disease *(144)*, and migraine *(145)*, where endothelin acting through ET_B receptors may play an important role in mediating neurogenic inflammation in the meninges of rats *(146)*. It is likely that over the next few years, clinical trials using novel ET-receptor antagonists will provide a better insight into the true importance of endothelin in the pathogenesis of different cardiovascular diseases.

3. Pulmonary Diseases

3.1. Asthma

Asthma is a chronic inflammatory disorder involving a number of pathologies in addition to bronchial constriction. Many of the activities of endothelin in experimental models mimic the clinical features of asthma including bronchoconstriction, airway hyperresponsiveness, mucus hypersecretion, bronchial edema, inflammatory cell activation and airway smooth-muscle hyperplasia *(8,11)*. In addition, a relationship between circulating endothelin and pulmonary function has been demonstrated in patients with asthma *(147)*. There have been numerous reports of increased endothelin levels in bronchoalveolar lavage fluid from patients with asthma *(8)* and there is a dramatic increase in endothelin expression in airways, epithelium and vascular endothelium in patients with asthma *(148)*. Both prepro-ET-1 and ET-1 mRNA are expressed in bronchial epithelial cells taken from asthmatics *(149,150)*. Endothelin receptors are expressed in the human lung *(11)*, however, asthma was not associated with any significant alterations in endothelin binding to alveolar-wall tissue *(151)*.

There is some evidence that endothelin may be involved in the chronic inflammation observed in asthma. Endothelin immunoreactivity is significantly increased in monocytes and alveolar macrophages from patients with stable, but not unstable, asthma *(152)*. In addition, when endothelin was administered intranasally to allergic and non-allergic individuals, it induced the symptoms relevant to inflammatory upper airway disease, and the responses of allergic subjects were more pronounced inasmuch as allergic individuals sneezed more and had significantly higher bilateral-secretion weights, contralateral-lysozyme secretion, and symptoms of rhinorrhea *(153)*. Blockade of endothelin with anti-endothelin antiserum has been shown to suppress the maximal reduction of specific airway conductance in both immediate and late asthmatic responses to antigen challenge in a guinea-pig model of asthma *(154)*. Interestingly, the two selective ET_B receptor antagonists, BQ788 and RES-701-1, have been shown to block the immediate but not the late asthmatic responses, whereas the two ET_A receptor antagonists, BQ123 and Shionogi 97-139, suppressed only the late asthmatic responses in guinea pigs *(154)*. Despite these experimental observations, the exact role of endothelin in the pathogenesis of asthma remains unknown and the utility of ET-receptor antagonists has yet to be proven.

3.2. Pulmonary Hypertension

Pulmonary hypertension is a relentless and progressive disease characterized by increased vascular tone and reactivity, vascular remodeling, and elevated pulmonary vascular resistance, which leads to right heart failure. A number of reports have demonstrated significant increases in circulating endothelin levels in patients with primary and secondary pulmonary hypertension *(8)*. Endothelin is also elevated in normal volunteers with high altitude-induced pulmonary hypertension *(155)* and is increased sevenfold in patients with acute respiratory failure *(156)*. Studies in patients with pulmonary hypertension owing to ventricular-septal or atrial-septal defects indicated that pressure overload to the pulmonary circulation is an important stimulus for endothelin release *(157)*. ET-1 mRNA is increased in patients with primary and secondary pulmonary hypertension *(158)* and lung ET-1 production is increased in rats with idiopathic pulmonary hypertension *(159)*. The expression of ET-1 mRNA is increased in the lungs of rats with congestive heart failure *(160)* and in rats with pulmonary hypertension induced by hypoxia, ET-mediated vasoconstriction of pulmonary arteries is enhanced *(161)*.

There is growing evidence that endothelin may also be involved in airway remodeling associated with pulmonary hypertension and asthma. Endothelin can stimulate pulmonary smooth muscle cell proliferation *(162,163)* and induce fibronectin expression in bronchial endothelial cells *(164)*. In monocrotaline-treated rats demonstrating medial hypertrophy and perivascular fibrosis of pulmonary arteries, endothelin levels and its mRNA expression in the lung were increased *(165)*.

A number of animal studies have demonstrated the efficacy of ET-receptor antagonists in pulmonary hypertension. BQ123 and/or bosentan have been shown to prevent pulmonary hypertension associated with hypoxia *(8,11)* and coronary-artery ligation *(160)* in rats and FR139317 decreases pulmonary-artery pressure in beagles with dehydromonocrotaline-induced pulmonary hypertension *(166)*. There have been only a few studies on the effects of endothelin or ET-receptor antagonists on the pulmonary system. When endothelin was infused intravenously into healthy volunteers, no major changes in the pulmonary circulation were observed *(167)*, however, studies in patients with congestive heart failure have demonstrated that intravenous bosentan can acutely reduce pulmonary artery pressure *(38)*.

4. Renal Diseases

The kidney is exquisitely sensitive to the vasoconstrictor actions of endothelin and intravenous administration of endothelin to normal volunteers will cause a substantial reduction in renal-blood flow and glomerular-filtration rate with little change in systemic arterial pressure *(3,168)*. In addition, endothelin has potent effects on renal tubular and mesangial cell function and, as such, has been implicated in a number of renal diseases.

4.1. Ischemia-Induced Acute Renal Failure

Acute renal failure remains one of the most daunting problems associated with acute critical-care medicine. Despite advances in the treatment of critically ill patients, there are currently no proven therapies for the treatment of established acute renal failure in humans and this disorder continues to be associated with a high mortality rate and extended hospitalizations. Acute renal failure most frequently develops in response to reduced renal perfusion, rhabdomyolysis secondary to major trauma or crush syndrome, or various nephrotoxins.

There is compelling evidence that endothelin is involved in ischemia-induced acute renal failure and the associated acute tubular necrosis. There appears to be an increase in endothelin production in acute renal failure as evidenced by increased plasma-endothelin levels in patients with acute renal failure *(169)*, as well as in dogs *(170)* and rats *(171)* following renal ischemia. In addition, there are increased tissue levels of endothelin as well as endothelin mRNA in postischemic kidneys *(171,172)*. Interestingly, expression of ET-3 decreases following ischemia *(172)*, however, the significance of this is unclear.

Endothelin binding to renal cortical membranes and its receptors is increased following renal ischemia, however, this response involved an increase in affinity rather than an increase in receptor number *(173,174)*. The increase in endothelin binding in renal cortical membrane may be to structures other than glomeruli because glomeruli taken from ischemic kidneys do not demonstrate any change in endothelin binding *(175)*.

Studies in which endothelin activity has been blocked with the converting enzyme inhibitor, phosphoramidon *(176)*, endothelin antibodies *(171,177,178)*, or ET-receptor antagonists such as BQ123 *(179–181)*, SB 209670 *(182,183)*, Ro-46-2005 *(184)*, or TAK 044 *(185)* have all demonstrated that blockade of endothelin activity can prevent and/or reverse ischemia-induced changes in renal function. There are two different reports demonstrating that an ET-receptor antagonist given 24 or 48 h following renal ischemia/reperfusion can acutely *(177)* or chronically *(181,183)* reverse acute renal failure. Interestingly, two studies in the dog using BQ123 have demonstrated that selective blockade of the ET_A receptor antagonist had no effect on ischemia-induced acute renal failure induced by aortic cross-clamping *(186)* or selective renal ischemia *(182)*; however, under identical conditions, Brooks et al. *(182)* was able to demonstrate that the mixed ET_A/ET_B receptor antagonist, SB 209670, could significantly attenuate ischemia-induced reductions in glomerular-filtration rate and increases in fractional sodium excretion. Thus, there appears to be differences in the effectiveness of ET-receptor antagonists to block ischemia-induced acute renal failure in dogs and rats. These differences may be owing to species differences in the roles of ET_A and ET_B receptors. In the dog, ET_A receptors mediate renal vasoconstrictor effects of endothelin, whereas ET_B receptors mediate endothelin's tubular actions and in the rat, the reverse may be true *(187,188)*. Based on these observations, some investigators have suggested that mechanisms other than blockade of endothelin-induced vasoconstriction, such as renal tubular effects, may contribute to the beneficial effect observed with ET-receptor antagonists in these disease models *(181,182)*. Consistent with this hypothesis is the observation that acute moderate hypoxia can be associated with significant increases in urinary endothelin excretion, urine flow and urine sodium excretion in dogs and that immunohistochemistry indicates increased endothelin staining in proximal and distal tubules following hypoxia *(189)*.

An increase in endothelin binding is also observed following renal failure induced by glycerol, a model of crush syndrome. The increased binding, however, involved an upregulation of ET-receptors *(190)* rather than the increased affinity as observed following renal ischemia *(see* Section 4.1.). Nonetheless, consistent with the effects of ET-receptor antagonists in ischemia-induced acute renal failure, the ET-receptor antagonist, bosentan, was shown to prevent rhabdomyolysis-induced acute renal failure in rats *(191)*.

There are some reports in the literature of agents that can prevent ischemia-induced acute renal failure in animals, especially when the intervention is made prior to or during the ischemic event. In contrast, some of the studies evaluating the effect of ET-receptor antagonists in acute renal failure have involved protocols involving administration of agents following the ischemic insult and establishment of renal dysfunction. Because most cases of acute renal failure cannot be predicted and patients often present with established deficits in renal function, ET-receptor antagonists represent an exciting new potential therapy.

4.2. Cyclosporine A- and FK506-Induced Nephrotoxicity

Cyclosporine A and FK506 are potent immunosuppressant agents used to prevent allograft rejection and treat certain immunopathogenic diseases. Their use, however, can be complicated by a number of side effects including hypertension, acute and chronic renal failure, and vasculopathy. Cyclosporine A-induced vasoconstriction and subsequent development of arteriolopathy and interstitial fibrosis have been reported and there is growing evidence that endothelin plays an important role in this disorder.

Administration of cyclosporine A can result in both increased systemic and renal production of endothelin and has been shown to result in increased endothelin release from cultured human endothelial cells *(192)* as well as cultured renal tubular and mesangial cells *(193,194)*. Plasma-endothelin concentrations are elevated in patients treated with cyclosporine A *(195–197)* and increased urinary endothelin excretion is induced by cyclosporine in humans *(198)* and rats *(199–202)*. In rats, treatment with nifedipine can attenuate both cyclosporine A-induced renal dysfunction and reduce urinary endothelin excretion *(202)*. Cyclosporine A-induced renal insufficiency in rats is also associated with increased ET-1 but not ET-3 or ET-converting enzyme mRNA in the renal medulla *(201)*.

In addition to producing increased renal production of endothelin, cyclosporine A causes an upregulation of endothelin binding *(203,204)* and increased gene expression of endothelin receptors in the kidney *(205)*. Interestingly, increased endothelin binding in cardiac tissue is observed in cyclosporine A-induced cardiac fibrosis in rats *(206)* as well as increased expression of ET_A receptor mRNA in aortic cells from cyclosporine-induced hypertensive rats *(207)*.

A number of studies have demonstrated that blockade of endothelin activity with either endothelin antibodies *(208–210)* or ET-receptor antagonists *(201,211–215)* can ameliorate the renal effects of cyclosporine A. Using a model of chronic cyclosporine A nephrotoxicity that elaborates the histological changes observed clinically *(216)*, Kon and colleagues demonstrated that blockade of endothelin receptors can abrogate the renal functional effects of cyclosporine treatment, but not the structural damage *(217,218)*. Interestingly, blockade of angiotensin II was able to block cyclosporine A-induced fibrosis, but not the functional deficits *(218)*. In addition to preventing cyclosporine A-induced reductions in renal function, ET-receptor blockade can prevent cyclosporine-induced hypertension in rats *(219)*. These data suggest that an endothelin receptor antagonist could be therapeutic in patients with cyclosporine A-induced renal complications and a preliminary report indicates that bosentan can attenuate cyclosporine A-induced reductions in renal plasma flow in healthy volunteers *(220)*.

The use of FK-506, another potent immunosuppressant agent, is beset with similar renal-complications as observed with cyclosporine A. Studies on renal endothelin production *(194,221)* and the use of an ET-receptor antagonist *(222)* provide evidence that endothelin also plays a role in FK-506-induced renal complications.

4.3. Radiocontrast Nephropathy

Administration of radiocontrast material can be associated with acute renal failure, especially in older patients and patients with pre-existing renal disease. Renal vasoconstriction and medullary hypoxia appear to be important in the development of radiocontrast-induced renal insufficiency, and there is growing evidence that endothelin may be an important mediator of these responses.

Radiocontrast agents have been shown to induce endothelin release, both in vitro and in vivo. Incubation of cultured endothelial cells with both high osmolar (iothalamate) and low osmolar (iohexol) radiocontrast agents resulted in enhanced endothelin release *(223)*. The increased endothelin release was not related to the increased osmolality because neither hypertonic saline nor hypertonic glucose had any effect *(223)*. In a study using porcine aortic endothelial cells, not only was ET-1 production stimulated by radiocontrast agents, but an increase in ET-1 mRNA expression was also observed *(224)*. When administered intravenously to rats, various radiocontrast agents increased plasma endothelin concentrations and this effect was once again not a consequence of changes in plasma osmolality because infusion of various hypertonic solutions failed to alter plasma endothelin release *(223)*. In a separate study in dogs, radiocontrast material was shown to increase both plasma and urinary endothelin *(225)*.

In addition to stimulating endothelin release, radiocontrast material appears to lead to increased production of vasodilator prostaglandins, such that in normal animals, it is difficult to observe ET-mediated radiocontrast-induced renal vasoconstriction without prior inhibition of prostaglandin production *(226–228)*. This observation is consistent with the clinical observation that radiocontrast nephrotoxicity is most commonly observed in older patients, diabetic patients, and patients with underlying renal disease, i.e., individuals who are likely to have reduced renal-vasodilator capacity.

In vitro studies using isolated perfused rat kidneys demonstrated that both high and low osmolar-radiocontrast agents caused a reduction in glomerular-filtration rate and renal-plasma flow in the presence of indomethacin and that this could be abolished by coadministration with the ET_A selective antagonist, BQ123 *(227)*. When given intravenously to rats, both contrast agents resulted in renal vasoconstriction that could also be inhibited by pretreatment with BQ123 *(227)*. Similar observations were made in rats using the ET-receptor antagonist, CP-170687 *(226)*, and in dogs using SB 209670 *(228)*. The ability of the mixed ET_A/ET_B receptor antagonist, SB 209670, to attenuate radiocontrast-induced nephropathy was confirmed in rats by investigators who also demonstrated that the ET_A selective antagonist, BMS-182874, was effective *(229)*.

Radiocontrast administration is an elective procedure and, as such, concomitant administration of an agent that reduces nephrotoxicity would be of value. Currently, the only maneuver thought to reduce radiocontrast nephrotoxicity is hydration of the patient, however, the development of ET-receptor antagonists may provide additional therapeutic opportunities.

4.4. Hepatorenal Syndrome

Hepatorenal syndrome is a relatively uncommon yet serious condition, which is a complication of advanced liver disease involving intense renal vasoconstriction, leading to oliguric acute renal failure. A number of different investigators have reported increased plasma-endothelin levels in patients with hepatorenal syndrome and/or liver cirrhosis *(8,188)*. It has been reported that plasma endothelin levels in patients with liver cirrhosis correlates with the presence of ascites, however, this is not a consistent finding *(8)*. Increased endothelin expression or tissue levels of endothelin have been observed in cirrhotic liver tissue from both humans *(230)* and rats *(231)*. Hepaticstellate cells appear to be the major site for endothelin synthesis *(230)* and these cells demonstrate increased endothelin-induced contractility in cirrhosis *(232)*. It is likely that the increased circulating endothelin levels observed in cirrhosis are hepatic in origin because the concentration of endothelin is increased in hepatic-venous blood from patients with cirrhosis *(233)*. In addition to changes in hepaticendothelin production, increased renal-tissue endothelin and renal ETreceptor binding has been observed in rats with cirrhosis *(231)*. One study evaluating the effect of an ET-receptor antagonist demonstrated that bosentan could reduce carbon tetrachloride-induced hepatotoxicity *(234)*. An interesting study in three patients with hepatorenal syndrome demonstrated that acute infusions of BQ123 resulted in increased inulin and PAH clearances, indicating improved glomerular-filtration rate and renal plasma flow *(235)*.

4.5. Chronic Renal Disease

Chronic renal disease is a progressive disease involving an inexorable decline in renal function until the development of endstage renal failure, at which time dialysis or renal transplantation is required to prevent death. Regardless of the initiating insult, the subsequent progression of this disease involves glomerulosclerosis. A number of different factors appear to contribute to glomerulosclerosis and these include glomerular hypertension, thrombosis, and hypertrophy, as well as mesangial cell matrix deposition and proliferation. Endothelin may be an important factor in the progression of renal disease because it has effects on many if not all of these processes.

Endothelin has a potent effect on the renal vasculature, including the ability to increase intraglomerular pressure *(236)*, stimulate mesangial-cell proliferation *(237)* as well as mediate angiotensin II-induced mitogenesis *(238)*. Endothelin can also increase the expression of various matrix proteins in mesangial cells *(239,240)* as well as increase fibronectin synthesis *(240)*. In addition, transforming growth-factor β, an important mediator of glomerular-matrix production, increases ETgene expression in mesangial cells *(241,242)*. Endothelin can affect the coagulation system, leading to decrements in renal function *(243)*.

A number of groups have demonstrated increased renal production of endothelin in models of renal failure, including 5/6 nephrectomy and streptozotocin-induced diabetes *(244–246)*. ET-gene expression is also increased in a number of models of renal failure, including 5/6 nephrectomy *(245,247)*, streptozotocin-induced diabetes *(248)*, aminonucleoside-induced nephrosis *(249)*, and hereditary polycystic kidney disease *(250)*. Furthermore, renal ET-gene expression correlates with disease progression in the rat remnant kidney model *(247)*. It is interesting that in transgenic rats expressing the human ET-2 gene, renal tissue ET-2 concentrations are significantly increased and gene expression was almost exclusively observed within the glomeruli *(251)*. Furthermore, glomerular transgene expression of ET-2 resulted in a glomerular injury and proteinuria *(251)*.

Numerous clinical studies have demonstrated increased urinary endothelin excretion or increased circulating endothelin in patients with chronic renal disease, including diabetic patients with microalbuminuria or vascular complications and patients with glomerulonephritis *(8,188)*. The effects of ET-receptor antagonists in models of chronic renal disease have suggested a therapeutic benefit of blocking endothelin activity. Benigni et al. *(252)* demonstrated that the selective ET_A receptor antagonist, FR-139317, could limit glomerular injury and reduce the proteinuria and hypertension in the rat remnant kidney model. These studies were provocative because this antagonist is rapidly metabolized and was given intraperitoneally once a day. This compound, given in a similar fashion, has also been shown to attenuate the proteinuria, hypertension, and accumulation of matrix proteins in a murine model of lupus nephritis *(253)*. More recently, a different ET-receptor antagonist, bosentan, has been shown to be therapeutic in rats with partial nephrectomy-induced progressive renal disease *(254,255)*, whereas A-127722 was ineffective *(256)*.

4.6. Renal Summary

Endothelin may be involved in a number of different renal diseases in addition to those described. These would include cisplatin-induced nephrotoxicity *(257)*, amphotericin B-induced nephrotoxicity *(258)*, sepsis-induced renal failure *(259)*, and ureteric obstruction-induced nephropathy *(260)*. The potential involvement of endothelin in all these different renal diseases suggests that under conditions where renal function or structure is compromised, endothelin production is increased. Clearly, there is a significant potential for ET-receptor antagonists in the treatment of renal disease of various etiologies.

5. Prostate Diseases

5.1. Benign Prostatic Hypertrophy

Benign prostatic hypertrophy (BPH) is a common problem in the aging male population and involves an increased resistance to bladder outflow. Two components are involved in this increased resistance; a static component involving hypertrophy of the prostate tissues and a dynamic component determined by the tone of the prostatic smooth muscle. Control of these two components is likely to be multifactorial, however, androgen-induced hypertrophy and sympathetic nervous system-induced prostate contraction appear to play important roles. Treatment with steroid 5-α-reductase inhibitors have shown limited efficacy, whereas it is known that α-adrenoceptor antagonists are beneficial for symptomatic relief in patients with BPH. Growing evidence suggests that an ET-receptor antagonist could provide additional therapeutic benefit in BPH because endothelin may be involved in these processes. Endothelin-like immunoreactivity is found in the prostate and is localized primarily to the secretory-glandular epithelium, suggesting that endothelin may be a paracrine factor mediating smooth-muscle contraction *(261)*. In addition, endothelin converting enzyme mRNA has been shown to be present in both stromal and glandular-prostate tissue *(262)* and endothelin receptors are present *(263)*. Quantitative autoradiography has demonstrated that ET_A receptors predominate in the stroma and ET_B receptors in glandular epithelium *(264)*, however, ET-induced contraction of prostate tissue can be mediated by both receptors *(265)*. Interestingly, endothelin binding is increased significantly in patients with BPH *(266)*, however, one report has indicated that despite an increased binding of endothelin, there is a reduced contractile activity in hyperplastic prostate tissue *(267)*. The demonstration of endothelin and endothelin receptors in prostate tissue and the ability of endothelin to induce contraction indicates a potential role for endothelin in BPH and a possible utility for ET-receptor antagonists.

5.2. Prostate Cancer

A number of different human cancer-cell lines have been shown to produce endothelin and/or express the ET-1 gene *(268–271)*. One human cancer cell line has been shown to contain a metalloproteinase, which can process endogenous big ET-1 to ET-1 *(272)*.

Plasma levels of endothelin immunoreactivity are increased in some patients with cancer. For example, plasma endothelin is markedly higher in patients with hepatocellular carcinoma than in patients with hepatic cirrhosis and the plasma endothelin levels reflected tumor size *(273)*. Endothelin receptors have also been located in cancer-cell lines *(274)* and cancerous tumors and these receptors are not present just in blood vessels. For example, autoradiographic localization of ET-binding sites in human colonic-cancer tissues demonstrated endothelin receptors over tumor vessels as well as stromal tissue surrounding cancer-cell nests *(275)*.

The most intriguing reports on endothelin and cancer involve advanced prostate cancer and metastatic adenocarcinoma of the prostate. It is well established that the prostate produces endothelin and contains numerous ET-binding sites (*see* Section 5.1.). Exogenous endothelin, however, induces prostate cancer-cell proliferation directly as well as enhancing the mitogenic effects of a number of different growth factors in vitro *(276)*. In addition to being a mitogenic factor for a variety of cell types, endothelin can also stimulate osteoblast proliferation *(277)*. It is interesting, therefore, that plasma immunoreactive endothelin concentrations are significantly elevated in men with metastatic prostate cancer and endothelin can increase alkaline phosphatase activity, suggesting that atopic ET-1 may be a mediator of the osteoblastic response of bone to metastatic prostate cancer *(278)*.

Much of the data regarding endothelin and cancer is circumstantial and, to date, there have been no reports of the use of an ET-receptor antagonist in an animal model or in humans with prostate cancer. The data implicating endothelin in prostate and other cancers, however, are intriguing and clearly warrant further evaluation.

6. Other Diseases

Endothelin has been implicated in a number of diseases other than those previously described. Endothelin may play a role in diabetes because both insulin and glucose can modulate endothelin synthesis and receptor expression *(279)* and plasma or urinary endothelin has been shown to be increased in patients *(280)* and in animals with diabetes *(281)*. Endothelin-induced vasoconstriction may contribute to some of the vascular complications associated with diabetes as described earlier in this chapter. One report, however, suggests that there is an impaired vasoconstriction to endothelin in patients with noninsulin-dependent diabetes mellitus *(282)*.

Endothelin's receptors are also present in the eye and retina and there have been suggestions that endothelin may be involved in both diabetic retinopathy *(283)* as well as glaucoma *(284)*.

Circulating endothelin levels are also increased in patients with systemic sclerosis *(8)* and endothelin production from fibroblasts taken from patients with systemic sclerosis is elevated *(285)*. It is possible therefore that endothelin may also be involved in this disease. Measurement of circulating endothelin and tissue endothelin mRNA levels in patients as well as animals have indicated that endothelin may be involved in organ rejection *(286)*.

Endothelin has been implicated in gastric disease because endothelin can be ulcerogenic in rats *(287)* and investigators have reported ET-1 expression and increased circulating endothelin in patients with Crohn's disease and ulcerative colitis *(288,289)*. It is interesting that ET_B receptors may be important in the development of the gastrointestinal tract because targeted disruption of the ET_B receptor *(290)* or the ET_B receptor ligand, ET-3 *(291)*, as well as natural mutations of the ET_B receptor (Piebald-Lethal) *(290)* are associated with aganglionic megacolon. Yanagisawa and his colleagues *(290,291)* postulated that defects in human ET-B receptor gene may cause a hereditary form of Hirschsprung's disease, because this disease is associated with colonic aganglionosis and has been mapped to chromosome 13, the chromosome on which the ET-B receptor gene is located. Subsequent studies in patients with Hirschsprung's disease support this suggestion *(292,293)*.

Endothelin may also have been involved in skin disease. Endothelin stimulates keratinocyte proliferation *(294,295)* and plasma-endothelin levels are elevated in psoriatics *(296)*. In addition, endothelin production and expression is increased in seborrheic keratosis *(297)*. Finally, it is clear that endothelin is involved in embryonic development beyond the intestines, because mice deficient in ET-1 have morphological abnormalities of the pharyngeal-arch-derived craniofacial tissues and organs *(298)*.

7. Summary

The list of potential of diseases in which endothelin may be involved continues to grow. Some of the data indicating the involvement of endothelin is controversial, however, there does appear to be some consistency in the data supporting the use of ET-receptor antagonists in vascular, cardiac, pulmonary, and renal diseases. In the next few years, two important questions are likely to be answered. One is whether endothelin is indeed important in these diseases, and the second is whether selective ET_A receptor or mixed ET_A/ET_B receptor antagonists will have different effects. Because of significant species differences in the involvement of ET_A and ET_B receptors in mediating the physiological and pathophysiological effects of endothelin, preclinical studies have not provided a clear insight into whether one or both receptors need to be blocked. Because a number of different organs are being targeted with ET-receptor antagonists, it is possible, indeed even likely, that different diseases will require receptor antagonists with different profiles.

Acknowledgments

The authors are grateful to Sue Tirri for expert secretarial assistance.

References

1. Yanagisawa, M., Kurihara, H., Kimura, S., Tomobe, Y., Kobayashi, M., Mitsui, Y., Yazaki, Y., Goto, K., and Masaki, T. (1988) A novel potent vasoconstrictor peptide produced by vascular endothelial cells. *Nature (Lond)* **332:**411–415.
2. Vierhapper, H., Wagner, O., Nowotny, P., and Waldhausl, W. (1990) Effect of endothelin-1 in man. *Circulation* **81:**1415–1418.
3. Sorensen, S. S., Madsen, J. K., and Pedersen, E. B. (1994) Systemic and renal effect of intravenous infusion of endothelin-1 in healthy human volunteers. *Am. J. Physiol.* **266:**F411–F418.
4. Rabelink, T. J., Kaasiager, K. A. H., Boer, P., Stroes, E. G., Braam, B., and Koomans, H. A. (1994) Effects of endothelin-1 on renal function in humans: implications for physiology and pathophysiology. *Kidney Int.* **46:**376–381.
5. Yokokawa, K., Tahara, H., Kohno, M., Murakawa, K., Yasunari, K., Nakagawa, K., Hamada, T., Otani, S., Yanagisawa, M., and Takeda, T. (1991) Hypertension associated with endothelin-secreting malignant hemangioendothelioma. *Ann. Intern. Med.* **114:**213–215.
6. Wilkes, F. C., Jr., Alberola, A., Mizelle, H. L., Opgenorth, T. J., and Granger, J. P. (1993) Chronic pathophysiological circulating endothelin levels produce hypertension in conscious dogs. *J. Cardiovasc. Pharmacol.* **22(Suppl. 8):**S325–S327.
7. Niranjan, V., Telemaque, S., Dewit, D., Gerard, R. D., and Yanagisawa, M. (1996) Systemic hypertension induced by hepatic overexpression of human prepro-endothelin-1 in rats. *J. Clin. Invest.* **98:**2364–2372.
8. Jorkasky, D. K., Hay, D. W. P. and Freed, M. I. (1995) The role of endothelin in human disease: implications and potential therapeutic

intervention, in *Endothelin Receptors: From the Gene to the Human* (Ruffolo, R. R., Jr., ed.), CRC, Boca Raton, FL, pp. 215–271.

9. Letizia, C., Cerci, S., De Ciocchis, A., D'Ambrosio, C., Scuro, L., and Scavo, D. (1995) Plasma endothelin-1 levels in normotensive and borderline hypertensive subjects during a standard cold pressor test. *J. Hum. Hypertens.* **9:**903–907.

10. Ergul, S., Parish, D. C., Puett, D., and Ergul, A. (1996) Racial differences in plasma endothelin-1 concentrations in individuals with essential hypertension. *Hypertension* **28:**652–655.

11. Ohlstein, E. H., Douglas, S. A., Brooks, D. P., Hay, D. W. P., Feuerstein, G. Z., and Ruffolo, R. R., Jr. (1995) Functions mediated by peripheral endothelin receptors, in *Endothelin Receptors: From the Gene to the Human* (Ruffolo, R. R., Jr., ed.), CRC, Boca Raton, FL, pp. 109–185.

12. Larivière, R., Thibault, G., and Schiffrin, E. (1993) Increase endothelin-1 content in blood vessels of deoxycorticosterone acetate-salt hypertension but not in spontaneously hypertensive rats. *Hypertension* **21:**294–300.

13. Wong, M. and Jeng, A. Y. (1989) Parallel increases in cardiac endothelin and blood pressure of spontaneously hypertensive rats. *Pharmacologist* **31:**374P.

14. Fujita, K., Matsumura, Y., Miyazaki, Y., Hashimoto, N., Takaoka, M., and Morimoto, S. (1996) ET_A receptor-mediated role of endothelin in the kidney of DOCA-salt hypertensive rats. *Life Sci.* **58:**PL1–PL7.

15. Takada, K., Matsumura, Y., Dohmen, S., Mitsutomi, N., Takaoka, M., and Morimoto, S. (1996) Endothelin-1 secretion from cultured vascular endothelial cells of DOCA-salt hypertensive rats. *Life Sci.* **59:**PL111–PL116.

16. Schiffrin, E. L., Lariviere, R., and Touyz, R. M. (1995) ETA and ETB receptors on vascular smooth muscle cells from mesenteric vessels of spontaneously hypertensive rats. *Clin. Exp. Pharmacol. Physiol.* **22(Suppl. 1),** S193,S194.

17. Hocher, B., Rohmeiss, P., Zart, R., Diekmann, F., Vogt, V., Metz, D., Fakhury, M., Gretz, N., Bauer, C., Koppenhagen, K., Neumayer, H. H., and Distler, A. (1996) Function and expression of endothelin receptor subtypes in the kidneys of spontaneously hypertensive rats. *Cardiovasc. Res.* **31:**499–510.

18. Hiraoka, J., Arai, H., Yoshimasa, T., Takaya, K., Miyamoto, Y., Yamashita, J., Suga, S., Ogawa, Y., Shirakami, G., and Itoh, H. (1995) Augmented expression of the endothelin-A receptor gene in cultured mesangial cells from stroke-prone spontaneously hypertensive rats. *Clin. Exp. Pharmacol. Physiol.* **22(Suppl. 1):**S191–S192.

19. Gellai, M., DeWolf, R., Pullen, M., and Nambi, P. (1994) Distribution and functional role of renal ET receptor subtypes in normotensive and hypertensive rats. *Kidney Int.* **46:**1287–1294.

20. Gu, X.-H., Casley, D. J., Cincotta, M., and Nayler, W. G. (1990) ^{125}I-Endothelin-1 binding to brain and cardiac membranes from normotensive and spontaneously hypertensive rats. *Eur. J. Pharmacol.* **177:**205–209.

21. Evangelista, S., Maggi, C.A., and Castellucci, A. (1992) Effect of endothelin (ET)-1, ET-3 and ET-(16–21) on the isolated and perfused rat

kidney from normotensive and spontaneously hypertensive rats. *Jpn. J. Pharmacol.* **59:**239–241.

22. Goligorsky, M. S., Iijima, K., Morgan, M., Yanagisawa, M., Masaki, T., Lin, L., Nasjletti, A., Kaskel, F., Frazer, M., and Badr, K. F. (1991) Role of endothelin in the development of Dahl hypertension. *J. Cardiovasc. Pharmacol.* **17(Suppl. 7):**S484–S491.

23. Ohno, A., Naruse, M., Kato, S., Hosaka, M., Karuse, K., and Demura, H. (1992) Endothelin-specific antibodies decrease blood pressure and increase glomerular filtration rate and renal plasma flow in spontaneously hypertensive rats. *J. Hypertens.* **10:**781–785.

24. Kato, T., Kassab, S., Wilkins, F. C., Jr., Kirchner, K. A., Keiser, J., and Granger, J. P. (1995) Endothelin antagonists improve renal function in spontaneously hypertensive rats. *Hypertension* **25(part 2):**883–887.

25. McMahon, E. G., Palomo, M. A., and Moore, W. M. (1991) Phosphoramidon blocks the pressor activity of big endothelin (1–39) and lowers blood pressure in spontaneously hypertensive rats. *J. Cardiovasc. Pharmacol.* **17(Suppl. 7):**S29–S33.

26. Sogabe, K., Nirei, H., Shoubo, M., Nomoto, A., Ao, S., Notsu, Y., and Ono, T. (1992) Pharmacological profile of FR139317, a novel, potent endothelin ET_A receptor antagonist. *J. Pharmacol. Exp. Ther.* **264:**1040–1044.

27. Nishikibe, M., Tsuchida, S., Okada, M., Fukuroda, R., Shimamoto, K., and Yano, M. (1993) Antihypertensive effect of a newly synthesized endothelin antagonist, BQ-123, in a genetic hypertensive model. *Life Sci.* **52:**717–724.

28. Ohlstein, E. H., Douglas, S. A., Ezekiel, M., and Gellai, M. (1993) Antihypertensive effects of the endothelin antagonist BQ-123 in conscious spontaneously hypertensive rats. *J. Cardiovasc. Pharmacol.* **22(Suppl. 8):**S321–S324.

29. Ohlstein, E. H., Nambi, P., Douglas, S. A., Edwards, R. M., Gellai, M., Lago, A., Leber, J. D., Cousins, R. D., Gao, A., Frazee, J. S., Peishoff, C. E., Bean, J. W., Eggleston, D. S., Elshourbagy, N. A., Kumar, C., Lee, J. A., Brooks, D. P., Ruffolo, R. R., Jr., Feuerstein, G. Z., Weinstock, J., Gleason, J. G., and Elliott, J. D. (1994) SB 209670, rationally designed potent nonpeptide endothelin receptor antagonist. *Proc. Natl. Acad. Sci. USA* **9:**8052–8056.

30. Douglas, S. A., Gellai, M., Ezekiel, M., and Ohlstein, E. H. (1994) BQ123, a selective endothelin (ET_A) receptor antagonist, lowers blood pressure in different models of hypertension. *J. Hypertens.* **12:**561–567.

31. Verma, S., Bhanot, S. and McNeill, J. H. (1995) Effect of chronic endothelin blockade in hyperinsulinemic hypertensive rats. *Am. J. Physiol.* **269:**H2017–H2021.

32. Stasch, J. P., Hirth-Dietrich, C., Frobel, K., and Wegner, M. (1995) Prolonged endothelin blockade reduces hypertension and cardiac hypertrophy in SHR-SP. *J. Cardiovasc. Pharmacol.* **26(Suppl. 3):**S436–S438.

33. Schiffrin, E. L., Sventek, P., Li, J.-S., Turgeon, A., and Reudelhuber, T. (1995) Antihypertensive effect of an endothelin receptor antagonist in DOCA-salt spontaneously hypertensive rats. *Br. J. Pharmacol.* **115:**1377–1381.

34. Bird, J. E., Moreland, S., Waldron, T. L., and Powell, J. R. (1995) Anti-hypertensive effects of a novel endothelin-A receptor antagonist in rats. *Hypertension* **25**:1191–1195.

35. Li, J.-S. and Schiffrin, E. L. (1995) Effect of chronic treatment of adult spontaneously hypertensive rats with an endothelin receptor antagonist. *Hypertension* **25(part 1)**:495–500.

36. Clozel, M. and Breu, V. (1996) The role of ET(B) receptors in normo-tensive and hypertensive rats as revealed by the non-peptide selective ET(B) receptor antagonist Ro 46-8443. *FEBS Lett.* **383**:42–45.

37. Donckier, J., Stoleru, L., Hayashida, W., Van Mechelen, H., Selvais, P., Galanti, L., Clozel, J.-P., Ketelslegers, J.-M., and Pouleur, H. (1995) Role of endogenous endothelin-1 in experimental renal hypertension in dogs. *Circulation* **92**:106–113.

38. Kiowski, W., Sutsch, G., Hunziker, P., Muller, P., Kim, J., Oechslin, E., Schmitt, R., Jones, R., and Bertel, O. (1995) Evidence for endothelin-1-mediated vasoconstriction in severe chronic heart failure. *Lancet* **346**:732–736.

39. Haynes, W. G. and Webb, D. J. (1994) Contribution of endogenous gen-eration of endothelin-1 to basal vascular tone. *Lancet* **344**:852–854.

40. Haynes, W. G., Ferro, C. J., O'Kane, K. P., Somerville, D., Lomax, C. C., and Webb, D. J. (1996) Systemic endothelin receptor blockade decreases peripheral vascular resistance and blood pressure in humans. *Circulation* **93**:1860–1870.

41. Freed, M. I., Thompson, K. A., Wilson, D. E., Ohlstein, E. H., Dennis, M., and Jorkasky, D. K. (1996) Effects of SB 217242, a non-selective endothelin (ET-A and ET-B receptor antagonist, in healthy humans. *J. Am. Soc. Nephrol.* **7,** 1561.

42. Wei, C. M., Lerman, A., Rodeheffer, R. J., McGregor, C. G. A., Brandt, R. R., Wright, S., Kao, P. C., Edwards, W. D., Burnett, J. C., and Heublein, D. M. (1994) Endothelin in human congestive heart failure. *Circulation* **89**:1580–1586.

43. Pacher, R., Stanek, B., Hulsmann, M., Koller-Strametz, J., Berger, R., Schuller, M., Hartter, E., Ogris, E., Frey, B., Heinz, G., and Maurer, G. (1996) Prognostic impact of big endothelin-1 plasma concentrations com-pared with invasive hemodynamic evaluation in severe heart failure. *J. Am. Coll. Cardiol.* **27**:633–641.

44. Omland, T., Lie, R. T., Aakvaag, A., Aarsland, T., and Dickstein, K. (1994) Plasma endothelin determinations as a prognostic indication of one year mortality after acute myocardial infarction. *Circulation* **89**:1573–1579.

45. Krum, H. and Itescu, S. (1994) Spontaneous endothelin production by circulating mononuclear cells from patients with chronic heart fail-ure but not from normal subjects. *Clin. Exp. Pharmacol. Physiol.* **21**:311–313.

46. Cavero, P. G., Miller, W. L., Heublein, D. M., Margulies, K. B., and Burnett, J. C. (1990) Endothelin in experimental congestive heart failure in the anesthetized dog. *Am. J. Physiol.* **259**:F312–F317.

47. Yorikane, R., Sakai, S., Miyauchi, T., Sakurai, T., Sugishita, Y., and Goto, K. (1993) Increased production of endothelin-1 in the hypertrophied rat heart due to pressure overload. *FEBS Lett.* **332:**31–34.

48. Miyauchi, T., Sakai, S., Ihara, M., Kasuya, Y., Yamaguchi, I., Goto, K., and Sugishita, Y. (1995) Increased endothelin-1 binding sites in the cardiac membranes in rats with chronic heart failure. *J. Cardiovasc. Pharmacol.* **26(Suppl. 3):**S448–S451.

49. Yamazaki, T., Komuro, I., Kudoh, S., Zou, Y., Shiojima, I., Hiroi, Y., Mizuno, T., Maemura, K., Kurihara, H., Aikawa, R., Takano, H., and Yazaki, Y. (1996) Endothelin-1 is involved in mechanical stress-induced cardiomyocyte hypertrophy. *J. Biol. Chem.* **271:**3221–3228.

50. Ito, H., Hiroe, M., Hirata, Y., Fujisaki, H., Adachi, S., Akimoto, H., Ohta, Y., and Marumo, F. (1994) Endothelin ET_A receptor antagonist blocks cardiac hypertrophy provoked by hemodynamic overload. *Circulation* **89:**2198–2203.

51. Teerlink, J. R., Loffler, B.-M., Hess, P., Maire, J.-P., Clozel, M., and Clozel, J.-P. (1994) Role of endothelin in the maintenance of blood pressure in conscious rats with chronic heart failure. Acute effects of the endothelin receptor antagonist Ro 47-0203 (bosentan). *Circulation* **90:**2510–2518.

52. Sakai, S., Miyauchi, T., Kobayashi, M., Yamaguchi, I., Goto, K., and Sugishita, Y. (1996) Inhibition of myocardial endothelin pathway improves long-term survival in heart failure. *Nature* **384:**353–355.

53. Shimoyama, H., Sabbah, H. N., Borzak, S., Tanimura, M., Shevlyagin, S., Scicli, G., and Goldstein, S. (1996) Short-term hemodynamic effects of endothelin receptor blockade in dogs with chronic heart failure. *Circulation* **94:**779–784.

54. Tohmo, H., Karanko, M., Korpilahti, K., Scheinin, M., Viinamaki, O., and Neuvonen, P. (1994) Enalaprilat in acute intractable heart failure after myocardial infarction: a prospective, consecutive sample, before and after. *Crit. Care Med.* **22:**965–973.

55. Davidson, N. C., Coutie, W. J., Webb, D. J., and Struthers, A. D. (1996) Hormonal and renal differences between low dose and high dose angiotensin converting enzyme inhibitor treatment in patients with chronic heart failure. *Heart* **75:**576–581.

56. Grenier, O., Pousset, F., Isnard, R., Kalotka, H., Carayon, A., Maistre, G., Lechat, P., Guerot, C., Thomas, D., and Komajda, M. (1996) Captopril does not acutely modulate plasma endothelin-1 concentration in human congestive heart failure. *Cardiovasc. Drugs Ther.* **10:**561–565.

57. Krum, H., Gu, A., Wilshire-Clement, M., Sackner-Bernstein, J., Goldsmith, R., Medina, N., Yushak, M., Miller, M., and Packer, M. (1996) Changes in plasma endothelin-1 levels reflect clinical response to beta-blockade in chronic heart failure. *Am. Heart J.* **131:**337–341.

58. Martin-Nizard, F., Houssaini, H. S., Lestavel-Delattre, S., Duriez, P., and Fruchart, J.-C. (1991) Modified low density lipoproteins activate human macrophages to secrete immunoreactive endothelin. *FEBS Lett.* **293:**127–130.

59. Salomone, O. A., Elliott, P. M., Calvino, R., Holt, D., and Kaski, J. C. (1996) Plasma immunoreactive endothelin concentration correlates with severity of coronary artery disease in patients with stable angina pectoris and normal ventricular function. *J. Am. Coll. Cardiol.* **28:**14–19.

60. Ihling, C., Gobel, H. R., Lippoldt, A., Wessels, S., Paul, M., Schaefer, H. E., and Zeiher, A. M. (1996) Endothelin-1-like immunoreactivity in human atherosclerotic coronary tissue: a detailed analysis of the cellular distribution of endothelin-1. *J. Pathol.* **179:**303–308.

61. Mangiafico, R. A., Malatino, L. S., Santonocito, M., Spada, R. S., Polizzi, G., and Tamburino, G. (1996) Raised plasma endothelin-1 concentrations in patients with primary hypercholesterolemia without evidence of atherosclerosis. *Int. Angiol.* **15:**240–244.

62. Lerman, A., Webster, M. W., Chesebro, J. H., Edwards, W. D., Wei, C. M., Fuster, V., and Burnett, J. C., Jr. (1993) Circulating and tissue endothelin immunoreactivity in hypercholesterolemic pigs. *Circulation* **88:**2923–2928.

63. Azuma, H., Hamasaki, H., Niimi, Y., Terada, T., and Matsubara, O. (1994) Role of endothelin-1 in neointima formation after endothelial removal in rabbit carotid arteries. *Am. J. Physiol.* **267:**H2259–H2267.

64. Wang, X., Douglas, S. A., and Ohlstein, E. H. (1996) The use of quantitative RT-PCR to demonstrate the increased expression of endothelin-related mRNAs following angioplasty-induced neointima formation in the rat. *Circ. Res.* **78:**322–328.

65. Lopez, J. A. G., Armstrong, M. L., Piegors, D. J., and Heistad, D. D. (1990) Vascular responses to endothelin-1 in atherosclerotic primates. *Artheriosclerosis* **10:**1113.

66. Prat, L., Carrió, I., Roca, M., Riambau, V., Berné, L., Estorch, M., Ferrer, I., and Garcia, C. (1993) Polyclonal ^{111}In-IgG, ^{125}I-LDL and ^{125}I-endothelin-1 accumulation in experimental arterial wall injury. *Eur. J. Nucl. Med.* **20:**1141–1145.

67. Dashwood, M., Barker, S. G. E., Muddle, J. R., Yacoub, M. H., and Martin, J. F. (1993) [^{125}I]-Endothelin-1 binding to vasa vasorum and regions of neovascularization in human and porcine blood vessels: a possible role for endothelin in intimal hyperplasia and atherosclerosis. *J. Cardiovasc. Pharmacol.* **22(Suppl. 8):**S343–S347.

68. Dashwood, M. R., Allen, S. P., Luu, T. N., and Muddle, J. R. (1994) The effect of the ET_A receptor antagonist, FR 139317, on [^{125}I]-ET-1 binding to the atherosclerotic human coronary artery. *Br. J. Pharmacol.* **112:**386–389.

69. Kurata, C., Callahan, R. J., Molea, N., Wilkinson, R., Fischman, A. J., and Strauss, H. W. (1995) Localization of [^{125}I] endothelin-1 in injured aorta of rabbits. *Eur. J. Pharmacol.* **293:**109–114.

70. Bacon, C. R., Cary, N. R., and Davenport, A. P. (1995) Distribution of endothelin receptors in atherosclerotic human coronary arteries. *J. Cardiovasc. Pharmacol.* **26(Suppl. 3):**S439–S441.

71. Douglas, S. A. and Ohlstein, E. H. (1993) Endothelin-1 promotes neointima formation after balloon angioplasty in the rat. *J. Cardiovasc. Pharmacol.* **22(Suppl. 8):**S371–S373.

72. Trachtenberg, J. D., Sun, S., Choi, E. T., Callow, A. D., and Ryan, U. S. (1993) Effect of endothelin-1 infusion on the development of intimal hyperplasia after balloon catheter injury. *J. Cardiovasc. Pharmacol.* **22 (Suppl. 8):**S355–359.

73. Douglas, S. A., Vickery-Clark, L. M., Storer, B. L., Hart, T., Louden, C., Elliott, J. D., and Ohlstein, E. H. (1994) A role for endogenous endothelin-1 in neointima formation following rat carotid artery balloon angioplasty: antiproliferative effects of the non-peptide endothelin receptor antagonist SB 209670. *Circ. Res.* **75:**190–197.

74. Ferrer, P., Valentine, M., Jenkins-West, T., Weber, H., Goller, N. L., Durham, S. K., Molloy, C. J., and Moreland, S. (1995) Orally active endothelin receptor antagonist BMS-182874 suppresses neointimal development in balloon-injured rat carotid arteries. *J. Cardiovasc. Pharmacol.* **26:**908–915.

75. Kowala, M. C., Rose, P. M., Stein, P. D., Goller, N., Recce, R., Beyer, S., Valentine, M., Barton, D., and Durham, S. K. (1995) Selective blockade of the endothelin subtype A receptor decreases early atherosclerosis in hamsters fed cholesterol. *Am. J. Pathol.* **146:**819–826.

76. Larkin, S. W., Clarke, J. G., Keogh, B. E., Araujo, L., Rhodes, C., Davies, G. J., Taylor, K. M., and Maseri, A. (1989) Intracoronary endothelin induces myocardial ischemia by small vessel constriction in the dog. *Am. J. Cardiol.* **64:**956–958.

77. Lee, S.-Y., Lee, C. Y., Chen, Y. M., and Kochva, E. (1986) Coronary vasospasm as the primary cause of death due to the venom of the burrowing asp, Atractaspis engaddensis. *Toxicon* **24:**285–291.

78. Setsuta, K., Seino, Y., Tomita, Y., Nejima, J., Takano, T., and Hayakawa, H. (1995) Origin and pathophysiological role of increased plasma endothelin-1 in patients with acute myocardial infarction. *Angiology* **46:**557–565.

79. Tonnessen, T., Giaid, A., Saleh, D., Naess, P. A., Yanagisawa, M., and Cristensen, G. (1995) Increased *in vivo* expression and production of endothelin-1 by porcine cardiomyocytes subjected to ischemia. *Circ. Res.* **76:**767–772.

80. Kyriakides, Z. S., Markianos, M., Iliodromitis, E. K., and Kremastinos, D. T. (1995) Vein plasma endothelin-1 and cyclic GMP increase during coronary angioplasty is related to myocardial ischaemia. *Eur. Heart J.* **16:**894–898.

81. Franco-Cereceda, A., Grip, L. G., Moor, E., Velander, M., Liska, J., and Lundberg, J. M. (1995) Influence of percutaneous transluminal coronary angioplasty on cardiac release of endothelin, neuropeptide Y and noradrenaline. *Int. J. Cardiol.* **48:**231–233.

82. Nelson, R. A., Burke, S. E., and Opgenorth, T. (1994) Endothelin receptor antagonist fr 139317 reduces infarct size in a rabbit coronary artery occlusion model. *FASEB J.* **8:**A854.

83. Lee, J. Y., Warner, R. B., Adler, A. L., and Opgenorth, T. J. (1994) The ET_A receptor antagonist FR 139317 reduces myocardial infarction induced by coronary artery occlusion and reperfusion in the rat. *FASEB J.* **8:**A854.

84. Wang, Q. D., Li, X. S., and Pernow, J. (1995) The nonpeptide endothelin receptor antagonist bosentan enhances myocardial recovery and endothelial function during reperfusion of the ischemic rat heart. *J. Cardiovasc. Pharmacol.* **26(Suppl. 3):**S445–S447.

85. McMurdo, L., Thiemermann, C., and Vane, J. R. (1994) The effects of the endothelin ET_A receptor antagonist, FR 139317, on infarct size in a rabbit model of acute myocardial ischemia and reperfusion. *Br. J. Pharmacol.* **112:**75–80.

86. Vitola, J. V., Forman, M. B., Holsinger, J. P., Kawana, M., Atkinson, J. B., Quertermous, T., Jackson, E. K., and Murray, J. J. (1996) Role of endothelin in a rabbit model of acute myocardial infarction—effects of receptor antagonists. *J. Cardiovasc. Pharmacol.* **28:**774–783.

87. Erikson, J. M. and Velasco, C. E. (1996) Endothelin-1 and myocardial preconditioning. *Am. Heart J.* **132:**84–90.

88. Mertz, T. E., McClanahan, T. B., Flynn, M. A., Juneau, P., Reynolds, E. E., Hallak, H., Bradford, L., and Gallagher, K. P. (1996) Endothelin$_A$ receptor antagonism by PD 156707 does not reduce infarct size after coronary artery occlusion/reperfusion in pigs. *J. Pharmacol. Exp. Ther.* **278:**42–49.

89. Wang, Q. D., Li, X. S., Lundberg, J. M., and Pernow, J. (1995) Protective effects of non-peptide endothelin receptor antagonist bosentan on myocardial ischaemic and reperfusion injury in the pig. *Cardiovasc. Res.* **29:**805–812.

90. Grover, G. J., Dzwonczyk, S., and Parham, C. S. (1993) The endothelin-1 receptor antagonist BQ123 reduces infarct size in a canine model of coronary occlusion and reperfusion. *Cardiovasc. Res.* **27:**1613–1618.

91. Kojima, M., Kusumoto, K., Fujiwara, S., Watanabe, T., and Fujino, M. (1995) Role of endogenous endothelin in the extension of myocardial infarct size studies with the endothelin receptor antagonist, TAK-044. *J. Cardiovasc. Pharmacol.* **26(Suppl. 3),** S365–S368.

92. Watanabe, T., Awane, Y., Ikeda, S., Fujiwara, S., Kubo, K., Kikuchi, T., Kusumoto, K., Wakimasu, M., and Fujino, M. (1995) Pharmacology of a non-selective ET_A and ET_B receptor antagonist TAK-044, and the inhibition of myocardial infarct size in rats. *Br. J. Pharmacol.* **114:**949–954.

93. Illing, B., Horn, M., Han, H., Hahn, S., Bureik, P., Ertl, G., and Neubauer, S. (1996) Protective effect of the specific endothelin-1 antagonist BQ610 on mechanical function and energy metabolism during ischemia/reperfusion injury in isolated perfused rat hearts. *J. Cardiovasc. Pharmacol.* **27:**487–494.

94. Garjani, A., Wainwright, C.L., Zeitlin, I. J., Wilson, C., and Slee, S.-J. (1995) Effects of endothelin-1 and the ET_A-receptor antagonist, BQ123, on ischemia arrhythmias in anesthetized rats. *J. Cardiovasc. Pharmacol.* **25:**634–642.

95. Omland, T., Bonarjee, V.V., Lie, R.T., and Caidahl, K. (1995) Neurohumoral measurements as indicators of long-term prognosis after acute myocardial infarction. *Am. J. Cardiol.* **76:**230–235.

96. Asano, T., Ikegaki, I., Suzuki, Y., Satoh, S.-I., and Shibuya, M. (1989) Endothelin and the production of cerebral vasospasm in dogs. *Biochem. Biophys. Res. Commun.* **159:**1345–1351.

97. Ohlstein, E. H. and Storer, B. L. (1992) Oxyhemoglobin stimulated endothelin production in cultured endothelial cells. *J. Neurosurg.* **77**:274–278.

98. Masaoka, H., Suzuki, R., Hirata, Y., Emori, T., Marumo, F., and Hirakawa, K. (1989) Raised plasma endothelin in aneurysmal subarachnoid haemorrhage. *Lancet* **2**:1402.

99. Wang, X., Zhu, C., Zhang, G., and Lu, Y. (1995) Changes of endothelin during cerebral vasospasm after experimental subarachnoid hemorrhage. *Chin. Med. J. Engl.* **108**:586–590.

100. Seifert, V., Loffler, B. M., Zimmermann, M., Roux, S., and Stolke, D. (1995) Endothelin concentrations in patients with aneurysmal subarachnoid hemorrhage. Correlation with cerebral vasospasm, delayed ischemic neurological deficits, and volume of hematoma. *J. Neurosurg.* **82**:55–62.

101. Papadopoulos, S. M., Gilbert, L. L., Webb, R. C., and D'Amato, C. J. (1990) Characterization of contractile responses to endothelin in human cerebral arteries: implications for cerebral vasospasm. *Neurosurgery* **26**:810–815.

102. Zimmerman, M., Seifert, V., Loffler, B. M., Stolke, D., and Stenzel, W. (1996) Prevention of cerebral vasospasm after experimental subarachnoid hemorrhage by RO 47-0203, a newly developed orally active endothelin receptor antagonist. *Neurosurgery* **38**:115–120.

103. Itoh, S., Sasaki, T., Asai, A., and Kuchino, Y. (1994) Prevention of delayed vasospasm by an endothelin ET_A receptor antagonist BQ123: change of ET_A receptor mRNA expression in a canine subarachnoid hemorrhage model. *J. Neurosurg.* **81**:759–764.

104. Matsumura, Y., Ikegawa, R., Suzuki, Y., Takaoka, M., Uchida, T., Kido, H., Shinyama, H., Hayashi, K., Watanabe, M., and Morimoto, S. (1991) Phosphoramidon prevents cerebral vasospasm following subarachnoid hemorrhage in dogs: the relationship to endothelin-1 levels in the cerebrospinal fluid. *Life Sci.* **49**:841–848.

105. Itoh, S., Sasaki, T., Ide, K., Ishikawa, K., Nishikibe, M., and Yano, M. (1993) A novel endothelin ET_A receptor antagonist, BQ-485, and its preventive effect on experimental vasospasm in dogs. *Biochem. Biophys. Res. Commun.* **195**:969–975.

106. Clozel, M. and Watanabe, H. (1994) BQ-123, a peptidic endothelin ET_A receptor antagonist, prevents the early cerebral vasospasm following subarachnoid hemorrhage after intracisternal but not intravenous injection. *Life Sci.* **52**:825–834.

107. Foley, P. L., Caner, H. H., Kassell, N. F., and Lee, K. S. (1994) Reversal of subarachnoid hemorrhage-induced vasoconstriction with an endothelin receptor antagonist. *Neurosurgery* **34**:108–113.

108. Hino, A., Weir, B. K. A., Macdonald, R. L., Thisted, R. A., Kim, C.-J., and Johns, L. M. (1995) Prospective, randomized, double-blind trial of BQ123 and bosentan for prevention of vasospasm following subarachnoid hemorrhage in monkeys. *J. Neurosurg.* **83**:503–509.

109. Cosentino, F., Mcmahon, E. G., Carter, J. S., and Katusic, Z. S. (1993) Effect of endothelin$_A$-receptor antagonist BQ-123 and phosphoramidon on cerebral vasospasm. *J. Cardiovasc. Pharmacol.* **22(Suppl. 8)**:S332–S335.

110. Caner, H. H., Kwan, A. L., Arthur, A., Jeng, A. Y., Lappe, R. W., Kassell, N. F., and Lee, K. S. (1996) Systemic administration of an inhibitor of endothelin converting enzyme for attenuation of cerebral vasospasm following experimental subarachnoid hemorrhage. *J. Neurosurg.* **85:**917–922.

111. Clozel, M., Breu, V., Gray, G. A., and Löffler, B. M. (1993) *In vivo* pharmacology of Ro 46-2005, the first synthetic nonpeptide endothelin receptor antagonist: implications for endothelin physiology. *J. Cardiovasc. Pharmacol.* **22(Suppl. 8):**S377–S379.

112. Nirei, H., Hamada, K., Shoubo, M., Sogabe, K., Notsu, Y., and Ono, T. (1993) An endothelin ET$_A$ receptor antagonist, FR139317, ameliorates cerebral vasospasm in dogs. *Life Sci.* **52:**1869–1874.

113. Roux, S., Loffler, B. M., Gray, G. A., Sprecher, U., Clozel, M., and Clozel, J. P. (1995) The role of endothelin in experimental cerebral vasospasm. *Neurosurgery* **37:**78–86.

114. Shigeno, T., Clozel, M., Sakai, S., Saito, A., and Goto, K. (1995) The effect of bosentan, a new potent endothelin receptor antagonist, on the pathogenesis of cerebral vasospasm. *Neurosurgery* **37:**87–90.

115. Zuccarello, M., Soattin, G. B., Lewis, A., Breu, V., Hallak, H., and Rapoport, R. M. (1996) Prevention of subarachnoid hemorrhage-induced cerebral vasospasm by oral administration of endothelin receptor antagonists. *J. Neurosurg.* **84:**503–507.

116. Willette, R. N., Zhang, H., Mitchell, M. P., Sauermelch, C. F., Ohlstein, E. H., and Sulpizio, A. C. (1994) Nonpeptide endothelin antagonist. Cerebrovascular characterization and effects on delayed cerebral vasospasm. *Stroke* **25:**2450–2456.

117. Willette, R. N., Feuerstein, G. Z., and Barone, F. C. (1995) Endothelin in the central nervous system, in *Endothelin Receptors: From the Gene to the Human* (Ruffolo, R. R., Jr., ed.), CRC, Boca Raton, FL, pp. 187–213.

118. Barone, F. C., Willette, R. N., Yue, T.-L., and Feuerstein, G. (1995) Therapeutic effects of endothelin receptor antagonists in stroke. *Neurol. Res.* **17:**259–264.

119. Sharkey, J. and Butcher, S. P. (1995) Characterization of an experimental model of stroke produced by intracerebral microinjection of endothelin-1 adjacent to the rat middle cerebral artery. *J. Neurosci. Methods* **60:**125–131.

120. Agnati, L. F., Zoli, M., Kurosawa, M., Benfenati, F., Biagini, G., Zini, I., Hallstrom, A., Ungerstedt, U., Toffano, G., and Fuxe, K. (1991) A new model of focal brain ischemia based on the intracerebral injection of endothelin-1. *Ital. J. Neurol. Sci.* **12(3 Suppl. 11):**49–53.

121. Ziv, I., Fleminger, G., Djaldetti, R., Achiron, A., Melamed, E., and Sokolovsky, M. (1992) Increased plasma endothelin-1 in acute ischemic stroke. *Stroke* **23:**1014–1016.

122. Wei, G. Z., Zhang, J., Sheng, S. L., Ai, H. X., Ma, J. C., and Lui, H. B. (1993) Increased plasma endothelin-1 concentration in patients with acute cerebral infarction and actions of endothelin-1 on pial arterioles of rat. *Chin. Med. J. Engl.* **106:**917–921.

123. Giuffrida, R., Bellomo, M., Polizzi, G., and Malatino, L. S. (1992) Ischemia-induced changes in he immunoreactivity for endothelin and other vasoactive peptides in the brain of the Mongolian gerbil. *J. Cardiovasc. Pharmacol.* **20(Suppl. 12):**S41–S44.

124. Willette, R. N., Ohlstein, E. H., Pullen, M., Sauermelch, C. F., Cohen, A., and Nambi, P. (1993) Transient forebrain ischemia alters acutely endothelin receptor density and immunoreactivity in gerbil brain. *Life Sci.* **52:**35–40.

125. Viossat, I., Duverger, D., Chapelat, M., Pirotzky, E., Chabrier, P. E., and Braquet, P. (1993) Elevated tissue endothelin content during focal cerebral ischemia in the rat. *J. Cardiovasc. Pharmacol.* **22(Suppl. 8):**S306–S309.

126. Barone, F. C., Globus, M. Y., Price, W. J., White, R. F., Storer, B. L., Feuerstein, G. Z., Busto, R., and Ohlstein, E. H. (1994) Endothelin levels increase in rat focal and global ischemia. *J. Cereb. Blood Flow Metab.* **14:**337–342.

127. Yamashita, K., Kataoka, Y., Niwa, M., Shigematsu, K., Himeno, A., Koizumi, S., and Taniyama, K. (1993) Increased production of endothelins in the hippocampus of stroke-prone spontaneously hypertensive rats following transient forebrain ischemia: histochemical evidence. *Cell Mol. Neurobiol.* **13:**15–23.

128. Kohzuki, M., Onodera, H., Yasujima, M., Itoyama, Y., Kanazawa, M., Sato, T., and Abe, K. (1995) Endothelin receptors in ischemic rat brain and Alzheimer brain. *J. Cardiovasc. Pharmacol.* **26(Suppl. 3):**S329–S331.

129. Feuerstein, G. Z., Gu, J.-L., Ohlstein, E. H., Barone, F. C., and Yue, T. L. (1994) Selective endothelin receptor (ETA) antagonist is neuroprotective in gerbil transient forebrain ischemia. *Stroke* **25:**264.

130. Barone, F. C., White, R. F., Elliott, J. D., Feuerstein, G. Z., and Ohlstein, E. H. (1995) The endothelin receptor antagonist SB 217242 reduces cerebral focal ischemic brain injury. *J. Cardiovasc. Pharmacol.* **26(Suppl. 3):**S404–S407.

131. Patel, T. R. and McCulloch, J. (1996) Failure of an endothelin antagonist to modify hypoperfusion after transient global ischaemia in the rat. *J. Cereb. Blood Flow Metab.* **16:**490–499.

132. Patel, T. R., McAuley, M. A., and McCulloch, J. (1994) Effects on feline pial arterioles in situ of bosentan, a non-peptide, endothelin receptor antagonist. *Eur. J. Pharmacol.* **260:**65–71.

133. Patel, T. R., Galbraith, S., Graham, D. I., Hallak, H., Doherty, A. M., and McCulloch, J. (1996) Endothelin receptor antagonist increases cerebral perfusion and reduces ischaemic damage in feline focal cerebral ischaemia. *J. Cereb. Blood Flow Metab.* **16:**950–958.

134. Wilkes, B. M., Susin, M., and Mento, P. F. (1993) Localization of endothelin-1-like immunoreactivity in human placenta. *J. Histochem. Cytochem.* **41:**535–541.

135. Nova, A., Sibai, B. M., Barton, J. R., Mercer, B. M., and Mitchell, M. D. (1991) Maternal plasma level of endothelin is increased in preeclampsia. *Am. J. Obstet. Gynecol.* **165:**724–727.

136. Benigni, A., Orisio, S., Gaspari, F., Frusca, T., Amuso, G., and Remuzzi, G. (1992) Evidence against a pathogenetic role for endothelin in preeclampsia. *Br. J. Obstet. Gynecol.* **99:**798–802.

137. Cervar, M., Kainer, F., Jones, C. J., and Desoye, G. (1996) Altered release of endothelin-1,2 and thromboxane B2 from trophoblastic cells in pre-eclampsia. *Eur. J. Clin. Invest.* **26:**30–37.

138. McMahon, L. P., Redman, C. W., and Firth, J. D. (1993) Expression of the three endothelin genes and plasma levels of endothelin in pre-eclampsia and normal gestations. *Clin. Sci. Colch.* **85:**417–424.

139. Schiff, E., Galron, R., Ben-Baruch, G., Mashiach, S., and Sokolovsky, M. (1993) Endothelin-1 receptors on the human placenta and fetal membranes: evidence for different binding properties in pre-eclamptic pregnancies. *Gynecol. Endocrinol.* **7:**67–72.

140. Cervar, M., Kainer, F., and Desoye, G. (1995) Pre-eclampsia and gestational age differently alter binding of endothelin-1 to placental and trophoblast membrane preparations. *Mol. Cell Endocrinol.* **110:**65–71.

141. Vedernikov, Y. P., Belfort, M. A., Saade, G. R., and Moise, K. J., Jr. (1995) Pre-eclampsia does not alter the response to endothelin-1 in human omental artery. *J. Cardiovasc. Pharmacol.* **26(Suppl. 3):**S233–S235.

142. Morel, D. R., Lacroix, J. S., Hemsen, A., Steinig, D. A., Pittet, J-F., and Lundberg, J. M. (1989) Increased plasma and pulmonary lymph levels of endothelin during endotoxin shock. *Eur. J. Pharmacol.* **167:**427,428.

143. Nambi, P., Pullen, M., Slivjak, M. J., Ohlstein, E. H., Storer, B., and Smith, E. F., III (1994) Endotoxin-mediated changes in plasma endothelin concentrations, renal endothelin receptor and renal function. *Pharmacology* **48:**147–156.

144. Smits, P., Hofman, H., Rosmalen, F., Wollersheim, H., and Thien, T. (1991) Endothelin-1 in patients with Raynaud's phenomenon. *Lancet* **337:**236.

145. Farkkila, M., Palo, J., Saijonmaa, O., and Fyhrquist, F. (1992) Raised plasma endothelin during acute migraine attack. *Cephalalgia* **12:**383,384.

146. Brandli, P., Loffler, B. M., Breu, V., Osterwalder, R., Maire, J. P., and Clozel, M. (1996) Role of endothelin in mediating neurogenic plasma extravasation in rat dura mater. *Pain* **64:**315–322.

147. Aoki, T., Kojima, T., Ono, A., Unishi, G., Yoshijima, S., Kameda-Hayashi, N., Yamamoto, C., Hirata, Y., and Kobayashi, Y. (1994) Circulating endothelin-1 levels in patients with bronchial asthma. *Ann. Allergy* **73:**365–369.

148. Springall, D. R., Howarth, P. H., Counihan, H., Djukanovic, R., Holgate, S. T., and Polak, J. M. (1991) Endothelin immunoreactivity of airway epithelium in asthmatic patients. *Lancet* **337:**697–701.

149. Vittori, E., Marini, M., Fasoli, A., De Franchis, R., and Mattoli, S. (1992) Increased expression of endothelin in bronchial epithelial cells of asthmatic patients and effect of corticosteroids. *Am. Rev. Respir. Dis.* **146:**1320–1325.

150. Ackerman, V., Carpi, S., Bellini, A., Vassalli, G., Marini, M., and Mattoli, S. (1995) Constitutive expression of endothelin in bronchial epithelial cells of patients with symptomatic and asymptomatic asthma and modulation by histamine and interleukin-1. *J. Allergy Clin. Immunol.* **96:**618–627.

151. Knott, P. G., D'Aprile, A. C., Henry, P. J., Hay, D. W., and Goldie, R. G. (1995) Receptors for endothelin-1 in asthmatic human peripheral lung. *Br. J. Pharmacol.* **114**:1–3.
152. Chanez, P., Vignola, A. M., Albat, B., Springall, D. R., Polak, J. M., Godard, P., and Bousquet, J. (1996) Involvement of endothelin in mononuclear phagocyte inflammation in asthma. *J. Allergy Clin. Immunol.* **98**:412–420.
153. Riccio, M. M., Reynolds, C. J., Hay, D. W., and Proud, D. (1995) Effects of intranasal administration of endothelin-1 to allergic and nonallergic individuals. *Am. J. Respir. Crit. Care Med.* **152**:1757–1764.
154. Uchida, Y., Jun, T., Ninomiya, H., Ohse, H., Hasegawa, S., Nomura, A., Sakamoto, T., Sardessai, M. S., and Hirata, F. (1996) Involvement of endothelins in immediate and late asthmatic responses of guinea pigs. *J. Pharmacol. Exp. Ther.* **277**:1622–1629.
155. Goerre, S., Wenk, M., Bartsch, P., Luscher, T. F., Niroomand, F., Hohenhaus, E., Oelz, O., and Reinhart, W. H. (1995) Endothelin-1 in pulmonary hypertension associated with high-altitude exposure. *Circulation* **90**:359–364.
156. Mitaka, C., Hirata, Y., Nagura, T., Tsunoda, Y., and Amaha, K. (1993) Circulating endothelin-1 concentrations in acute respiratory failure. *Chest* **104**:476–480.
157. Ishikawa, S., Miyauchi, T., Ueno, H., Ushinohama, H., Sagawa, K., Fusazaki, N., Sunagawa, H., Honda, S., Sakai, S., and Yamaguchi, I. (1995) Influence of pulmonary blood pressure and flow on endothelin-1 production in humans. *J. Cardiovasc. Pharmacol.* **26(Suppl. 3)**:S429–S433.
158. Giaid, A., Yanagisawa, M., Langleben, D., Michel, R. P., Levy, R., Shennib, H., Kimura, S., Masaki, T., Duguid, W. P., and Stewart, D. J. (1993) Expression of endothelin-1 in the lungs of patients with pulmonary hypertension. *New Engl. J. Med.* **328**:1732–1739.
159. Stelzner, T. J., O'Brien, R. F., Yanagisawa, M., Sakurai, T., Sato, K., Webb, S., Zamora, M., McMurtry, I. F., and Fisher, J. H. (1992) Increased lung endothelin-1 production in rats with idiopathic pulmonary hypertension. *Am. J. Physiol.* **262**:L614–L618.
160. Sakai, S., Miyauchi, T., Sakurai, T., Yamaguchi, I., Kobayashi, M., Goto, K., and Sugishita, Y. (1996) Pulmonary hypertension caused by congestive heart failure is ameliorated by long-term application of an endothelin receptor antagonist. *J. Am. Coll. Cardiol.* **28**:1580–1588.
161. MacLean, M. R., McCulloch, K. M., and Baird, M. (1995) Effects of pulmonary hypertension on vasoconstrictor responses to endothelin-1 and sarafotoxin S6c and on inherent tone in rat pulmonary arteries. *J. Cardiovasc. Pharmacol.* **26**:822–830.
162. Stewart, A. G., Grigoriadis, G., and Harris, T. (1994) Mitogenic actions of endothelin-1 and epidermal growth factor in cultured airway smooth muscle. *Clin. Exp. Pharmacol. Physiol.* **21**:277–285.
163. Panettieri, R. A., Jr., Goldie, R. G., Rigby, P. J., Eszterhas, A. J., and Hay, D. W. (1996) Endothelin-1-induced potentiation of human airway

smooth muscle proliferation: an ET_A receptor-mediated phenomenon. *Br. J. Pharmacol.* **118**:191–197.

164. Marini, M., Carpi, S., Bellini, A., Patalano, F., and Mattoli, S. (1996) Endothelin-1 induces increased fibronectin expression in human bronchial epithelial cells. *Biochem. Biophys. Res. Commun.* **220**:896–899.

165. Mansoor, A. M., Honda, M., Saida, K., Ishinaga, Y., Kuramochi, T., Maeda, A., Takabatake, T., and Mitsui, Y. (1995) Endothelin-induced collagen remodeling in experimental pulmonary hypertension. *Biochem. Biophys. Res. Commun.* **215**:981–986.

166. Okada, M., Yamashita, C., Okada, M., and Okada, K. (1995) Role of endothelin-1 in beagles with dehydromonocrotaline-induced pulmonary hypertension. *Circulation* **92**:114–119.

167. Wagner, O. F., Vierhapper, H., Gasic, S., Nowotny, P., and Waldhausl, W. (1992) Regional effects and clearance of endothelin-1 across pulmonary and splanchnic circulation. *Eur. J. Clin. Invest.* **22**:277–282.

168. Kaasjager, K. A. H., Shaw, S., Koomans, H. A., and Rabelink, T. J. (1997) Role of endothelin receptor subtypes in the systemic and renal responses to endothelin-1 in humans. *J. Am. Soc. Nephrol.* **8**:32–39.

169. Tomita, K., Ujiie, K., Nakanishi, T., Tomura, S., Matsuda, O., Ando, K., Shichiri, M., Hirata, Y., and Marumo, F. (1989) Plasma ET levels in patients with acute renal failure. *Eur. J. Med.* **32**:1127.

170. Sandok, E. K., Lerman, A., Stingo, A. J., Perrella, M. A., Gloviczki, P., and Burnett, J. C., Jr. (1992) Endothelin in a model of acute ischemic renal dysfunction: modulating action of atrial natriuretic factor. *J. Am. Soc. Nephrol.* **3**:196–202.

171. Shibouta, Y., Suzuki, N., Shino, A., Matsumoto, H., Terashita, Z.-I., Kondo, K., and Nishikawa, K. (1990) Pathophysiological role of ET in acute renal failure. *Life Sci.* **46**:1611–1618.

172. Firth, J. D. and Ratcliffe, P. J. (1992) Organ distribution of the three rat ET messenger RNAs and the effects of ischemia on renal gene expression. *J. Clin. Invest.* **90,** 1023–1031.

173. Clozel, M., Löffler, B. M. and Gloor, H. (1991) Relative preservation of the responsiveness to ET-1 during reperfusion following renal ischemia in the rat. *J. Cardiovasc. Pharmacol.* **17(Suppl. 7)**:S313–S315.

174. Nambi, P., Pullen, M., Jugus, M., and Gellai, M. (1993) Rat kidney ET receptors in ischemia-induced acute renal failure. *J. Pharmacol. Exp. Ther.* **264**:345–348.

175. Wilkes, B. M., Pearl, A. R., Mento, P. F., Maita, M. E., Macica, C. M., and Girardi, E. P. (1991) Glomerular ET receptors during initiation and maintenance of ischemic acute renal failure in rats. *Am. J. Physiol.* **260**:F110–F118.

176. Vemulapalli, S., Chiu, P. J. S., Chintala, M., and Bernardino, V. (1993) Attenuation of ischemic acute renal failure by phosphoramidon in rats. *Pharmacology* **47**:188–193.

177. Kon, V., Yoshioka, T., Fogo, A., and Ichikawa, I. (1989) Glomerular actions of ET *in vivo. J. Clin. Invest.* **83**:1762–1767.

178. López-Farré, A., Gómez-Garre, D., Bernabeu, F., and López-Novoa, J. (1991) A role for ET in the maintenance of post-ischaemic renal failure in the rat. *J. Physiol.* **444:**513–522.

179. Mino, N., Kobayashi, M., Nakajima, A., Amano, H., Shimamoto, K., Ishikawa, K., Watanabe, K., Nishikebe, M., Yano, M., and Ikemoto, F. (1992) Protective effect of a selective ET receptor antagonist, BQ123, in ischemic acute renal failure in rats. *Eur. J. Pharmacol.* **221:**77–83.

180. Chan, L., Chittinandana, A., Shapiro, J. I., Shanley, P. F., and Schrier, R. W. (1994) Effect of an ET-receptor antagonist on ischemic acute renal failure. *Am. J. Physiol.* **266:**F135–F138.

181. Gellai, M., Jugus, M., Fletcher, T. A., DeWolf, R., and Nambi, P. (1994) Reversal of postischemic acute renal failure with a selective ET_A receptor antagonist in the rat. *J. Clin. Invest.* **93:**900–906.

182. Brooks, D. P., DePalma, P. D., Gellai, M., Nambi, P., Ohlstein, E. H., Elliott, J. D., Gleason, J., and Ruffolo, R. R., Jr. (1994) Non-peptide ET receptor antagonists. III. Effect of SB 209670 and BQ123 on acute renal failure in anesthetized dogs. *J. Pharmacol. Exp. Ther.* **271:**769–775.

183. Gellai, M., Jugus, M., Fletcher, T., Nambi, P., Ohlstein, E. H., Elliott, J. D., and Brooks, D. P. (1995) Nonpeptide endothelin receptor antagonists. V: prevention and reversal of acute renal failure in the rat by SB 209670. *J. Pharmacol. Exp. Ther.* **275:**200–206.

184. Clozel, M., Breu, V., Burri, K., Cassal, J.-M., Fischli, W., Gray, G. A., Hirth, G., Löffler, B.-M., Müller, M., Neidhart, W., and Ramuz, H. (1993) Pathophysiological role of ET revealed by the first orally active ET receptor antagonist. *Nature* **365:**759–761.

185. Kusumoto, K., Kubo, K., Kandori, H., Kitayoshi, T., Sato, S., Wakimasu, M., Watanabe, T., and Fujino, M. (1994) Effects of a new endothelin antagonist, TAK-044, on post-ischemic acute renal failure in rats. *Life Sci.* **55:**301–310.

186. Stingo, A. J., Clavell, A. L., Aarhus, L. L., and Burnett, J. C., Jr. (1993) Biological role for the ET-A receptor in aortic cross-clamping. *Hypertension* **22:**62–66.

187. Brooks, D. P., DePalma, P. D., Pullen, M., and Nambi, P. (1994) Characterization of canine renal ET receptor subtypes and their function. *J. Pharmacol. Exp. Ther.* **268:**1091–1097.

188. Brooks, D. P. (1996) Role of endothelin in renal function and dysfunction. *Clin. Exp. Pharmacol. Physiol.* **23:**345–348.

189. Nir, A., Clavell, A. L., Heublein, D., Aarhus, L. L., and Burnett, J. C., Jr. (1994) Acute hypoxia and endogenous renal ET. *J. Am. Soc. Nephrol.* **4:**1920–1924.

190. Roubert, P., Gillard-Roubert, V., Pourmarin, L., Cornet, S., Guilmard, C., Plas, P., Pirotzky, E., Chabrier, P. E., and Braquet, P. (1993) Endothelin receptor subtypes A and B are up-regulated in an experimental model of acute renal failure. *Mol. Pharmacol.* **45:**182–188.

191. Karam, H., Bruneval, P., Clozel, J.-P., Loffler, B.-M., Bariety, J., and Clozel, M. (1995) Role of endothelin in acute renal failure due to rhabdomyolysis in rats. *J. Pharmacol. Exp. Ther.* **274:**481–486.

192. Bunchman, T. E. and Brookshire, C. A. (1991) Cyclosporine-induced synthesis of ET by cultured human endothelial cells. *J. Clin. Invest.* **88:**310–314.

193. Nakahama, H. (1990) Stimulatory effect of cyclosporine A on ET secretion by a cultured renal epithelial cell line, LLC-PK1 cells. *Eur. J. Pharmacol.* **180:**191,192.

194. Moutabarrik, A., Ishibashi, M., Fukunaga, M., Kameoka, H., Takano, Y., Kokado, Y., Takahar, S., Jiang, H., Sonoda, T., and Okuyama, A. (1991) FK506 mechanism of nephrotoxicity: stimulatory effect on ET secretion by cultured kidney cells. *Transplant. Proc.* **23:**3133–3136.

195. Edwards, B. S., Hunt, S. A., Fowler, M. B., Valentine, H. A., Anderson, L. M., and Lerman, A. (1991) Effect of cyclosporine on plasma ET levels in humans after cardiac transplantation. *Am. J. Cardiol.* **67:**782–784.

196. Grieff, M., Loertscher, R., Shohaib, S. A., and Stewart, D. J. (1993) Cyclosporine-induced elevation in circulating ET-1 in patients with solid-organ transplants. *Transplantation* **56:**880–884.

197. Haug, C., Duell, T., Lenich, A., Kolb, H. J., and Grunert, A. (1995) Elevated plasma endothelin concentrations in cyclosporine-treated patients after bone marrow transplantation. *Bone Marrow Transplant.* **16:**191–194.

198. Textor, S. C., Burnett, J. C., Jr., Romero, C., Canzanello, V. J., Taler, S. J., Wiesner, R., Porayko, M., Krom, R., Gores, G., and Hay, E. (1995) Urinary endothelin and renal vasoconstriction with cyclosporine or FK506 after liver transplantation. *Kidney Int.* **47:**1426–1433.

199. Tanda, K., Seki, T., Kobayashi, S., Kanagawa, K., Chikaraishi, T., Togashi, M., Nonomura, K., and Koyanagi, T. (1994) *In vivo* effect of a selective endothelin receptor antagonist, BQ123, on renal function in cyclosporin A-treated rats. *Int. J. Urol.* **1:**309–315.

200. Benigni, A., Perico, N., Ladny, J. R., Imberti, O., Bellizzi, L., and Remuzzi, G. (1991) Increased urinary excretion of ET-1 and its precursor, big-ET-1, in rats chronically treated with cyclosporine. *Transplantation* **52:**175–177.

201. Abassi, Z. A., Pieruzzi, F., Nakhoul, F., and Keiser, H. R. (1996) Effects of cyclosporin A on the synthesis, excretion and metabolism of endothelin the rat. *Hypertension* **27:**1140–1148.

202. Brooks, D. P., Ohlstein, E. H., Contino, L. C., Storer, B., Pullen, M., Caltabiano, M., and Nambi, P. (1991) Effect of nifedipine on cyclosporine A-induced nephrotoxicity, urinary ET excretion and renal ET receptor number. *Eur. J. Pharmacol.* **194:**115–117.

203. Nambi, P., Pullen, M., Contino, L. C., and Brooks, D. P. (1990) Upregulation of renal ET receptors in rats with cyclosporine A-induced nephrotoxicity. *Eur. J. Pharmacol.* **187:**113–116.

204. Awazu, M., Sugiura, M., Inagami, T., Ichikawa, I., and Kon, V. (1991) Cyclosporine promotes glomerular ET binding *in vivo*. *J. Am. Soc. Nephrol.* **1:**1253–1258.

205. Takeda, M., Iwasaki, S., Hellings, S. E., Yoshida, H., Homma, T., and Kon, V. (1994) Divergent expression of ET_A and ET_B receptors in response to cyclosporine in mesangial cells. *Am. J. Pathol.* **144:**473–479.

206. Nayler, W. G., Gu, X. H., Casley, D. J., Panagiotopoulos, S., Liu, J., and Mottram, P. L. (1989) Cyclosporine increases ET-1 binding site density in cardiac cell membranes. *Biochem. Biophys. Res. Commun.* **163**:1270–1274.

207. Iwai, J., Kanayama, Y., Negoro, N., Okamura, M., and Takeda, T. (1995) Gene expression of endothelin receptors in aortic cells from cyclosporine-induced hypertensive rats. *Clin. Exp. Pharmacol. Physiol.* **22**:404–409.

208. Kon, V., Sugiura, M., Inagami, T., Harvie, B. R., Ichikawa, I., and Hoover, R. L. (1990) Role of ET in cyclosporine-induced glomerular dysfunction. *Kidney Int.* **37**:1487–1491.

209. Perico, N., Dadan, J., and Remuzzi, G. (1990) Endothelin mediates the renal vasoconstriction induced by cyclosporine in the rat. *J. Am. Soc. Nephrol.* **1**:76–83.

210. Bloom, I. T. M., Bentley, F. R., and Garrison, R. N. (1993) Acute cyclosporine-induced renal vasoconstriction is mediated by ET-1. *Surgery* **114**:480–488.

211. Brooks, D. P. and Contino, L. C. (1995) Prevention of cyclosporine A-induced renal vasoconstriction by the endothelin receptor antagonist SB 209670. *Eur. J. Pharmacol.* **294**:571–576.

212. Fogo, A., Hellings, S. E., Inagami, T., and Kon, V. (1992) Endothelin receptor antagonism is protective in in vivo acute cyclosporine toxicity. *Kidney Int.* **42**:770–774.

213. Bartholomeusz, B., Hardy, K. J., Nelson, A. S., and Phillips, P. A. (1996) Bosentan ameliorates cyclosporin A-induced hypertension in rats and primates. *Hypertension* **27**:1341–1345.

214. Conger, J. D., Kim, G. E., and Robinette, J. B. (1994) Effects of ANG II, ET_A and TxA2 receptor antagonists on cyclosporin A renal vasoconstriction. *Am. J. Physiol.* **267**:F443–F449.

215. Davis, L. S., Haleen, S. J., Doherty, A. M., Cody, W. L., and Keiser, J. A. (1994) Effects of selective endothelin antagonists on the hemodynamic response to cyclosporin A. *J. Am. Soc. Nephrol.* **4**:1448–1454.

216. Elzinga, L. W., Rosen, S., and Bennett, W. M. (1993) Dissociation of glomerular filtration rate from tubulointerstitial fibrosis in experimental chronic cyclosporine nephropathy: role of sodium intake. *J. Am. Soc. Nephrol.* **42**:214–221.

217. Hunley, T. E., Fogo, A., Iwasaki, S., and Kon, V. (1995) Endothelin A receptor mediates functional but not structural damage in chronic cyclosporine nephrotoxicity. *J. Am. Soc. Nephrol.* **5**:1718–1723.

218. Kon, V., Hunley, T. E., and Fogo, A. (1995) Combined antagonism of endothelin A/B receptors links endothelin to vasoconstriction whereas angiotensin II effects fibrosis. *Transplantation* **60**:89–95.

219. Takeda, Y., Miyamori, I., Wu, P., Yoneda, T., Furukawa, K., and Takeda, R. (1995) Effects of an endothelin receptor antagonist in rats with cyclosporine-induced hypertension. *Hypertension* **26**:932–936.

220. Binet, I., Wallnofer, A., Jones, R., and Thiel, G. (1996) Renal hemodynamic effects of an endothelin antagonist bosentan, and interaction with cyclosporin A: a placebo controlled double-blind study. *J. Am. Soc. Nephrol.* **7**:1578.

221. Goodall, T., Kind, C. N., and Hammond, T. G. (1995) FK506-induced endothelin release by cultured rat mesangial cells. *J. Cardiovasc. Pharmacol.* **26(Suppl. 3):**S482–S485.

222. Kumano, K., Chen, J., He, M., Endo, T., and Masaki, Y. (1995) Role of endothelin in FK 506-induced renal hypoperfusion in rats. *Transplant. Proc.* **27:**550–553.

223. Heyman, S. N., Clark, B. A., Kaiser, N., Spokes, K., Rosen, S., Brezis, M., and Epstein, F. H. (1992) Radiocontrast agents induce ET release *in vivo* and *in vitro. J. Am. Soc. Nephrol.* **3:**58–65.

224. Sung, J.-M., Shu, G. H. F., Tsai, J.-C., and Huang, J.-J. (1995) Radiocontrast media induced endothelin-1 mRNA expression and peptide release in porcine aortic endothelial cells. *J. Formos. Med. Assoc.* **94:**77–86.

225. Margulies, K. B., Hildebrand, F. L., Heublein, D. M., and Burnett, J. C., Jr. (1991) Radiocontrast increases plasma and urinary ET. *J. Am. Soc. Nephrol.* **2:**1041–1045.

226. Cantley, L. G., Spokes, K., Clark, B., McMahon, E. G., Carter, J., and Epstein, F. H. (1993) Role of ET and prostaglandins in radiocontrast-induced renal artery constriction. *Kidney Int.* **44:**1217–1223.

227. Oldroyd, S., Slee, S.-J., Haylor, J., Morcos, S. K., and Wilson, C. (1994) Role for endothelin in the renal responses to radiocontrast media in the rat. *Clin. Sci.* **87:**427–434.

228. Brooks, D. P. and DePalma, P. D. (1996) Blockade of radiocontrast-induced nephrotoxicity by the endothelin receptor antagonist, SB 209670. *Nephron* **72:**629–636.

229. Bird, J. E., Giancarli, M. R., Megill, J. R., and Durham, S. K. (1996) Effects of endothelin in radiocontrast-induced nephropathy in rats are mediated through endothelin-A receptors. *J. Am. Soc. Nephrol.* **7:**1153–1157.

230. Pinzani, M., Milani, S., DeFranco, R., Grappone, C., Caligiuri, A., Gentilini, A., Tosti-Guerra, C., Maggi, M., Failli, P., Ruocco, C., and Gentilini, P. (1996) Endothelin 1 is overexpressed in human cirrhotic liver and exerts multiple effects on activated hepatic stellate cells. *Gastroenterology* **110:**534–548.

231. Hocher, B., Zart, R., Diekmann, F., Slowinski, T., Thone-Reineke, C., Lutz, J., and Bauer, C. (1995) Role of the paracrine liver endothelin system in the pathogenesis of CC14-induced liver injury. *Eur. J. Pharmacol.* **293:**361–368.

232. Rockey, D. C. and Weisiger, R. A. (1996) Endothelin-induced contractility of stellate cells from normal and cirrhotic rat liver: implications for regulation of portal pressure and resistance. *Hepatology* **24:**233–240.

233. Moller, S., Gulberg, V., Henriksen, J. H., and Gerbes, A. L. (1995) Endothelin-1 and endothelin-3 in cirrhosis: relations to systemic and splanchnic haemodynamics. *J. Hepatol.* **23:**135–144.

234. Hocher, B., Zart, R., Diekmann, F., Slowinski, T., Thone-Reineke, C., Lutz, J., and Bauer, C. (1996) Protective effects of the mixed endothelin receptor antagonist bosentan in rats with CCL4-induced liver injury. *J. Cardiovasc. Pharmacol.* **26(Suppl. 3):**S130,S131.

235. Soper, C. P. R., Latif, A. B., and Bending, M. R. (1996) Amelioration of hepatorenal syndrome with selective endothelin-A antagonist. *Lancet* **347**:1842–1843.

236. King, A. J., Brenner, B. M., and Anderson, S. (1989) Endothelin: a potent renal and systemic vasoconstrictor peptide. *Am. J. Physiol.* **256**:F1051–F1058.

237. Simonson, M. S., Wann, S., Mené, P., Dubyak, G. R., Kester, M., Nakazato, Y., Sedor, J. R., and Dunn, M. J. (1989) Endothelin stimulates phospholipase C, Na$^+$/H$^+$ exchange, c-fos expression, and mitogenesis in rat mesangial cells. *J. Clin. Invest.* **83**:708–712.

238. Bakris, G. L. and Re, R. N. (1993) Endothelin modulates angiotensin II-induced mitogenesis of human mesangial cells. *Am. J. Physiol.* **264**:F937–F942.

239. Ishimura, E., Shouji, S., Nishizawa, Y., Morii, H., and Kashgarian, M. (1991) Regulation of mRNA expression for extracellular matrix (ECM) by cultured rat mesangial cells (MCs). *J. Am. Soc. Nephrol.* **2**:546 (abst.).

240. Gomez-Garre, D., Ruiz-Ortega, M., Ortego, M., Largo, R., Lopez-Armada, M. J., Plaza, J. J., Gonzalez, E., and Egido, J. (1996) Effects and interactions of endothelin-1 and angiotensin II on matrix protein expression and synthesis and mesangial cell growth. *Hypertension* **27**:885–892.

241. Zoja, C., Orisio, S., Perico, N., Benigni, A., Morigi, M., Benatti, L., Rambaldi, A., and Remuzzi, G. (1991) Constitutive expression of ET gene in cultured human mesangial cells and its modulation by transforming growth factor-β, thrombin, and a thromboxane A$_2$ analog. *Lab. Invest.* **64**:16–20.

242. Horie, M., Uchida, C., Yanagisawa, M., Matsushita, Y., Kurokawa, K., and Ogata, E. (1991) Mechanisms of ET-1 mRNA and peptides induction by TGFβ and TPA in MDCK cells. *J. Cardiovasc. Pharmacol.* **17(Suppl. 7)**:S222–S225.

243. Schulz, E., Ruschitzka, F., Lueders, S., Heydenbluth, R., Schrader, J., and Muller, G. A. (1995) Effects of endothelin on hemodynamics, prostaglandins, blood coagulation and renal function. *Kidney Int.* **47**:795–801.

244. Brooks, D. P., Contino, L. C., Storer, B., and Ohlstein, E. H. (1991) Increased ET excretion in rats with renal failure induced by partial nephrectomy. *Br. J. Pharmacol.* **104**:987–989.

245. Benigni, A., Perico, N., Gaspari, F., Zoja, C., Bellizzi, L., Gabanelli, M., and Remuzzi, G. (1991) Increased renal ET production in rats with reduced renal mass. *Am. J. Physiol.* **260**:F331–F339.

246. Morabito, E., Corsico, N., and Arrigoni-Martelli, E. (1994) Endothelins urinary excretion is increased in spontaneously diabetic rats: BB/BB. *Life Sci.* **25**:PL13–18.

247. Orisio, S., Benigni, A., Bruzzi, I., Corna, D., Perico, N., Zoja, C., Benatti, L., and Remuzzi, G. (1993) Renal ET gene expression is increased in remnant kidney and correlates with disease progression. *Kidney Int.* **43**:354–358.

248. Fukui, M., Nakamura, T., Ebihara, I., Osada, S., Tomino, Y., Masaki, T., Goto, K., Furuichi, Y., and Koide, H. (1993) Gene expression for ETs and their receptors in glomeruli of diabetic rats. *J. Lab. Clin. Med.* **122**:149–156.

249. Nakamura, T., Ebihara, I., Fukui, M., Osada, S., Tamino, Y., Masaki, T., Goto, K., Furuichi, Y., and Koide, H. (1995) Modulation of glomerular endothelin and endothelin receptor gene expression in aminonucleoside-induced nephrosis. *J. Am. Soc. Nephrol.* **5:**1585–1590.

250. Nakamura, T., Ebihara, I., Fukui, M., Osada, S., Tomino, Y., Masaki, T., Goto, K., Furuichi, Y., and Koide, H. (1993) Increased ET and ET receptor mRNA expression in polycystic kidneys of cpk mice. *J. Am. Soc. Nephrol.* **4:**1064–1072.

251. Hocher, B., Liefeldt, L., Thone-Reineke, C., Orzechowski, H.-D., Distler, A., Bauer, C., and Paul, M. (1996) Characterization of the renal phenotype of transgenic rats expressing the human endothelin-2 gene. *Hypertension* **28:**196–201.

252. Benigni, A., Zoja, C., Corna, D., Orisio, S., Longaretti, L., Bertani, T., and Remuzzi, G. (1993) A specific ET subtype A receptor antagonist protects against injury in renal disease progression. *Kidney Int.* **44:**440–444.

253. Nakamura, T., Ebihara, I., Tomino, Y., and Koide, H. (1995) Effect of a specific endothelin A receptor antagonist on murine lupus nephritis. *Kidney Int.* **47:**481–489.

254. Benigni, A., Zoja, C., Corna, D., Orisio, S., Facchinetti, D., Benatti, L., and Remuzzi, G. (1996) Blocking both type A and B endothelin receptors in the kidney attenuates renal injury and prolongs survival in rats with remnant kidney. *Am. J. Kid. Dis.* **27:**416–423.

255. Nabokov, A., Amann, K., Wagner, J., Gehlen, F., Munter, K., and Ritz, E. (1996) Influence of specific and non-specific endothelin receptor antagonists on renal morphology in rats with surgical renal ablation. *Nephrol. Dial. Transplant.* **11:**514–520.

256. Pollock, D. M. and Polakowski, J. S. (1997) ET$_A$ receptor blockade prevents hypertension associated with exogenous ET-1 but not renal mass reduction in the rat. *J. Am. Soc. Nephrol.* **8:**1054–1060.

257. Ohta, K., Hirata, Y., Shichiri, M., Ichioka, M., Kubota, T., and Marumo, F. (1991) Cisplatin-induced urinary ET excretion. *JAMA* **265:**1391,1392.

258. Heyman, S. N., Clark, B. A., Kaiser, N., Epstein, F. H., Spokes, K., Rosen, S., and Brezis, M. (1992) *In vivo* and *in vitro* studies on the effect of amphotericin B on ET release. *J. Antimicrob. Chemother.* **29:**69–77.

259. Morise, Z., Ueda, M., Aiura, K., Endo, M., and Kitajima, M. (1994) Pathophysiologic role of endothelin-1 in renal function in rats with endotoxin shock. *Surgery* **115:**199–204.

260. Kelleher, J. P., Shah, V., Godley, M. L., Wakefield, A. J., Gordon, I., Ransley, P. G., Snell, M. E., and Risdon, R. A. (1992) Urinary endothelin (ET1) in complete ureteric obstruction in the miniature pig. *Urol. Res.* **20:**63–65.

261. Langenstroer, P., Tang, R., Shapiro, E., Divish, B., Opgenorth, T., and Lepor, H. (1993) Endothelin-1 in the human prostate: tissue levels, source of production and isometric tension studies. *J. Urol.* **149:**495–499.

262. Rossi, G. P., Albertin, G., Franchin, E., Sacchetto, A., Cesari, M., Palu, G., and Pessina, A. C. (1995) Expression of the endothelin-converting

enzyme gene in human tissues. *Biochem. Biophys. Res. Commun.* **211**:249–253.

263. Kondo, S., Morita, T., and Tashima, Y. (1995) Benign prostatic hypertrophy affects the endothelin receptor density in the human urinary bladder and prostate. *Urol. Int.* **54**:198–203.

264. Kobayashi, S., Tang, R., Wang, B., Opgenorth, T., Langenstoer, P., Shapiro, E., and Lepor, H. (1994) Binding and functional properties of endothelin receptor subtypes in the human prostate. *Mol. Pharmacol.* **45**:306–311.

265. Le Brun, G., Moldovan, F., Aubin, P., Ropiquet, F., Cussenot, O., and Fiet, J. (1996) Identification of endothelin receptors in normal and hyperplasic human prostate tissues. *Prostate* **28**:379–384.

266. Kondo, S., Morita, T., and Tashima, Y. (1994) Endothelin receptor density in human hypertrophic and non-hypertrophic prostate tissue. *J. Exp. Med.* **172**:381–384.

267. Moriyama, N., Kurimoto, S., Miyata, N., Yamaura, H., Yamazaki, R., Sudoh, K., Inagaki, O., Takenaka, T., and Kawabe, K. (1996) Decreased contractile effect of endothelin-1 on hyperplastic prostate. *Gen. Pharmacol.* **6**:1061–1065.

268. Kusuhara, M., Yamaguchi, K., Nagasaki, K., Hayashi, C., Suzaki, A., Hori, S., Handa, S., Nakamura, Y., and Abe, K. (1990) Production of endothelin in human cancer cell lines. *Cancer Res.* **50**:3257–3261.

269. Giaid, A., Hamid, Q. A., Springall, D. R., Yanagisawa, M., Shinmi, O., Sawamura, T., Masaki, T., Kimura, S., Corrin, B., and Polak, J. M. (1990) Detection of endothelin immunoreactivity and mRNA in pulmonary tumors. *J. Pathol.* **162**:15–22.

270. Shichiri, M., Hirata, Y., Nakajima, T., Ando, K., Imai, T., Yanagisawa, M., Masaki, T., and Marumo, F. (1991) Endothelin-1 is an autocrine/paracrine growth factor for human cancer cell lines. *J. Clin. Invest.* **87**:1867–1871.

271. Oikawa, T., Kushuhara, M., Ishikawa, S., Hitomi, J., Kono, A., Iwanaga, T., and Yamaguchi, K. (1994) Production of endothelin-1 and thrombomodulin by human pancreatic cancer cells. *Br. J. Cancer* **69**:1059–1064.

272. Patel, K. V. and Schrey, M. P. (1995) Human breast cancer cells contain a phosphoramidon-sensitive metalloproteinase which can process exogenous big endothelin-1 to endothelin-1: a proposed mitogen for human breast fibroblasts. *Br. J. Cancer* **71**:442–447.

273. Nakamuta, M., Ohashi, M., Tabata, S., Tanabe, Y., Goto, K., Naruse, M., Naruse, K., Hiroshe, K., and Nawata, H. (1993) High plasma concentration of endothelin-like immunoreactivities in patients with hepatocellular carcinoma. *Am. J. Gastroenterol.* **88**:248–252.

274. Economos, K., MacDonald, P. C., and Casey, M. L. (1992) Endothelin-1 gene expression and biosynthesis in human endometrial HEC-1A cancer cells. *Cancer Res.* **52**:554–557.

275. Inagaki, H., Bishop, A. E., Eimoto, T., and Polak, J. M. (1992) Autoradiographic localization of endothelin-1 binding sites in human colonic cancer tissue. *J. Pathol.* **168**:263–267.

276. Nelson, J. B., Chan-Tack, K., Hedican, S. P., Magnuson, S. R., Opgenorth, T. J., Bova, G. S., and Simons, J. W. (1996) Endothelin-1 production and decreased endothelin B receptor expression in advanced prostate cancer. *Cancer Res.* **56:**663–668.

277. Takuwa, Y., Masaki, T., and Yamashita, K. (1990) The effects of the endothelin family peptides on cultured osteoblastic cells from rat calvariae. *Biochem. Biophys. Res. Commun.* **170:**998–1005.

278. Nelson, J. B., Hedican, S. P., George, D. J., Reddi, A. H., Piantadosi, S., Eisenberger, M. A., and Simons, J. W. (1995) Identification of endothelin-1 in the pathophysiology of metastatic adenocarcinoma of the prostate. *Nature* **1:**944–949.

279. Oliver, F. J., de la Rubia, G., Feener, E. P., Lee, M. E., Loeken, M. R., Shiba, T., Quertermous, T., and King, G. L. (1991) Stimulation of endothelin-1 gene expression by insulin in endothelial cells. *J. Biol. Chem.* **266:**23251–23256.

280. Takahashi, K., Ghatei, M. A., Lam, H.-C., O'Halloran, D. J., and Bloom, S. R. (1990) Elevated plasma endothelin in patients with diabetes mellitus. *Diabetologia* **33:**306–310.

281. Totsune, K., Sone, M., Takahashi, K., Ohneda, M., Itoi, K., Murakami, O., Saito, T., Mouri, T., and Yoshinaga, K. (1991) Immunoreactive endothelin in urine of patients with and without diabetes mellitus. *J. Cardiovasc. Pharmacol.* **17(Suppl. 7):**S423–S424.

282. Nugent, A. G., McGurk, C., Hayes, J. R., and Johnston, G. D. (1996) Impaired vasoconstriction to endothelin-1 in patients with NIDDM. *Diabetes* **45:**105–107.

283. Kawamura, M., Ohgawara, H., Naruse, M., Suzuki, N., Iwasaki, N., Naruse, K., Hori, S., Demura, H., and Omori, Y. (1992) Increased plasma endothelin in NIDDM patients with retinopathy. *Diabetes Care* **15:**1396,1397.

284. Kaiser, H. J., Flammer, J., Wenk, M., and Luscher, T. (1995) Endothelin-1 plasma levels in normal-tension glaucoma: abnormal response to postural changes. *Graefes. Arch. Clin. Exp. Ophthalmol.* **233:**484–488.

285. Kawaguchi, Y., Suzuki, K., Hara, M., Hidaka, T., Ishizuka, T., Kawagoe, M., and Nakamura, H. (1994) Increased endothelin-1 production in fibroblasts derived from patients with systemic sclerosis. *Ann. Rheum. Dis.* **53:**506–510.

286. Watschinger, B., Vychytil, A., Schuller, M., Hartter, E., and Traindl, O. (1991) The pathophysiologic role of ET in acute vascular rejection after renal transplantation. *Transplantation* **52:**743–746.

287. Wallace, J. L., Cirino, G., De Nucci, G., McKnight, W., and MacNaughton, W. K. (1989) Endothelin has potent ulcerogenic and vasoconstrictor actions in the stomach. *Am. J. Physiol.* **256:**G661–G666.

288. Murch, S. H., Braegger, C. P., Sessa, W. C., and MacDonald, T. T. (1992) High endothelin-1 immunoreactivity in Crohn's disease and ulcerative colitis. *Lancet* **339:**381–385.

289. Rachmilewitz, D., Eliakim, R., Ackerman, Z., and Karmeli, F. (1992) Colonic endothelin-1 immunoreactivity in active ulcerative colitis. *Lancet* **339:**1062.

290. Hosoda, K., Hammer, R. E., Richardson, J. A., Greenstein Baynash, A., Cheung, J. C., Giaid, A., and Yanagisawa, M. (1994) Targeted and natural (piebald-lethal) mutations of endothelin-B receptor gene produce megacolon associated with spotted coat color in mice. *Cell* **79**:1267–1276.

291. Baynash, A. G., Hosoda, K., Giaid, A., Richardson, J. A., Emotom, N., Hammer, R. E., and Yanagisawa, M. (1994) Interaction of endothelin-3 with endothelin B receptor is essential for development of epidermal melanocytes and enteric neurons. *Cell* **79**:1277–1285.

292. Hofstra, R. M., Osinga, J., Tan Sindhunata, G., Wu, Y., Kamsteeg, E. J., Stulp, R. P., van Ravenswaaij, A. C., Majoor Krakauer, D., Angrist, M., Chakravarti, A., Meijers, C., and Buys, C. H. (1996) A homozygous mutation in the endothelin-3 gene associated with a combined Waardenburg type 2 and Hirschsprung phenotype (Shah-Waardenburg syndrome). *Nat. Genet.* **12**:445–447.

293. Edery, P., Attie, T., Amiel, J., Pelet, A., Eng, C., Hofstra, R. M., Martelli, H., Bidaud, C., Munnich, A., and Lyonnet, S. (1996) Mutation of the endothelin-3 gene in the Waardenburg-Hirschsprung disease (Shah-Waardenburg syndrome). *Nat. Genet.* **12**:442–444.

294. Tsuboi, R., Sato, C., Shi, C.-M., Nakamura, T., Sakurai, T., and Ogawa, H. (1994) Endothelin-1 acts as an autocrine growth factor for normal human keratinocytes. *J. Cell Physiol.* **159**:213–220.

295. Bagnato, A., Venuti, A., DiCastro, V., and Marcante, M. L. (1995) Identification of the ETA receptor subtype that mediates endothelin induced autocrine proliferation of normal human keratinocytes. *Biochem. Biophys. Res. Commun.* **209**:80–86.

296. Zachariae, H., Heickendorff, L., and Bjerring, P. (1996) Plasma endothelin in psoriasis—possible relations to therapy and toxicity. *Acta. Dermatol. Venereol.* **76**:442,443.

297. Teraki, E., Tajima, S., Manaka, I., Kawashima, M., Miyagishi, M., and Imokawa, G. (1996) Role of endothelin-1 in hyperpigmentation in seborrheic keratosis. *Br. J. Dermatol.* **96**:918–923.

298. Kurihara, Y., Kurihara, H., Suzuki, H., Kodama, T., Maemura, K., Nagai, R., Oda, H., Kuwaki, T., Cao, W.-H., Kamada, N., Jishage, K., Ouchi, Y., Azuma, S., Toyoda, Y., Ishikawa, T., Kumada, M., and Yazaki, Y. (1994) Elevated blood pressure and craniofacial abnormalities in mice deficient in endothelin-1. *Nature* **368**:703–710.

Index

A

5-α-reductase inhibitors, 243
α-adrenoceptor, 243
A-127722, 242
ACE inhibitors, 227
Acute renal failure, 236, 237, 240
Acute respiratory failure, 235
Acute tubular necrosis, 236
Adrenal gland, 16
Amphotericin B-induced, 242
Angina pectoris, 229
Angioplasty, 205, 228
Angiotensin II, 167, 171, 172, 239, 241
Antibodies, 226
AP-1, 135
Arterial pressure, 228, 236
Asthma, 234
Astrocytes, 232
ATF-2, 139
Atherosclerosis, 205, 228

B

βγ subunits, 130
Bacteriorhodopsin (BR), 53
Benign prostatic hypertrophy (BHP), 243
Big endothelin analog, 81

Big ET, 76, 176, 179, 233
Binding site model, 60
Blood pressure, 224, 226, 227, 233
Blood–brain barrier, 231
BMS-182874, 195, 229, 240
Bone, 244
Bosentan, 197, 226, 228, 232, 235, 237, 239
BQ-123, 192, 200, 226, 229, 231, 232, 234, 235, 237, 240, 241
BQ-153, 193
BQ-485, 231
BQ-610, 193, 230
BQ-788, 196, 226, 234
Bronchoconstriction, 234

C

C-9526303, 231
Calcium, 175
Calcium activated chloride channels, 105
Calcium mobilization, 101
Cancer cell, 244
Cardiac, 225, 226, 227, 228
Cardiac hypertrophy, 227
Cardiac output, 226
Cardiomyocyte, 227, 229

Carvedilol, 228
Central nervous system, 15
Cerebrospinal fluid, 230, 231
Cerebrovascular disease, 206
c-*fos*, 135
CGS-27830, 198
Chronic renal disease, 242
Circulating endothelin, 228, 234, 235, 242
Cirrhosis, 240, 244
Cisplatin, 242
c-Jun N-terminal kinases (JNKs), 138, 150
c-*jun*, 135, 137
c-*myc*, 135, 137, 138
Coronary, 227, 235
CP-170687, 240
c-Raf-1/ERK, 127, 128
c-Raf-1/extracellular-signal regulated kinase (ERK), 121
Crohn's disease, 245
Cyclin-dependent kinase 4 and 6, 141
Cyclins, 141
Cyclosporine A, 238, 239
Cytoskeletal reorganization, 144

D
DAG levels, 100
Diabetes, 241, 244
Diabetic retinopathy, 245
Diacylglycerol, 94
DOCA-salt hypertensive, 225

E
ECE, 75, 81, 192, 228, 230
ECE inhibitor, 81, 226
ECE intracellular localization, 88
ECE-1 cDNA, 81
ECE-1α, 85
ECE-1β, 85
ECE-1-gene knockout mice, 86
ECE-2 gene knockout mice, 86
Edema, 232, 234
Egr-1, 135, 138
Elk-1, 136, 137
Endothelial cells, 225, 238, 239
Endothelin antibodies, 190, 237, 238
Endotoxic shock, 233
Epithelial cells, 234
Erk-1/-2, 151
ET, 31, 167, 223, 224, 227
ET binding, 228, 232, 233, 236, 237
ET mRNA, 229, 233, 236
ET receptor subtypes, 2, 31, 95
ET receptors, 31, 168, 177
ET-receptor antagonists, 223, 226, 230, 231, 233, 234, 235, 237, 239, 241, 242
ET_A receptor, 2, 191, 225, 231
ET_A receptor mRNA, 225, 231
ET_B receptor, 2, 191, 225, 226, 229
ET_C receptor, 5, 191
Extracellular calcium influx, 102
Extracellular signal regulated kinases (ERKs), 127, 138

F

Female reproductive system, 16
Fibronectin, 235, 241
Fibrosis, 238
FK-506, 238, 239
Focal adhesion kinase (FAK), 122, 126
Focal adhesions, 144
FR-139317, 193, 226, 230, 231, 235
Furin, 77

G

G protein, 130
G protein-coupled receptor, 31
Gastric disease, 245
Gastrointestinal system, 17
Gastrointestinal tract, 245
Glaucoma, 245
Glomerular filtration, 174, 226, 236, 237, 240, 241
Glomeruli, 225, 236, 242
Glomerulonephritis, 242
Glomerulosclerosis, 241
GPCR models, 53
Green fluorescence protein (GFP), 87
Growth factor receptor bound protein 2 (Grb2), 128, 129, 143
Guanine nucleotide regulatory proteins/G proteins, 97

H

Heart, 9
Heart disease, 201
Heart failure, 226, 227, 235

Hemangioendothelioma, 224
Hemodynamics, 169
Hemoglobin, 230
Hepatorenal syndrome, 240
Heterotrimeric G proteins, 99
Hirschsprung's disease, 17, 245
Hypercholesterolemia, 228
Hypertension, 203, 224, 225, 246
Hypothalamus, 15
Hypoxia, 235, 237

I

In situ hybridization, 229
Indomethacin, 240
Infarct size, 229
Inflammation, 233
Inositol 1,4,5-triphosphate (IP$_3$), 94, 99
Intracellular localization of ECE, 88
IRL-1038, 196
Ischemia, 229, 232, 236

J

Jak/STAT, 147
Janus kinase (Jak/Jaks), 122, 126

K

Keratinocyte, 245
Kidney, 12, 171, 174, 224, 226, 236, 242
Kinase-1 (MEK-1), 133

L

Left ventricular hypertrophy, 227

L-type calcium channels, 103
Lung, 13
Lupus nephritis, 242

M
Macrophages, 228, 234
MAP/ERK, 132
MEK kinase (MEKK), 128
MEKK-1, 133
Mesangial cells, 225, 238, 241
Metastatic adenocarcinoma, 244
Migraine, 233
Mitogen, 233
Mitogen-activated protein (MAP) kinases, 121, 122, 127
MKP-1 (MAP kinase phosphatase-1), 140
Molecular cloning, 39
Mononuclear cells, 227
mRNA, 228
mSOS, 128, 129, 143
Mutagenesis, 53
Myocardial infarction, 201, 227, 229
Myofibroblasts, 228

N
Na^+-H^+ exchanger, 109
Neointimal, 229
NEP-ECE-Kell family, 84, 86
Nephrotoxicity, 238, 239, 242
Nephrotoxins, 236
Neuroprotective, 232
Neutral endopeptidase (NEP), 84

Nitric oxide, 192
Non ET_A/ET_B receptors, 192
Non-selective cation channels, 106

O
Organ rejection, 245
Osteoblast, 244
Oxidized low density lipoprotein (LDL), 228

P
p38, 122, 150, 151
PD-142893, 196
PD-145065, 197, 230
PD-156707, 195, 230, 232
PDGF, 127
Peripheral nervous system, 15
Phosphoinositide-3 kinases, 122
Phospholipase C (PLC), 94, 98, 108
Phospholipase D (PLD), 100, 108
Phosphoramidon, 77, 79, 226, 230, 231, 237
Pituitary, 15
Placenta, 233
Plasma endothelin, 168, 224, 229, 230, 232, 233, 236, 238, 239, 240, 244
Polycystic kidney disease, 242
Pre-eclampsia, 232, 233
Pregnancy, 232, 233
Prepro-ET-1 gene expression, 233
Prepro-ET-1 mRNA, 227

Prepro-ET-1, 224, 226
Prostaglandins, 240
Prostate, 17, 243
Protein kinase A, 132
Protein kinase C (PKC), 121, 125, 128, 131
Protein kinase C signaling, 106
Proteinuria, 232, 242
Psoriatics, 245
Pulmonary, 229
Pulmonary hypertension, 190, 204, 235
Pulmonary vascular resistance, 235

R
Racial differences, 225
Ras, 128, 129
Raynaud's disease, 233
Receptor chimeras, 48
Receptor models, 53
Receptor operated Ca^{2+} channels (ROC), 104
Regulation of transcription, 134
Renal blood flow (RBF), 169, 172, 232, 236
Renal disease, 202, 236
Renal plasma flow, 240, 241
Renal prepro-ET-1 mRNA, 225
Renal transplantation, 241
Renal vasoconstriction, 225, 240
RES-701-1, 196, 234
Restenosis, 205
Rhabdomyolysis, 236, 237
Rhinorrhea, 234
Ro-46-2005, 197, 231, 237

Ro-47-0203 (bosentan), 197
Ryanodine receptor, 101

S
Sarafotoxin 6c, 229
SB-209670, 198, 229, 231, 232, 237, 240
SB-217242, 232, 226
Serum response element (SRE), 136, 137
Serum response factor (SRF), 136, 137
Shc, 143
Shock, 207
Signal transduction, 6, 124
Site-directed mutagenesis, 53
Skin, 245
Smooth muscle, 235
Sodium excretion, 178
Spontaneously hypertensive rats, 225, 232
Src homology 2 (SH2) domains, 128
Src, 122, 126, 128, 141, 143, 144
STAT (signal transducers and activators of transcription), 122, 126
Stress-activated protein kinases (SAPKs), 122, 133, 138, 150, 151
Stroke-prone spontaneously hypertensive rats, 225, 232
Subarachnoid hemorrhage, 206, 230, 231
Systemic actions, 179
Systemic sclerosis, 245

T
TAK-044, 197, 200, 226, 230, 237
Ternary complex factors (TCF), 136
Thiorphan, 77
Thrombosis, 241
Tissue distribution of ET, 8
Transforming growth factor β, 241
T-type calcium channels, 103
Tumor, 224
Tyrosine kinase, 126, 128, 141

U
Ulcerative colitis, 245
Ulcerogenic, 245

Urinary endothelin, 225, 233, 240
Urine flow, 178

V
Vascular restenosis, 228
Vasoactive intestinal contractor, 17
Vasoconstriction, 224, 226, 237, 240
Vasospasm, 228, 229, 230, 231
Voltage dependent Ca^{2+} channels (VDCC), 103

W
WS-79089B, 87